Erectile Dysfunction

Guest Editor

CULLEY C. CARSON III, MD, FACS

UROLOGIC CLINICS
OF NORTH AMERICA

www.urologic.theclinics.com

May 2011 • Volume 38 • Number 2

SAUNDERS an imprint of ELSEVIER, Inc.

W.B. SAUNDERS COMPANY
A Division of Elsevier Inc.

1600 John F. Kennedy Blvd. • Suite 1800 • Philadelphia, PA 19103-2899

http://www.theclinics.com

UROLOGIC CLINICS OF NORTH AMERICA Volume 38, Number 2
May 2011 ISSN 0094-0143, ISBN-13: 978-1-4557-0517-7

Editor: Stephanie Donley

Urologic Clinics of North America (ISSN 0094-0143) is published quarterly by Elsevier Inc., 360 Park Avenue South, New York, NY 10010-1710. Months of issue are February, May, August, and November. Business and Editorial Offices: 1600 John F. Kennedy Blvd., Suite 1800, Philadelphia, PA 19103-2899. Periodicals postage paid at New York, NY and additional mailing offices. Subscription prices are $311.00 per year (US individuals), $519.00 per year (US institutions), $363.00 per year (Canadian individuals), $636.00 per year (Canadian institutions), $451.00 per year (foreign individuals), and $636.00 per year (foreign institutions). Foreign air speed delivery is included in all *Clinics* subscription prices. All prices are subject to change without notice. **POSTMASTER:** Send address changes to *Urologic Clinics of North America*, Elsevier Health Sciences Division, Subscription Customer Service, 3251 Riverport Lane, Maryland Heights, MO 63043. Customer Service: 1-800-654-2452 (US). From outside the United States, call 1-314-447-8871. Fax: 1-314-447-8029. E-mail: JournalsCustomerServiceusa@elsevier.com (for print support) and JournalsOnlineSupport-usa@elsevier.com (for online support).

Reprints. For copies of 100 or more, of articles in this publication, please contact the Commercial Reprints Department, Elsevier Inc., 360 Park Avenue South, New York, New York 10010-1710. Tel.: 212-633-3813; Fax: 212-462-1935; E-mail: reprints@elsevier.com.

Urologic Clinics of North America is covered in MEDLINE/PubMed (*Index Medicus*), *Excerpta Medica, Current Contents/Clinical Medicine, Science Citation Index,* and *ISI/BIOMED.*

Printed and bound by CPI Group (UK) Ltd, Croydon, CR0 4YY
Transferred to Digital Print 2011

Contributors

GUEST EDITOR

CULLEY C. CARSON III, MD, FACS
Chief, John Sloan Rhodes and John Flint
Rhodes Distinguished Professor, Division
of Urologic Surgery, Department of Surgery,
University of North Carolina, Chapel Hill,
North Carolina

AUTHORS

STANLEY E. ALTHOF, PhD
Executive Director, Center for Marital and
Sexual Health of South Florida, West Palm
Beach, Florida; Professor Emeritus, Case
Western Reserve University School of
Medicine, Cleveland, Ohio

TRINITY J. BIVALACQUA, MD, PhD
Assistant Professor of Urology and
Oncology, Department of Urology,
The James Buchanan Brady Urological
Institute, Johns Hopkins Medical
Institutions, Johns Hopkins Hospital,
Baltimore, Maryland

GREGORY A. BRODERICK, MD
Professor of Urology, Department of Urology,
Mayo Clinic Florida, Jacksonville, Florida

ARTHUR L. BURNETT, MD, MBA
Professor of Urology and Director, Division
of Sexual Medicine, Department of
Urology, The James Buchanan Brady
Urological Institute, Johns Hopkins
Medical Institutions, Johns Hopkins
Hospital, Baltimore, Maryland

STEVEN E. CANFIELD, MD
Assistant Professor of Surgery, Division of
Urology, Department of Surgery, University
of Texas Health Science Center and MD
Anderson Cancer Center, Houston, Texas

CULLEY C. CARSON III, MD, FACS
Chief, John Sloan Rhodes and John Flint
Rhodes Distinguished Professor, Division
of Urologic Surgery, Department of Surgery,
University of North Carolina, Chapel Hill,
North Carolina

PHILIPP DAHM, MD, MHSc
Associate Professor of Urology; and Director
of Clinical Research, Department of Urology,
College of Medicine, University of Florida,
Gainesville, Florida

CRAIG F. DONATUCCI, MD
Professor of Surgery, Division of Urology,
Department of Surgery, Duke University
Medical Center, Durham, North Carolina

ANDRE T. GUAY, MD
Center for Sexual Function/Department
of Endocrinology, Lahey Clinic, Peabody;
Professor, Tufts University School of Medicine,
Boston, Massachusetts

DIANA KANG, MD
Urology Resident, Department of Urology,
College of Medicine, University of Florida,
Gainesville, Florida

RAJEEV KUMAR, MD, MCh
Associate Professor of Urology, Department of
Urology, All India Institute of Medical Sciences,
New Delhi, India

JOSHUA P. LANGSTON, MD
Division of Urologic Surgery, Department of Surgery, University of North Carolina, Chapel Hill, North Carolina

STEPHEN M. LARSEN, MD
Resident in Urology, Department of Urology, Rush University Medical Center, Chicago, Illinois

TIMOTHY J. LEROY, MD
Chief Resident of Urology, Department of Urology, Mayo Clinic Florida, Jacksonville, Florida

LAURENCE A. LEVINE, MD
Professor in Urology, Department of Urology, Rush University Medical Center, Chicago, Illinois

CLARISSE MAZZOLA, MD
Male Sexual & Reproductive Medicine Program, Division of Urology, Memorial Sloan-Kettering Cancer Center, New York, New York

ERIN R. MCNAMARA, MD
Senior Resident, Division of Urology, Department of Surgery, Duke University Medical Center, Durham, North Carolina

DROGO K. MONTAGUE, MD
Professor of Surgery, Cleveland Clinic Lerner College of Medicine of Case Western Reserve University; Director, Center for Genitourinary Reconstruction, Department of Urology, Glickman Urological and Kidney Institute, Cleveland Clinic, Cleveland, Ohio

ABRAHAM MORGENTALER, MD
Director, Men's Health Boston, Brookline; Associate Clinical Professor of Surgery (Urology), Beth Israel Deaconess Medical Center, Harvard Medical School, Boston, Massachusetts

JOHN P. MULHALL, MD
Director, Male Sexual & Reproductive Medicine Program, Division of Urology, Memorial Sloan-Kettering Cancer Center, New York, New York

RACHEL B. NEEDLE, PsyD
Staff Psychologist, Center for Marital and Sexual Health of South Florida, West Palm Beach; Assistant Professor, Coordinator of Clinical Experiences, South University, West Palm Beach; Adjunct Professor, Nova Southeastern University, Florida; Director of Health Information Services, Positive Friends, Palm Beach, Florida

AJAY NEHRA, MD, FACS
Professor of Urology, Department of Urology, Mayo Clinic College of Medicine, Mayo Clinic, Rochester, Minnesota

MICHAEL A. PERELMAN, PhD
Co-Director, Human Sexuality Program, Payne Whitney Clinic, The New York Presbyterian Hospital, New York; Clinical Associate Professor of Psychiatry, Reproductive Medicine and Urology, New York Weill Medical College of Cornell University, New York, New York

J. PATRICK SELPH, MD
Resident Physician, Division of Urologic Surgery, Department of Surgery, University of North Carolina, Chapel Hill, North Carolina

TARYN L. STOFFS, MS
Research Assistant, Department of Urology, College of Medicine, University of Florida, Gainesville, Florida

ABDULMAGED TRAISH, PhD
Departments of Biochemistry and Urology, Boston University School of Medicine, Boston, Massachusetts

Contents

Several reported advantages of the robotic-assisted laparoscopic approach to the treatment of clinically localized prostate cancer include superior results for erectile function as one of the critical outcomes of radical prostate surgery. This article provides a critical assessment of the evidence that exists for erectile function outcomes based on a systematic literature review. We found that the low methodological and reporting quality of existing studies did not appear well suited to guide clinical practice. A new framework of prospective investigation using validated patient self-assessment instruments would seem critical to the future advancement of this field.

The number of patients diagnosed with prostate cancer was estimated to be 192,000 in 2009 according to the American Cancer Society. The prevalence of reported erectile dysfunction after radical prostatectomy has significant variance. Among the studies in which the nerve-sparing status was described, erectile function recovery adequate for sexual intercourse was achieved in 50% of patients. This article reviews the animal and human studies in this field and provides a useful penile rehabilitation algorithm.

With increased recognition of the benefits of testosterone (T) therapy for middle-aged men, there has been a concomitant reexamination of the historical fear that raising T will result in more prostate cancer (PCa). Studies have failed to show increased risk of PCa in men with higher serum T, and supraphysiologic T fails to increase prostate volume or prostate-specific antigen in healthy men. This apparent paradox is explained by the Saturation Model, which posits a finite capacity of androgen to stimulate PCa growth. Modern studies indicate no increased risk of PCa among men with serum T in the therapeutic range.

The comorbid conditions erectile dysfunction (ED) and depression are highly prevalent in men. Multiple regression analysis to control for all other predictors of ED indicate that men with high depression scores are nearly twice as likely to report ED than nondepressed men. Depression continues to be among the most common comorbid problems in men with ED, both in the community and in clinical samples. This article reviews the current knowledge about the relationship between ED and depression, the effect of treatments for depression on ED, ways to improve screening for depression, and treatment of ED in patients with this comorbidity.

> Male sexual dysfunctions, including erectile dysfunction, hypoactive sexual desire disorder, premature ejaculation, and delayed ejaculation, are a complex amalgam of interrelated biological, psychological, and contextual variables that can combine to produce distressing symptoms both for the male diagnosed with the dysfunction and for his partner. This article describes the assessment process for identifying the psychological concerns associated with the man's sexual complaint, and presents a stepwise algorithm for treating mild to moderate psychosocial issues. Physicians' awareness of psychological and interpersonal issues will help them better manage patients' ongoing medical treatment and limit discontinuation of efficacious therapies.

> The underlying processes in vasculogenic erectile dysfunction (ED) are arterial insufficiency, venoocclusive disease, or combinations of both. Doppler blood flow analysis is a diagnostic modality useful in elucidating the cause of ED and the magnitude of its severity. This article describes the procedural techniques, typical findings, and relevant pathophysiology for in-office Doppler studies. Specific conditions include arterial insufficiency, venous occlusive disease, Peyronie's disease, and priapism.

> Erectile dysfunction is defined as the consistent or recurrent inability to attain or maintain penile erection sufficient for sexual performance. Self-reported erectile dysfunction has increased significantly as men seek effective therapy, such as oral phosphodiesterase 5 inhibitors (PDE5i). PDE5i are now the drugs of choice in the initial therapy of erectile dysfunction. This review compares the currently available PDE5i with the second-generation PDE5i, which are soon to be available.

> Several centrally acting agents have shown potential to improve erectile function in men with ED. They still lack adequate data in efficacy and tolerability. Nasal formulations of apomorphine and bremelanotide seem to be the most likely candidates for future approval. They may play a role, specifically in men who fail phosphodiesterase 5 (PDE5) therapy, are unable to take PDE5 inhibitors because of side effects, or are on nitrate therapy. This article reviews the centrally acting agents and the data on their efficacy.

> The most common cause of erectile dysfunction (ED) is penile vascular insufficiency. This is usually part of a generalized endothelial dysfunction and is related to several

conditions, including type 2 diabetes mellitus, hypertension, hyperlipidemia, and obesity. These conditions underlie the pathophysiology of metabolic syndrome (MetS). Hypogonadism, or testosterone deficiency (TD), is an integral component of the pathology underlying endothelial dysfunction and MetS, with insulin resistance (IR) at its core. Testosterone replacement therapy for TD has been shown to ameliorate some of the components of the MetS, improve IR, and may serve as treatment for decreasing cardiovascular and ED risk.

Advances have recently been made in both medical and surgical management of priapism, and these offer improvements in the level of care afforded such patients. Further developments can be expected based on ongoing progress, particularly in the area of molecular science, which is the primary source for driving novel therapeutic approaches. Continued action to address the health care administrative concerns of those most commonly affected by priapism, specifically individuals with sickle cell disease, is also appropriate. All successes in these arenas ensure that afflicted individuals avoid the health burdens of priapism and preserve sexual function.

The purpose of this article is to review the contemporary literature on nonsurgical therapies for Peyronie's disease (PD); focus on randomized, placebo-controlled trials; and review the latest guidelines for the management of PD from the International Consultation on Sexual Medicine. A combination of oral agents or intralesional injection with traction therapy may provide a synergy between the chemical effects of the drugs and the mechanical effects of traction. Until a reliable treatment emerges, some of the nonsurgical treatments discussed can be used to stabilize the scarring process and may result in some reduction of deformity with improved sexual function.

Peyronie disease (PD) is an incurable, sexually debilitating disease resulting in penile deformity, coital failure, and significant psychological stress for patients and their partners. Appropriate treatment should be individualized and tailored to the patient's goals and expectations, disease history, physical examination findings, and erectile function. After medical therapy is considered and the disease has stabilized, surgical correction, including tunical shortening or lengthening procedures, is an excellent option for patients with functional impairment caused by PD. Outcomes are satisfactory when proper treatment decisions are made, with the goal being expected return to normal sexual function following PD treatment.

Penile prosthesis implantation, the oldest of the modern treatments for erectile dysfunction (ED), still plays an important role despite the advent of less invasive alternatives. For some men with ED, penile prosthesis implantation is the only effective or acceptable treatment. Penile prosthesis implantation remains a viable option in the contemporary management of ED as evidenced by annual penile prosthesis implantation cases in the United States rising from 17,540 in 2000 to 22,420 in 2009. Improvements in prosthesis design and implantation techniques have resulted in significant increases in device survival and patient satisfaction.

Epidemiologic studies have estimated that more than 50% of men ages 40 to 70 have some form of erectile dysfunction. Penile prosthesis implantation remains a mainstay for treatment of erectile dysfunction unresponsive to other less-invasive methods. Improvements in penile prosthesis design have extended the long-term survival of implants. As the improved design of prostheses has led to their increased mechanical survival, other complications, such as infection, have emerged as the leading causes of implant failure. This article focuses on approaches to prevention and treatment of penile prosthesis infection.

GOAL STATEMENT

The goal of *Urologic Clinics of North America* is to keep practicing urologists and urology residents up to date with current clinical practice in urology by providing timely articles reviewing the state of the art in patient care.

ACCREDITATION

The *Urologic Clinics of North America* is planned and implemented in accordance with the Essential Areas and Policies of the Accreditation Council for Continuing Medical Education (ACCME) through the joint sponsorship of the University of Virginia School of Medicine and Elsevier. The University of Virginia School of Medicine is accredited by the ACCME to provide continuing medical education for physicians.

The University of Virginia School of Medicine designates this educational activity for a maximum of 15 *AMA PRA Category 1 Credits*™ for each issue, 60 credits per year. Physicians should only claim credit commensurate with the extent of their participation in the activity.

The American Medical Association has determined that physicians not licensed in the US who participate in this CME activity are eligible for a maximum of 15 *AMA PRA Category 1 Credits*™ for each issue, 60 credits per year.

Credit can be earned by reading the text material, taking the CME examination online at http://www.theclinics.com/home/cme, and completing the evaluation. After taking the test, you will be required to review any and all incorrect answers. Following completion of the test and evaluation, your credit will be awarded and you may print your certificate.

FACULTY DISCLOSURE/CONFLICT OF INTEREST

The University of Virginia School of Medicine, as an ACCME accredited provider, endorses and strives to comply with the Accreditation Council for Continuing Medical Education (ACCME) Standards of Commercial Support, Commonwealth of Virginia statutes, University of Virginia policies and procedures, and associated federal and private regulations and guidelines on the need for disclosure and monitoring of proprietary and financial interests that may affect the scientific integrity and balance of content delivered in continuing medical education activities under our auspices.

The University of Virginia School of Medicine requires that all CME activities accredited through this institution be developed independently and be scientifically rigorous, balanced and objective in the presentation/discussion of its content, theories and practices.

All authors/editors participating in an accredited CME activity are expected to disclose to the readers relevant financial relationships with commercial entities occurring within the past 12 months (such as grants or research support, employee, consultant, stock holder, member of speakers bureau, etc.). The University of Virginia School of Medicine will employ appropriate mechanisms to resolve potential conflicts of interest to maintain the standards of fair and balanced education to the reader. Questions about specific strategies can be directed to the Office of Continuing Medical Education, University of Virginia School of Medicine, Charlottesville, Virginia.

The faculty and staff of the University of Virginia Office of Continuing Medical Education have no financial affiliations to disclose.

The authors/editors listed below have identified no professional or financial affiliations for themselves or their spouse/partner:
Trinity J. Bivalacqua, MD, PhD; Steven E. Canfield, MD; Philipp Dahm, MD, MHSc; Kerry Holland, (Acquisitions Editor); Diana Kang, MD; Joshua P. Langston, MD; Stephen M. Larsen, MD; Timothy J. LeRoy, MD; Clarisse Mazzola, MD; Erin R. McNamara, MD; Rachel B. Needle, PsyD; J. Patrick Selph, MD; Taryn L. Stoffs, MS; and Abdulmaged Traish, PhD.

The authors/editors listed below identified the following professional or financial affiliations for themselves or their spouse/partner:
Stanley E. Althof, PhD is a consultant and is on the Advisory Board/Committee for Eli Lilly, Palitan, and Shionogi; is on the Advisory Board/Committee for Bayer and Neurohealing; is an industry funded research/investigator for Endoceutics; is an industry funded research/investigator and consultant for Johnson & Johnson; and is an industry funded research/investigator, and is on the Speakers' Bureau and Advisory Board/Committee, for Boehringer Ingelheim.
Gregory A. Broderick, MD is an industry funded research/investigator for Vivus.
Arthur L. Burnett, MD, MBA is an industry funded research/investigator for Pfizer Inc. and Vivus, and is a consultant for Endo Pharmaceuticals and Abbott.
Culley C. Carson III, MD, FACS (Guest Editor) is a consultant and is on the Speakers' Bureau for AMS Coloplast, is an industry funded research/investigator, consultant, and is on the Speakers' Bureau for Auxilium, and is on the Speakers' Bureau for GSK, Lilly, and Pfizer.
Craig F. Donatucci, MD is on the Advisory Board/Committee for Lilly, Pfizer, Endo, and Abbott, and is on the Speakers' Bureau for Lilly and Pfizer.
Andre T. Guay, MD is a consultant and is on the Advisory Board/Committee for Auxilium, Abbott, Solvay, Endo Pharmaceuticals, and Repros Therapeutics.
Rejeev Kumar, MD, MCh is an industry funded research/investigator for Charak Pharmaceuticals, Mumbai, India.
Laurence A. Levine, MD is a consultant for Pfizer, is a consultant and is on the Speakers' Bureau for American Medical Systems and Coloplast, and is an industry funded research/investigator, consultant, and is on the Speakers' Bureau for Auxilium.
Drogo K. Montague, MD is a consultant and is on the Speakers' Bureau for American Medical Systems.
Abraham Morgentaler, MD is a consultant for Slate, is an industry funded research/investigator and is on the Speakers' Bureau for Auxilium and Endo, is on the Speakers' Bureau for Watson and Abbott, and is an industry funded research/investigator for GSK.
John P. Mulhall, MD is an industry funded research/investigator for Pfizer, Inc., and is on the Advisory Committee/Board for Auxilium.
Ajay Nehra, MD, FACS is a consultant for American Medical Systems, Coloplast, and Pfizer, Inc.
Michael A. Perelman, PhD is a consultant and is on the Speakers' Bureau for Bayer Schering Pharam; is a consultant and is on the Speakers' Bureau and Advisory Board for Boehringer Ingelheim, and Eli Lilly; is an industry funded research/investigator and consultant for GSK; is an industry funded research/investigator, consultant, and is on the Advisory Board for Johnson & Johnson; and is a consultant and is on the Advisory Board for Palatin Technologies and Scionogi.
William Steers, MD (Test Author) is employed by the American Urologic Association, is a reviewer and consultant for NIH, and is an investigator for Allergan.

Disclosure of Discussion of Non-FDA Approved Uses for Pharmaceutical Products and/or Medical Devices.
The University of Virginia School of Medicine, as an ACCME provider, requires that all faculty presenters identify and disclose any off-label uses for pharmaceutical and medical device products. The University of Virginia School of Medicine recommends that each physician fully review all the available data on new products or procedures prior to clinical use.

TO ENROLL

To enroll in the Urologic Clinics of North America Continuing Medical Education program, call customer service at 1-800-654-2452 or visit us online at www.theclinics.com/home/cme. The CME program is available to subscribers for an additional fee of $207.00.

Urologic Clinics of North America

THE CLINICS ARE NOW AVAILABLE ONLINE!

Access your subscription at:
www.theclinics.com

Preface

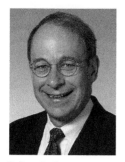

Culley C. Carson III, MD
Guest Editor

The field of men's health continues to gain momentum and interest around the world. An integral part of men's health is men's sexual health and erectile dysfunction (ED). This issue of *Urologic Clinics of North America* is focused on the issues facing men and their urologists when they suffer from ED. As several years have passed since the last issue discussing these difficult issues, many changes and advancements have occurred in the clinical and basic science understanding of ED. Increased investigation of the etiologies and risk factors for ED has clarified the association of ED and benign prostatic hyperplasia and lower urinary tract symptoms. The association with testosterone deficiency syndrome (TDS) and the benefits of normalizing testosterone in men with sexual problems is now more important than ever before. Recent treatment options have provided men with TDS with improved methods for supplementing testosterone. New understanding of the pathophysiology and treatment of premature ejaculation has lead to hope for the more than 30% of American men of all ages that suffer from this difficult and previously underappreciated condition.

The study of Peyronie's disease continues to search for better understanding and treatment for this debilitating sexual dysfunction that affects as many as 10% of American men over 40 years of age. While previously there were no effective treatment options, new medical therapy is on the horizon and surgical options continue to be refined with improved outcomes and patient selection.

Surgery for ED continues to be a last option for most patients, but the success and safety of these procedures are vastly better than a decade or two ago. The improved penile implants with longer survival, fewer mechanical malfunctions, and improved infection rates have made these implantable prostheses safer, better tolerated, and more widely implanted. Patients with these devices have excellent satisfaction rates and use their implants frequently.

In this issue of *Urologic Clinics of North America*, the contributing authors have provided outstanding reviews of the current state of the art in sexual medicine and have elucidated the latest understanding of important topics in ED. The contributors are among the world's experts in sexual medicine and have brought that expertise to this issue of *Urologic Clinics*.

I would like to thank the contributors for their hard work and for sharing their knowledge of ED. Their efforts are evident throughout this issue with their lucid and complete discussions. I am indebted to the editorial staff at *Urologic Clinics* for their expertise, assistance, and efficiency in publishing this outstanding issue.

Culley C. Carson III, MD
Division of Urologic Surgery
Department of Surgery
University of North Carolina
2113 Physician's Office Building
Chapel Hill, NC 27599-7235, USA

E-mail address:
culley_carson@med.unc.edu

Urol Clin N Am 38 (2011) xi
doi:10.1016/j.ucl.2011.02.008
0094-0143/11/$ – see front matter © 2011 Elsevier Inc. All rights reserved.

Recovery of Erectile Function After Robotic Prostatectomy: Evidence-Based Outcomes

Philipp Dahm, MD, MHSc[a,*], Diana Kang, MD[a],
Taryn L. Stoffs, MS[a], Steven E. Canfield, MD[b]

KEYWORDS

- Erectile dysfunction • Evidence-based medicine
- Systematic review • Radical prostatectomy
- Robotic-assisted radical prostatectomy

THE DIFFUSION OF ROBOTIC-ASSISTED LAPAROSCOPIC PROSTATECTOMY

One of the most remarkable developments in urology over the last decade has been the shift from open to robotic-assisted laparoscopic prostatectomy (RALP) for localized prostate cancer. This change has occurred particularly in the United States, but is also increasing in other wealthy countries of the world. At the time when Binder described the first RALP in the year 2000, the vast majority of radical prostatectomies were performed using a retropubic approach involving an infraumbilical midline incision.[1] Pioneering work by Walsh[2] and coworkers on the location and function of the neurovascular bundles had led to the introduction of the nerve-sparing retropubic approach in appropriately selected patients. Similar techniques were demonstrated to be effective with perineal radical prostatectomy but had never reached the widespread dissemination seen with the retropubic approach.[3–5] Laparoscopic prostatectomy, the third surgical treatment option prior to the advent of RALP, was developed

and technically perfected in centers of excellence in France, but for a variety of reasons, including surgical learning curve, was never widely used in the United States outside of select institutions.

Approval of the robotic-assist device, more accurately described as a master-slave system, by the US Food and Drug Administration (FDA) in 2001 and the events that followed dramatically changed the playing field for radical prostate surgery. Initially developed by the United States military, then purchased by a small start-up company called Intuitive, this technology offered the initial appeal of performing minimally invasive surgery from a remote location. It also promised to reduce blood loss and length of hospital stay and, most importantly, improve on the critical, patient-important outcomes of radical surgery, namely oncological control, urinary control, and erectile function.[6] From the surgeon's perspective the technique offered the advantages of 3-dimensional visualization, magnification, improved ergonomics, and (when compared with pure laparoscopic surgery) a shortened surgical learning curve. It is noteworthy that FDA approval was

Funding support: Departmental funding.
Disclosures/Conflict of interest: The authors have nothing to disclose.
[a] Department of Urology, College of Medicine, University of Florida, 1600 South West Archer Road, PO Box 100247, Rm N-203, Gainesville, FL 32610-0247, USA
[b] Division of Urology, Department of Surgery, University of Texas Health Science Center and MD Anderson Cancer Center, 6431 Fannin Street, MSB 6.018, Houston, TX 77030, USA
* Corresponding author.
E-mail address: Philipp.Dahm@urology.ufl.edu

Urol Clin N Am 38 (2011) 95–103
doi:10.1016/j.ucl.2011.02.001
0094-0143/11/$ – see front matter © 2011 Published by Elsevier Inc.

granted through the mechanism of a 501(k) premarket notification process. This approval process is open to technology that is perceived as sufficiently similar to other surgical devices that are already in the marketplace. The evidentiary standards for FDA approval in this framework are relatively low, in particular when compared with the hurdles faced by new drugs, which are ultimately subjected to head-to-head clinical trials to demonstrate superiority, equivalence, or at least noninferiority to an existing standard drug.[7] As a result, very limited evidence about the actual outcomes was required to receive FDA approval.

Since that time, the rate of uptake for RALP has been remarkable. Factors that have contributed to the rapid uptake have been the minimally invasive nature of the procedure and plausible advantages over open approaches in terms of blood loss and length of stay.[8] The rapid dissemination, however, is also a product of aggressive marketing by the manufacturer, with claims of superior oncological and functional outcomes.[6] It has undoubtedly benefited from a broad-based fascination for new technology, which has been labeled "gizmo idolatry."[9]

Although nerve-sparing radical prostatectomy was a major advance in preserving erectile function, it remains an imperfect technique because of various factors. The hope of a better method, which might "guarantee" preservation of erections, has been a major driver for the adoption of this new technology. The following sections review the guiding principle of evidence-based decision making and apply it to the assessment of erectile function outcomes after RALP, with special emphasis on the implications for future research in this field.

EVIDENCE-BASED CLINICAL DECISION MAKING

As it is understood today, clinical and health policy decision making should ideally be based on sound scientific research that provides high-quality evidence. For questions of therapy the highest quality of evidence is potentially provided by randomized controlled trials.[10,11] These studies stand out by using established methodological techniques such as randomization and allocation concealment to create groups that are comparable at baseline. Blinding, intention to treat analysis, and completeness of follow-up then provide assurance that the groups are treated similarly (with the exception of the intervention of interest) and the results remain balanced. As a result, high-quality randomized controlled trials stand at the top of the hierarchy of evidence for questions

of therapy. Observational studies are unable to offer the same safeguards against bias. Common issues of observational studies include the lack of comparability at baseline, and differential treatment and outcomes assessment of the groups being compared.[12] Only under select circumstances are observational studies considered to provide high-quality evidence, the most common of which relates to a very large effect size that would be unlikely to be invalidated by potential biases.[13] This particular scenario is exemplified by the example of the parachute, which has never been prospectively evaluated as an intervention to prevent death from falling from an airplane, but unquestionably works.[14] However, interventions with such a large magnitude of effectiveness are rare in medicine, which is why randomized controlled trials are needed in most settings.[15]

The reality is that the highest level of evidence is not often feasible for surgical interventions. Acknowledging the specific challenges of randomizing patients to different surgical approaches, prospectively designed, hypothesis-driven, nonrandomized observational studies provide the next highest category of evidence quality.

THE ROLE OF SYSTEMATIC REVIEW TO GUIDE EVIDENCE-BASED PRACTICE

Systematic reviews have a preeminent role in guiding evidence-based clinical practice by providing summaries of the totality of evidence.[16] Decisions ideally should not be made on the basis of individual studies but on the totality of evidence on a certain clinical question summarizing both the benefits and harms associated with an intervention. For questions of therapy, such as the comparative effectiveness of RALP to treat clinically localized prostate cancer, such data should be derived from several randomized controlled trials performed comparing RALP to more established approaches such as laparoscopic prostatectomy, radical retropubic prostatectomy, or radical perineal prostatectomy. The methodology of how to perform systematic reviews has been pioneered by the Cochrane Collaboration and may be considered well established. Defining quality characteristics include a focused clinical question that is being addressed, defined inclusion and exclusion criteria, a systematic literature search of the published and unpublished literature, as well as disclosure of any conflict of interest of both the individual trials that are incorporated in the systematic review and the authors of the systematic review themselves. Systematic reviews should furthermore consider the heterogeneity of study results across studies that can potentially be explained by differences in the clinical (patients, interventions, outcomes) and methodological (use of methodological safeguards against bias) study characteristics.

ASSESSING MALE SEXUAL DYSFUNCTION AFTER RADICAL PROSTATECTOMY

For a large proportion of men undergoing radical prostatectomy for clinically localized prostate cancer, erectile function is a critically important outcome that is only superseded by oncological control (overall survival, disease-specific survival, recurrence-free survival) and urinary control (absence of stress incontinence, urinary quality of life) in importance. In contrast to localized radiation therapy that is characterized by a slow but progressive loss of erectile function over the course of a year, patients undergoing radical surgery experience an immediate loss of their ability to achieve erections, followed by a potential recovery of function that may take up to 2 years. The recovery phase is characterized by the steepness of the recovery curve as well as the degree of sexual function that is ultimately regained. Both outcomes are influenced by several variables that should find consideration in well-designed studies that assess sexual function outcomes. These factors include the patients' baseline erectile function and level of sexual activity, age, and the extent to which—based on the surgeon's subjective assessment—the nerve-sparing was performed. To measure the recovery of function over time, frequent assessments are necessary to establish a time profile. Because sexual function may also be affected by urinary outcomes and pathologic features (such as stage and margin status) that may prompt postoperative radiation, erectile function outcomes should not be measured in isolation but in the context of other outcome variables.

In the absence of more objective end points such as tumescence studies, assessment of erectile function requires the use of a validated patient self-assessment questionnaire that is administered by an independent third party who is not involved in the analysis nor vested in the outcomes in any way other than the comprehensive and accurate collection of data. Examples of validated instruments that assess erectile function are the International Index of Erectile Function (IIEF) and the Sexual Health Inventory for Men (SHIM, or IIEF-5). Aside from accounting for adjuvant and salvage treatment, studies further need to account for the use of erection-enhancing interventions such as phosphodiesterase-5 inhibitors, injection therapies, and vacuum erection devices (VEDs).

Whereas much attention is given to a sample size as a (misleading) surrogate of study quality, completeness of follow-up is a much underappreciated methodological safeguard against bias that is highly relevant to observational studies of surgical interventions. It is well established that patients lost to follow-up frequently have a different prognosis to patients with complete follow-up. This scenario can thereby bias the results favorably if those lost to follow-up had worse outcomes. Well-designed studies should therefore aim to achieve a high proportion of patients with complete follow-up data and account for all patients who are lost in a flow diagram. In the commonly used Kaplan-Meier-type analysis, this requires not only the transparent reporting of the patients at risk but the clear distinction of patients who were censored because their follow-up ended or they were lost to follow-up.

Lastly, there is the issue of selective reporting and publication bias. Given the importance of erectile function to most patients undergoing radical prostatectomy as a critical outcome, one would expect most if not all studies assessing the outcomes of robotic-assisted prostatectomy to provide some assessment of the observed outcomes. Failure to do so raises the concern of selective reporting of only those sets of outcomes with favorable results, thereby biasing the body of literature toward better outcomes.

EVIDENCE-BASED OUTCOMES OF ROBOTIC-ASSISTED LAPAROSCOPIC PROSTATECTOMY

In 2010 the authors reported a systematic review of the published literature on RALP.[8] In brief, the published literature through MEDLINE and EMBASE was systematically searched, focusing on original research publications. Two reviewers independently performed the data abstraction using a standardized form derived from the Strengthening the Reporting of Observational Studies in Epidemiology (STROBE) criteria.[17] This systematic review identified 75 original research studies. The following analysis represents a secondary analysis of a subset of studies that addressed erectile function outcomes.

RANDOMIZED CONTROLLED TRIALS ON ROBOTIC-ASSISTED LAPAROSCOPIC PROSTATECTOMY

The systematic review by Kang and colleagues[8] identified two randomized controlled trials of RALP. Neither compared robotic surgery to alternative surgical approaches. Both studies focused on technical modifications of the robotic-assisted approach in terms of extraperitoneal versus intra-peritoneal access and bladder neck reconstruction. Neither study reported sexual function outcomes; therefore no level I evidence on this topic exists.

PROSPECTIVE COHORT STUDIES ON ROBOTIC-ASSISTED LAPAROSCOPIC PROSTATECTOMY

Well-designed prospective studies are protocol-driven investigations with predefined inclusion and exclusion criteria, active patient follow-up, blinded outcomes assessment, and an analysis plan that is triggered by a certain length of follow-up or event rate not dissimilar a randomized controlled trial. These types of prospective cohort studies need to be carefully distinguished from retrospective analyses of prospectively collected data, which have become the predominant study type reported in the urological literature yet represents retrospective case series nevertheless.

The systematic literature review identified 4 comparative studies that addressed erectile function outcome following RALP. Although some of these were labeled as prospective, none of them met the criteria of prospective study design as defined here. There are therefore currently no prospective and dedicated studies of erectile function outcomes for robotic-assisted laparo-scopic surgery to help define these outcomes or establish the comparative effectiveness of RALP to alternative surgical approaches.

HEALTH SERVICES RESEARCH ON ROBOTIC-ASSISTED LAPAROSCOPIC PROSTATECTOMY

In the absence of evidence stemming from either randomized controlled trials or prospective cohort studies, the best quality of evidence on the outcomes of RALP can be drawn from a single much criticized study, based on an administrative database, by Hu and colleagues.[18] In brief, these investigators used US Surveillance, Epidemiology, and End Results (SEER)/Medicare-linked data from 2003 to 2007 to compare the short-term complication rates and intermediate-term health-related quality of life outcomes for minimal-invasive (laparoscopic or robotic) prostatectomy and radical retropubic prostatectomy. In a propensity-score–adjusted analysis, the investigators found a significantly higher risk of being diagnosed with erectile dysfunction in the minimal-invasive than in the open surgery group (26.8% vs 19.2% per 100 person-years), thereby contradicting the widespread claims of superior outcomes of RALP compared with alternative approaches.[6]

Several methodological issues should be recognized when critically appraising this study. First, the investigators were unable to distinguish between patients undergoing RALP versus laparo-scopic prostatectomy, thereby leading to potential contamination of (superior) RALP outcomes by (inferior) laparoscopic results. However, given the low prevalence of laparoscopic prostatectomy in the United States, this contamination is unlikely to have exceeded 5% to 10%. Second, the study period likely represented the early learning curve for robotic surgery, which may not be reflective of contemporary outcomes. This is an important and valid argument but also raises serious ethical questions about how surgical procedures and devices are adopted in the urological community. Third, the study results were informed by data coded for billing purposes, rather than via patient query using validated patient self-assessment tools. In the absence of more objective data on the patients' actual sexual function, it is difficult to accurately characterize the effects of the different surgical approaches. The higher incidence of diagnoses codes of impotence may reflect unrealistic patient expectations rather than inferior outcomes, which relates back to how RALP has been marketed not only by the manufacturer but also by the hospitals and surgeons.[19] Recognizing all these issues, one might argue that the importance of this study stems less from its validity in assessing the erectile function outcomes, but from how it highlights the major limitations of the remaining body of evidence, which only provides very low-quality evidence for the outcome of erectile function recovery, as is now described.

EVIDENCE FROM UNCONTROLLED OBSERVATIONAL COHORT STUDIES AND CASE SERIES

The 23 original studies identified in the systematic review by Kang and colleagues[8] that addressed erectile function recovery were retrospective observational studies. All studies reported single-institution experiences and very few studies identified this institution as either an academic or community setting (**Table 1**). The median study sample size was 200 (interquartile range: 100–498). Ten of 23 studies (43.5%) did not provide information on institutional review board approval, and 6 of 23 studies (26.1%) did not identify the number of surgeons involved in the series. Also noteworthy was the concentration of authorship, with 3 centers contributing 8, 4, and 3 studies and thereby 15 of 23 (65.2%) published studies

Table 1
Characteristics of published RALP studies addressing the recovery of erectile function (N = 23) from 2001 to 2008

Year of Publication	
2001–2004	4 (17.4%)
2005–2008	19 (82.6%)
Study Design	
Case series	19 (82.6%)
Case-control/retrospective cohort	4 (17.4%)
Number of Centers	
Single	23 (100.0%)
Funding Source Addressed	
No	23 (100.0%)
Institutional Review Board Approval Specified	
Yes	13 (56.5%)
No	10 (43.5%)
Overall Sample Size	
1–99	2 (8.7%)
100–199	9 (39.1%)
≥200	12 (52.2%)
Research by Setting	
Academic	1 (4.3%)
Community	0 (0.0%)
Not specified	22 (95.7%)
Number of Surgeons	
1–4	15 (65.2%)
≥5	2 (8.7%)
Not specified	6 (26.1%)

during this time period, which raises questions about the generalizability of the results.

Table 2 summarizes the methodological and reporting quality of these studies based on the STROBE criteria. The most common reporting deficits regarding the study methods were related to sample size considerations, blinding of outcome assessors, and the standardization of perioperative care, which were reported by 4.3%, 26.1%, and 34.8% of studies, respectively. None of these studies made mention of an a priori protocol that defined the subsequent analyses. Approximately 74% of studies (17/23) used a validated instrument to assess functional outcomes. However, only 11 of 23 (47.8%) used a questionnaire that specifically addresses erectile function, most commonly the SHIM. The authors found only one study that used and explicitly reported baseline erectile function scores using a specific instrument.[20] Additional shortcomings (see **Table 2**) included the reporting of the average

length of follow-up and the percentage of study subjects lost to follow-up over time, which were reported by only 56.5% and 52.2% of studies, respectively. Less than half the investigators (43.5%) acknowledged the issues of missing data points in the discussion, and only 11 of 23 studies (47.8%) included a discussion of study limitations. In summary, this analysis revealed considerable methodological shortcomings in the quality and reporting of these studies, beyond the fact that they were all retrospective in nature. This raises further concerns about the validity of the results (as outlined below) when used as a guide to patient care.

ERECTILE FUNCTION OUTCOMES AFTER ROBOTIC-ASSISTED LAPAROSCOPIC PROSTATECTOMY

The reported outcomes for erectile function after RALP range from 61%[21] to 70%[22] at 6 months, 70%[23] to 81%[24] at 12 months, 84%[21] to 86%[23] at 24 months, 86%[23] at 36 months, and 100%[23] at 46 months, based on a single study with extended follow-up. Definitions for erectile function varied, and most of these studies did not use a validated and erectile function-specific questionnaire. A single-armed study specifically labeled as reflecting the early institutional learning curve with RALP meanwhile found that less than 20% of patients recovered their baseline sexual summary score as measured by the Expanded Prostate Cancer Index Composite questionnaire.[25] A study by Tewari and colleagues[26] stands out by providing Kaplan-Meier curves for time to recovery of erectile function for both radical retropubic prostatectomy (n = 100) and RALP (n = 200) patients as assessed by patient interview. The investigators found a median time to "return of erections" of 440 days versus 180 days that strongly favored the robotic group. Little assurance was provided that the patients were comparable at baseline and were treated and followed similarly, except for the procedure of interest. No efforts were made to adjust for potential confounding, thereby raising questions about the validity of these findings. Whereas the results of RALP in the hands of experienced surgeons may indeed be superior as claimed, the evidence base to support such claims is poor and unconvincing.

ADVANCING SURGICAL RESEARCH: THE IDEAL RECOMMENDATIONS

The poor-quality evidence that exists to accurately describe the expected erectile function outcomes

Table 2
Quality of reporting in published RALP studies (N = 23) from 2001 to 2008

| | Overall | Year of Publication | |
		2001–2004 (n = 4)	2005–2008 (n = 19)
Methods			
Scientific rationale/background explained	100% (23)	100.0% (4)	100.0% (19)
Inclusion/exclusion criteria described	56.5% (13)	100.0% (4)	47.4% (9)
Surgical technique described	78.3% (18)	100.0% (4)	73.7% (14)
Surgical learning curve addressed	56.5% (13)	100.0% (4)	47.4% (9)
Standardization of perioperative care	34.8% (8)	50.0% (2)	31.6% (6)
Methods of assessing outcome described	91.3% (21)	100.0% (4)	89.5% (17)
Standardized questionnaire for functional outcomes	73.9% (17)	50.0% (2)	78.9% (15)
Blinding of evaluators	26.1% (6)	25.0% (1)	26.3% (5)
Active follow-up	78.3% (18)	75.0% (3)	78.9% (15)
Considerations to justify sample size	4.3% (1)	0% (0)	5.3% (1)
Statistical methods described	65.2% (15)	100.0% (4)	57.9% (11)
Results			
Baseline demographic data given for each group	91.3% (21)	100.0% (4)	89.5% (17)
Timeline for cases clearly stated	91.3% (21)	100.0% (4)	89.5% (17)
Median/mean length of follow-up reported	56.5% (13)	75.0% (3)	52.6% (10)
Attrition of subjects and reason recorded	52.2% (12)	50.0% (2)	52.6% (10)
Number and nature of complications addressed	78.3% (18)	75.0% (3)	78.9% (15)
Discussion			
Authors discuss missing data	43.5% (10)	75.0% (3)	36.8% (7)
Addresses sources of potential bias	47.8% (11)	75.0% (3)	42.1% (8)
Interpretation of results reported	100.0% (23)	100.0% (4)	100.0% (19)
Explicitly addresses study hypothesis	95.7% (22)	100.0% (4)	94.7% (18)
Interpretation in context of current evidence	95.7% (22)	100.0% (4)	94.7% (18)

of RALP or to analyze its comparative effectiveness with alternative surgical approaches is not unique to the arena of sexual medicine. Previous publications have described how the published urological literature mainly consists of low-quality evidence that is ill suited to inform clinical practice.[27] In addition, there is a lack of transparent reporting of studies in the urological literature to make these issues apparent to the reader.[10,12,28,29] Aside from reporting established methodological safeguards against bias, this also refers to the use of validated questionnaires at baseline and at defined intervals in all prostatectomy series so as to provide meaningful outcome data.[30]

Recognizing the practical limitations faced by surgical research in general as it relates to procedures and devices, the Balliol Collaboration has recently developed the IDEAL model (Idea/Innovation, Development, Exploration, Assessment, Long-term study), which focuses on how to replace the largely unregulated and variable process of surgical innovation with a more structured approach. In contrast to innovations in drug therapy for which well-established regulatory frameworks exist, the introduction of innovative operative procedures is not integrated in any regulatory framework unless the investigators choose to do so. Urologists can perform highly innovative and untested surgical procedures if these are aimed at improving the outcomes of individual patients.[7] These clinicians can subsequently go on to publish the results of their innovative and previously untested efforts as noncomparative trials (usually case series) without the special institutional review board or ethics committee requirements that have become commonplace for randomized controlled trials. As a result, surgical procedures and devices can become established in the community in the absence of much information on their safety and therapeutic efficacy.

Aside from the lack of a regulatory framework to enforce higher quality research, it is important to acknowledge the challenges faced by surgical innovators. First, there is the issue of what represents "surgical innovation". An innovative procedure in surgery has been defined as "a new or modified surgical procedure that differs from currently accepted local practice, the outcomes of which have been not described, and which may entail risk to the patient."[31] Whereas it was clear in the early phase of RALP adoption that the application of robotic surgery to radical prostatectomy represented a major change in the way this procedure was being done and therefore clearly represented a "surgical innovation," many other developments are more subtle and may not be as clearly identifiable. It has also been argued that small incremental changes and therefore continued innovation is integral to the practice (and art) of surgery, and should not be stifled by increased regulatory burdens. Second, there is the challenge of the complexity of a surgical procedure (**Fig. 1**), which typically involves a surgical device or instrument, a surgeon with certain training, skill level, and experience, operating room personnel, as well as several individuals involved in preoperative and postoperative care pathways.[32,33] The complexity of the surgical procedure stands in stark contrast to the administration of a pharmaceutical agent with a certain dosing schedule. The phenomenon of the surgical learning curve itself poses multiple methodological issues in the evaluation of surgical procedures,[34] which raises the third issue: when it is appropriate to perform a randomized controlled trial. If done too early, the constraints of a randomized controlled trial may obstruct innovation and be impractical; if done too late, equipoise may be lost.[33] The dilemma of the appropriate time for rigorous evaluation of a randomized controlled trial is reflected in Burton's law of innovation in the context of technology assessment, which states that "it is always too early until, unfortunately, it is suddenly too late."[7]

The IDEAL framework seeks to address the challenges of surgical research in a 5-stage model (**Table 3**) that defines the role of various study

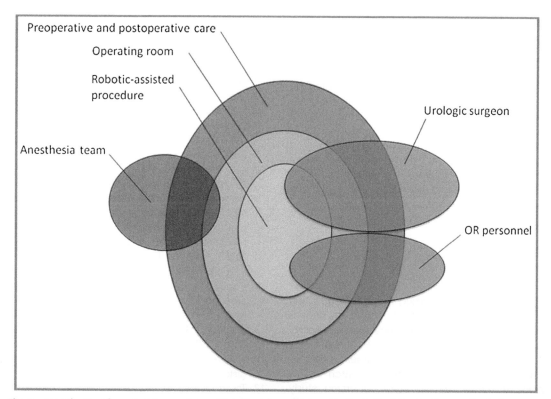

Fig. 1. Complexity of surgical innovations. (*Adapted from* Ergina PL, Cook JA, Blazeby JM, et al. Challenges in evaluating surgical innovation. Lancet 2009;374(9695):1097–104; with permission.)

Table 3
The IDEAL concept of surgical innovation

IDEAL Stages	Research Participants	Objective (Study Design)
Idea/Innovation (1)	Very few; innovators	Proof of concept (structured case reports)
Development (2a)	Few; innovators and early adopters	Procedure development (prospective studies)
Exploration (2b)	Many; early adopters and early majority	Refinement, community learning (randomized controlled trials)
Assessment (3)	Many; early majority	Comparison (randomized controlled trials)
Long-term study (4)	All eligible	Surveillance, safety, quality assurance (registries)

Data from McCulloch P, Altman DG, Campbell WB, et al. No surgical innovation without evaluation: the IDEAL recommendations. Lancet 2009;374(9695):1105–12.

designs to different phases of innovation analogous to that used for pharmaceutical agents. The IDEAL model begins with the proof of concept (Idea/Innovation), moves through stages of development at few, select centers (Development), further refinement at more centers for broader indications (Exploration), evaluation in large and robust studies (Assessment), and ultimately includes the study of long-term outcomes (Long-term study).[35] A critical aspect of this model of surgical innovation is the emphasis on a prospective (rather than retrospective) mode of investigation that identifies not only the role for randomized controlled trials but also for case series and prospective cohort studies, as well as registries. Rigorous prospective study design and data collection provide important protection against bias,[36] and detailed collection of all relevant clinical data points allows the use of advanced statistical techniques such as propensity scores to adjust for potential confounding effects. The IDEAL model therefore presents an important addition to surgical research that is attracting considerable interest from regulatory agencies, publishers, and funding agencies, and is highly applicable to urology.

SUMMARY

The evidence characterizing the erectile function outcomes of RALP is largely based on uncontrolled retrospective case series that are poorly suited to guide clinical practice or health policy decision making. There is an urgent need to improve the quality of surgical research in this arena using prospective, protocol-driven study designs as well as validated patient self-assessment tools.

REFERENCES

1. Binder J, Kramer W. Robotically-assisted laparoscopic radical prostatectomy. BJU Int 2001;87(4): 408–10.
2. Walsh PC. Radical prostatectomy, preservation of sexual function, cancer control. The controversy. Urol Clin North Am 1987;14(4):663–73.
3. Weldon VE, Tavel FR. Potency-sparing radical perineal prostatectomy: anatomy, surgical technique and initial results. J Urol 1988;140(3):559–62.
4. Kubler HR, Tseng TY, Sun L, et al. Impact of nerve sparing technique on patient self-assessed outcomes after radical perineal prostatectomy. J Urol 2007;178(2):488–92 [discussion: 492].
5. Wiygul JB, Harris MJ, Dahm P. Early patient self-assessed outcomes of nerve-sparing perineal prostatectomy. Urology 2005;66(3):582–6.
6. Mulhall JP, Rojaz-Cruz C, Muller A. An analysis of sexual health information on radical prostatectomy websites. BJU Int 2010;105(1):68–72.
7. Barkun JS, Aronson JK, Feldman LS, et al. Evaluation and stages of surgical innovations. Lancet 2009;374(9695):1089–96.
8. Kang DC, Hardee MJ, Fesperman SF, et al. Low quality of evidence for robot-assisted laparoscopic prostatectomy: results of a systematic review of the published literature. Eur Urol 2010;57(6):930–7.
9. Leff B, Finucane TE. Gizmo idolatry. JAMA 2008; 299(15):1830–2.
10. Scales CD Jr, Norris RD, Keitz SA, et al. A critical assessment of the quality of reporting of randomized, controlled trials in the urology literature. J Urol 2007;177(3):1090–5.
11. Scales CD Jr, Preminger GM, Keitz SA, et al. Evidence based clinical practice: a primer for urologists. J Urol 2007;178(3):775–82.
12. Tseng TY, Breau RH, Fesperman SF, et al. Evaluating the evidence: the methodological and reporting quality of comparative observational studies of

surgical interventions in urological publications. BJU Int 2008;103(8):1026–31.

13. Guyatt GH, Oxman AD, Kunz R, et al. What is "quality of evidence" and why is it important to clinicians? BMJ 2008;336(7651):995–8.

14. Smith GC, Pell JP. Parachute use to prevent death and major trauma related to gravitational challenge: systematic review of randomised controlled trials. BMJ 2003;327(7429):1459–61.

15. Glasziou P, Chalmers I, Rawlins M, et al. When are randomised trials unnecessary? Picking signal from noise. BMJ 2007;334(7589):349–51.

16. Dickersin K. Health-care policy. To reform U.S. health care, start with systematic reviews. Science 2010;329(5991):516–7.

17. Vandenbroucke JP, von Elm E, Altman DG, et al. Strengthening the Reporting of Observational Studies in Epidemiology (STROBE): explanation and elaboration. Ann Intern Med 2007;147(8): W163–94.

18. Hu JC, Gu X, Lipsitz SR, et al. Comparative effectiveness of minimally invasive vs open radical prostatectomy. JAMA 2009;302(14):1557–64.

19. Schroeck FR, Krupski TL, Sun L, et al. Satisfaction and regret after open retropubic or robot-assisted laparoscopic radical prostatectomy. Eur Urol 2008; 54(4):785–93.

20. Kaul S, Adnan S, Ketan B, et al. Functional outcomes and oncological efficacy of Vattikuti Institute prostatectomy with Veil of Aphrodite nerve-sparing: an analysis of 154 consecutive patients. BJU Int 2006;97(3):467–72.

21. Zorn KC, Ofer NG, Marcelo AO, et al. Robotic-assisted laparoscopic prostatectomy: functional and pathologic outcomes with interfascial nerve preservation. Eur Urol 2006;51(3):755–63.

22. Mottrie A, Peter Van M, Geert De N, et al. Robot-assisted laparoscopic radical prostatectomy: oncologic and functional results of 184 cases. Eur Urol 2007;52(3):746–51.

23. Mani M, Alok S, Sanjeev K, et al. Vattikuti institute prostatectomy: contemporary technique and analysis of results. Eur Urol 2006;51(3):648–58.

24. Joseph JV, Rosenbaum R, Madeb R, et al. Robotic extraperitoneal radical prostatectomy: an alternative approach. J Urol 2006;175(3):945–51.

25. Tseng TY, Kuebler HR, Cancel QV, et al. Prospective health-related quality-of-life assessment in an initial cohort of patients undergoing robotic radical prostatectomy. Urology 2006;68(5):1061–6.

26. Tewari A, Srivasatava A, Menon M. A prospective comparison of radical retropubic and robot-assisted prostatectomy: experience in one institution. BJU Int 2003;92(3):205–10.

27. Borawski KM, Norris RD, Fesperman SF, et al. Levels of evidence in the urological literature. J Urol 2007; 178(4):1429–33.

28. Breau RH, Gaboury I, Scales CD Jr, et al. Reporting of harm in randomized controlled trials published in the urological literature. J Urol 2010;183(5):1963–7.

29. MacDonald SL, Canfield SE, Fesperman SF, et al. Assessment of the methodological quality of systematic reviews published in the urological literature from 1998 to 2008. J Urol 2010;184(2):648–53.

30. Porst H, Vardi Y, Akkus E, et al. Standards for clinical trials in male sexual dysfunctions. J Sex Med 2010; 7(1 Pt 2):414–44.

31. Biffl WL, Spain DA, Reitsma AM, et al. Responsible development and application of surgical innovations: a position statement of the Society of University Surgeons. J Am Coll Surg 2008;206(3):1204–9.

32. Campbell M, Fitzpatrick R, Haines A, et al. Framework for design and evaluation of complex interventions to improve health. BMJ 2000;321(7262):694–6.

33. Ergina PL, Cook JA, Blazeby JM, et al. Challenges in evaluating surgical innovation. Lancet 2009; 374(9695):1097–104.

34. Cook JA. The challenges faced in the design, conduct and analysis of surgical randomised controlled trials. Trials 2009;10:9.

35. McCulloch P, Altman DG, Campbell WB, et al. No surgical innovation without evaluation: the IDEAL recommendations. Lancet 2009;374(9695): 1105–12.

36. Weil RJ. The future of surgical research. PLoS Med 2004;1(1):e13.

Penile Rehabilitation After Prostate Cancer Treatment: Outcomes and Practical Algorithm

Clarisse Mazzola, MD, John P. Mulhall, MD*

KEYWORDS
- Penile rehabilitation • Radical prostatectomy
- Erectile dysfunction • Prostate cancer

Erectile dysfunction (ED) is a recognized complication of radical prostatectomy (RP). The number of patients diagnosed with prostate cancer was estimated to be 192,000 in 2009 according to the American Cancer Society. The prevalence of ED after RP reported until now has significant variance, with a wide range of rates between 20% to 90%. The reasons for this discrepancy are numerous, mostly because of the lack of standardization of currently available literature. Roughly, three categories of variables can be considered as confounding issues in the assessment of erectile function recovery after RP: patient population, definition of ED, and means of data acquisition. Based on a comprehensive review of the literature performed recently by Tal and colleagues,[1] a prevalence rate among men following contemporary RP was 42%. Among the studies in which the nerve-sparing status was described, erectile function recovery adequate for sexual intercourse was achieved in 50%.

PATHOPHYSIOLOGY OF ED AFTER RP

The pathophysiology of ED after RP involves three major factors: neural injury, vascular injury, and corporal smooth muscle damage. Erectile function recovery is dependent on the degree and reversibility of these injuries.

Neural Trauma

It is recognized that a macroscopic injury to the cavernous nerves during RP, such as transection or thermal damage, will result in a permanent loss of erectile function after surgery. Consequently, the recovery of erectile function has been attributed largely to the success of the macroscopic preservation of the neurovascular bundle at the time of RP. It has been well demonstrated that the nerve-sparing status of a RP greatly influences erectile function recovery.[2,3] Bilateral nerve-sparing is associated with an increased spontaneous and phosphodiesterase type 5 (PDE5) inhibitor (PDE5i)-assisted recovery of erectile function compared with unilateral nerve sparing; both lead to a better erectile function recovery than non–nerve-sparing surgery.[4–6]

Nevertheless, the macroscopic integrity of the cavernous nerves at surgery does not guarantee their future function. In a recent study, Moskovic and colleagues[7] showed that the subjective characterization of nerve sparing, using a nerve-sparing grading system, represented an accurate means to predict erectile function recovery after

Male Sexual & Reproductive Medicine Program, Division of Urology, Memorial Sloan-Kettering Cancer Center, 1275 York Avenue, New York, NY 10065, USA
* Corresponding author.
E-mail address: mulhalj1@mskcc.org

Urol Clin N Am 38 (2011) 105–118
doi:10.1016/j.ucl.2011.03.002
0094-0143/11/$ – see front matter © 2011 Published by Elsevier Inc.

RP. In this study, a significant proportion of men who underwent RP with bilateral nerve sparing assessed as complete, still experienced a significant impairment of their erectile function, with a mean reduction in their International Index of Erectile Function (IIEF): Erectile Function Domain score of 7.2 points at 24 months after surgery.

Indeed, as was shown by Masterson and colleagues,[8] even minimal traction trauma of the cavernous nerves, is likely to cause long-term damage. In this study, a cohort of 275 RP patients (74%) operated on using a standard technique had their erectile function recovery compared with a simultaneous cohort of 97 patients (26%) treated with a technique avoiding the use of a Foley catheter as a tool to stretch the lateral pedicles. At 6 months after RP, 67% of the patients treated with the "no stretch" technique had recovery of functional erections compared with 45% in the standard technique group.

However, the ability of the surgeon to preserve the cavernous nerves at the time of surgery is not the only factor that influences erectile function outcomes after RP. As highlighted in a study by Katz and colleagues,[9] 25% of the patients who had functional erections with or without PDE5i within the first 3 months after surgery were nonfunctional by 6 months. These data suggest that postoperative factors such as edema and inflammation may lead to ongoing postoperative wallerian degeneration, which may in turn be responsible for delayed damage to the cavernous nerves.

The underlying pathophysiological mechanisms that lead from neuropraxia or neurotomy to ED have been well documented in animal studies and imply consequences on both smooth muscle cells and endothelial cells.

Corporal Smooth Muscle Alterations

Corporal smooth muscle alterations are the result of two mechanisms, each leading to increased deposition of collagen with decreased penile distensibility, which translates into venoocclusive dysfunction.

First, after RP, in the absence of erection due to neuropraxia, cavernosal oxygenation is diminished and, therefore, smooth muscle cells are exposed to a prolonged environment of decreased oxygen tension. This results in the inhibition of prostaglandin E1 (PGE1), which suspends its inhibiting effect on profibrotic substances, such as, transforming growth factor-β1 (TGF-β1) and TGF-β1–dependent endothelin-1 (ET-1). Consequently, TGF-β1 is permitted to promote connective tissue synthesis (especially collagen I and III), with the

subsequent replacement of trabecular smooth muscle. These data have been consistently demonstrated in the penile tissue of denervated rat models, in which a significant increase in collagen content and a decrease in the smooth muscle-collagen ratio compared with controls have been seen.[10–15]

Corporal smooth muscle alterations also happen through the apoptosis induced by the proapoptotic cytokines released by the damaged nerve axons. This was first shown by Klein and colleagues.[16] In their study, the penile tissue of 15 rats with bilateral cavernous neurotomy was compared with 15 sham-operated controls. In the glans penis and the cavernous tissue of the denervated rats elevated sulfated glycoprotein-2, intranuclear DNA fragmentation, and apoptotic nuclei were seen, all of which are characteristic of apoptotic cells. These elements were not present in the controls. In this study, however, the specific cell subtypes undergoing apoptosis were not identified.

In a subsequent study, User and colleagues[11] operated on male rats that were randomized to unilateral or bilateral cavernous nerve transection. Changes in wet penile weight, DNA, protein, and apoptotic cells of the penis were measured at different time points after injury. Penile wet weight was significantly decreased at all time points after bilateral neurotomy (P<.001). Unilateral neurotomy allowed much greater preservation of penile weight. DNA content was also significantly decreased in bilaterally denervated penes. Bilateral neurotomy induced significant apoptosis, whereas unilateral surgery caused significantly less apoptosis. Interestingly, the study showed that, in both cases, the apoptotic process affected mostly the smooth muscle cells located beneath the tunica albuginea. It was proposed by the investigators that this sudden and massive apoptosis of smooth muscle cells in the subtunical area might be a mechanism for the development of venoocclusive dysfunction observed after RP.

However, it was later shown by other investigators that the apoptotic process not only involved smooth muscle cells but also endothelial cells.[17,18] More precisely, in a study by Lysiak and colleagues,[17] mice were subjected to cavernous nerve resection or sham surgery and their penes were processed for the identification of apoptotic cells, changes in phosphorylation of several protein kinases, and immunolocalization of specific kinases. An increase in apoptotic cavernous smooth muscle and endothelial cells was evident by 2 weeks, which further increased by 4 and 6 weeks after cavernous nerve resection. Apoptosis coincided with an increase in the phosphorylation of c-jun N-terminal kinase and p38 mitogen activated protein kinase. Phospho-c-jun N-terminal kinase was immunolocalized to endothelial and smooth muscle cells. These findings are consistent with earlier findings by Podlasek and colleagues.[18]

Various types of cavernous nerve injury have been studied in an attempt to model RP-associated cavernous nerve injury using rodent models, including crush, freezing, transection, and excision of the cavernous nerve either unilaterally or bilaterally depending on the underlying aims of each particular experiment.[19] It was shown by many investigators that the apoptotic process in both smooth muscle and endothelium may be different according to the model used. The process was indeed shown to occur in a more delayed fashion in nerve crush injury model compared with the neurotomy model in a study by Mulhall and colleagues.[20] In another study by Jin and colleagues,[21] performed on four groups of 36 mice (control, sham operation, bilateral cavernous nerve crush, and bilateral cavernous neurotomy), erectile function was significantly less in the cavernous nerve crushing and neurotomy group than in the control or sham group. This difference was observed at the earliest time point assayed (day 3) and persisted up to 4 weeks after nerve crushing and to 12 weeks after neurotomy.

A study by Iacono and colleagues[22] showed that the same process is likely to happen in the corpora cavernosa of men after RP. Indeed, in their study, the preoperative histologic data of the corpora cavernosa biopsies of 19 men undergoing RP were compared with the data of the same biopsies performed at 2 and 12 months after surgery. Trabecular elastic fibers ($P<.0003$) and smooth muscle fibers were decreased and collagen content was significantly increased ($P<.0003$) compared with preoperative biopsies. One year after surgery elastic fibers ($P<.0003$) and smooth muscle fibers were decreased and collagen content was significantly increased ($P<.001$) compared with the first postoperative biopsy.

Many theories have been proposed to explain smooth muscle alterations and increased corpus cavernosum collagenization after RP. It is likely that these changes result from the combination of suppression of growth factor production by damaged cavernosal nerves as well as the subsequent production of proapoptotic and profibrotic factors within the corpora cavernosa.[12,14,23]

Arterial Injury

Accessory pudendal arteries (APAs) are vessels that arise from a source above the levator ani (usually obturator, femoral, vesical, or iliac arteries) and travels caudal toward the anterior perineum. The fact that they run in the periprostatic region puts them at risk for injury during RP.[24] More precisely, as shown by Secin and colleagues,[25,26] APAs can be divided into two distinct varieties. There are APAs that course along the lateral aspect of the prostate, termed lateral APAs, and APAs that emerge through the levator ani fibers near the apical region of the prostate, termed apical APAs.

Literature reports a variable prevalence of APAs, ranging from 4% to 75% depending upon their identification method: open surgery,[27–29] laparoscopic prostatectomy,[25,26,30] angiographically during an internal pudendal or internal iliac artery flush,[31,32] or during cadaveric studies.[29,33,34] APAs have been found to provide a significant blood supply to the corpora cavernosa in many studies. In a study by Rosen and colleagues,[31] where selective bilateral internal pudendal angiography was performed in 195 men suspected of having arteriogenic ED, APAs were the major source of inflow to the penis in all cases where they were identified (7%). In a cadaveric dissection study by Breza and colleagues,[34] APAs were identified in 7 cadavers out of 10. APAs were found to be the major source of arterial inflow to the corpora cavernosa in four cases, and the only source of erectile arterial inflow in one case. In a study by Benoit and colleagues,[33] where a total of 33 APAs were identified in 20 cadavers, in 15% of cases the penile arterial inflow originated exclusively from APAs.

It was later demonstrated by Droupy and colleagues,[29] that APAs are functional. In their study, preoperative transrectal color Doppler ultrasound was performed in 12 patients with normal erectile function who were undergoing radical pelvic surgery. APAs were identified in 75% of the patients. Pharmacologically-assisted erections (obtained after intracavernosal injection of papaverine) induced hemodynamic changes in APAs similar to those described in cavernous arteries, suggesting the functional role of APAs in penile erection.

In a study performed at the Johns Hopkins Hospital, with 52 patients with identified APAs undergoing bilateral nerve-sparing surgery between 1987 and 1994, the effect of artery preservation was shown to increase the likelihood of erectile function recovery more than twofold and significantly shorten median time to erectile function recovery—6 versus 12 months.[28]

Nevertheless, these conclusions have not been confirmed by other investigators. In a study by Box and colleagues,[35] for example, in a cohort of

200 patients undergoing robot-assisted laparoscopic RP, of which 80 patients (40%) were found to have APAs, multivariate analysis showed no significant correlation between the presence or absence of APAs and preoperative sexual function. Sacrificing APAs did not correlate with time of erectile function recovery, quality of postoperative erections, or mean IIEF-5 score.

Cavernosal Oxygenation

Neurapraxia may not be the only process by which smooth muscle integrity is affected. It was proposed that the absence of cavernosal oxygenation might play an important role as well. In the flaccid state, the penis acts as a large vein and during the erect state, as an artery. In the flaccid state, the Po_2 is approximately 35 to 40 mm Hg, which has a propensity to upregulate fibrogenic cytokines such as TGF-β, involved in collagen production and therefore in the genesis of fibrosis and venous leak. During oxygenation, Po_2 rises to 75 to 100 mm Hg, which instead upregulates production of endogenous prostanoids as well as cyclic adenosine monophosphate (cAMP).[36]

Moreland and colleagues,[36] have shown in a series of in vitro experiments that exposure of cultured corporal smooth muscle cells to low oxygen levels suppresses PGE1 and cAMP production. Upon returning oxygen tension to normoxic levels, measured levels of both PGE1 and cAMP are normalized. In a further series of experiments, the same investigators showed that, in the in vitro setting, prostanoids inhibit TGF-β activity and thus reduce collagen production.[37]

Therefore, in a healthy male it is plausible that the alternation between the flaccid and erect states, as long as it occurs with a certain frequency, allows preservation of erectile tissue. After RP, however, in a state of unantagonized flaccidity, the balance between flaccid and erect states may be shifted in favor of fibrogenic cytokine production, leading to structural changes and venous leak development.

In a study by Muller and colleagues,[38] in a rat cavernous-nerve-injury model, the potential benefit of the use of hyperbaric oxygen therapy (HBOT) on erectile function and cavernosal tissue has been demonstrated. Animals with bilateral nerve crush were divided into two groups: exposure to a 10 day course of 90 minute treatments with HBOT (3 atm) beginning the day of the cavernous nerve injury compared with animals exposed to room air within an identical chamber. Ten days after bilateral nerve crush, the animals underwent cavernous nerve stimulation measuring the maximal intracavernosal pressure (ICP) to mean arterial pressure (MAP) ratios. Rats exposed to HBOT had significantly higher ICP to MAP ratio recovery compared with the control group (55% vs 31%, $P<.01$). These data suggest that cavernosal oxygenation may be a significant factor in erectile tissue health and to recovery of erectile function.

Nevertheless, in a study by Vignozzi and colleagues,[39] in rats with bilateral cavernous neurotomy, sildenafil treatment was capable of counteracting penile hypo-oxygenation, and the over-expression of the profibrotic ET-1 type B receptor (associated with a 3 month period of hypoxia) with its effect being more evident the earlier it was administered. The threshold of oxygenation beyond which the balance is shifted in the penis from profibrogenic to the synthesis of prostanoids that inhibits TGF-β activity remains unclear, as well as the optimal level of erectile rigidity for cavernosal oxygenation.

Confirming a study by Kim and colleagues,[40] Tal and colleagues[41] have shown, in a study population of 13 patients undergoing cavernosometry, with blood specimens collected at various intracavernosal pressures, that significant increases in cavernosal oxygenation occur in the earliest stages of erection at relatively low ICP. In their study, blood specimens were collected at an ICP range of 6 to 90 mm Hg. Mean plus or minus SD Po_2 was 39 mm Hg at ICP less than 10 mm Hg, 87 at ICP 11 to 20 mm Hg, 89 at ICP 21 to 45 mm Hg, and 96 at ICP greater than 45 mm Hg. These findings suggest that partial erections may be sufficient to oxygenate erectile tissue and protect it from prolonged hypoxia-induced damage.

Reproducing in human subjects a study previously done on monkeys by Lue and colleagues,[42] Knispel and Andresen[43] have investigated the dynamic evolution of oxygen pressure within the penis during the flaccid state and the erection state. In their study, 34 patients with ED had their cavernous oxygen tension monitored, with an oxygen-sensitive Eppendorf needle electrode. The mean cavernous oxygen tension of 38 mm Hg during flaccidity was shown to undergo a continuous and gradual increase to 61 mm Hg a minute after injection of vasoactive agent 30 to 60 seconds lasting up to 8 minutes after the injection.[43] In this study, the duplex Doppler ultrasound peak arterial flow was shown to correlate with maximal cavernosal Po_2 in 71% of cases. However, no ICP was monitored to examine the correlation between the cavernous oxygen pressure and the degree of rigidity.

Finally, it is possible that each PDE5i does not have the same kinetics, tissue selectivity, and impact on tissue oxygenation. In a study by

Ghofrani and colleagues,[44] 60 consecutive patients with pulmonary artery hypertension were assigned to oral intake of 50 mg sildenafil (n = 19), 10 mg (n = 7), or 20 mg (n = 9) vardenafil, or 20 mg (n = 9), 40 mg (n = 8), or 60 mg (n = 8) tadalafil. Maximum effects on pulmonary artery vasorelaxation was obtained more rapidly for vardenafil (40–45 minutes) compared with 60 and 75 to 90 minutes for sildenafil and tadalafil respectively. Only sildenafil and tadalafil (but not vardenafil) allowed significant reduction in the pulmonary to systemic vascular resistance ratio. Significant improvement in arterial oxygenation (equally to nitric oxide [NO] inhalation) was only seen with sildenafil.

Venous Leak

The hemodynamic alterations that frequently underlie the development of long-term ED after RP is venous leak (corporovenocclusive dysfunction [CVOD]). During the erection process, as the smooth muscle expands in a three-dimensional fashion under NO control, it induces the compression of the subtunical venules that are positioned externally between the tunica albuginea and the corporal smooth muscle. Conditions in which the muscle fails to expand adequately leave subtunical venules in an noncompressed state, leading to venous leak. The two things that lead to failure of the corporal smooth muscle to expand are adrenaline and structural changes such as fibrosis. Nehra and colleagues[45] have shown, in human corporal tissue biopsy specimens taken at the time of cavernosometry, that when smooth muscle content in the penis drops below 40%, venous leak occurs. Indeed, the further this figure drops below 40%, the greater the magnitude of the leak. Iacono and colleagues[22] have shown that as early as 2 months after RP in an untreated man, there is a marked increase in collagen deposition and a marked increase in elastic fiber content in erectile tissue. This is in keeping with the finding of the animal data outlined above, which suggests that structural changes occur even in the earliest stages after cavernous nerve injury. Mulhall and Graydon[46] have shown, in a series of patients who had preoperative and postoperative hemodynamic assessment, that more than half of the men developed venous leak after surgery. In a more recent analysis by Mulhall and colleagues,[47] of men who had partner-corroborated excellent erectile function before surgery and who underwent duplex Doppler penile ultrasound after surgery, venous leak (based on elevated end-diastolic velocities) developed in a time-dependent fashion after RP. The incidence of venous leak less than 4 months after surgery was approximately 10% and rose to 35% between 8 to 12 months after surgery and 50% after 12 months. The importance of this information is that, in the same series, men with normal erectile hemodynamics were more likely to have recovery of natural erectile function. However, only 8% of men who had venous leak had recovery of naturally functioning erections (capable of sexual intercourse) after surgery. It is also known that men with venous leak are far less likely to respond to a PDE5i than men with arterial insufficiency.[48]

ANIMAL DATA SUPPORTING REHABILITATION

Several studies in animal models have demonstrated a positive effect of regular PDE5i use (tadalafil, sildenafil, or vardenafil) after cavernous nerve injury. It appears from those studies that this positive effect may result from a protective effect of PDE5i on various tissues involved in erectile function.

Firstly, it has been shown in rat models of stroke that the administration of PDE5i (sildenafil) increases brain levels of cyclic GMP, induces neurogenesis and reduces neurologic deficits when given to rats 2 or 24 hours after stroke.[48,49] This potential neuroprotective effect of chronic PDE5i was shown by Mulhall and colleagues[47] to occur also on cavernous nerves. In a cavernous injury model, chronic sildenafil treatment (20 mg/kg) was associated with an improvement in neural organization and greater density of myelin sheaths compared with the control group. In a recent study by Becher and colleagues,[50] caveolin-1 and alpha-smooth muscle actin expression in cavernous tissue was shown to be significantly reduced by pelvic nerve injury. The loss was related to the extent of the neural damage and the early administration of sildenafil elicited caveolin-1 expression, which appeared to preserve cavernous nerve function.

It has also been shown that PDE5i is effective in preventing fibrosis. Indeed, several studies have demonstrated a reduced amount of collagen deposition and fibrosis in penile tissues of animals chronically treated with PDE5i.[12–15,51,52] The underlying molecular mechanism for this appears to be related to the fact that PDE5i has been shown to have an antifibrotic effect at persistently high levels on a variety of tissues as well being a NO donor.[53,54] A study by Ferrini and colleagues,[12] suggested that the effect of a PDE5i such as vardenafil might be mediated by an increased inducible NO synthase (iNOS) expression and activity. In their study, rats exposed to nerve injury demonstrated a threefold increase in corporal smooth muscle apoptosis, a 60% reduction in the smooth muscle to collagen ratio, a twofold increase in iNOS expression, and development of CVOD compared with the sham group. When vardenafil was given daily for 45 days to the animals that underwent bilateral nerve resection, the iNOS was increased, the corporal smooth muscle to collagen ratio was normalized, and the subsequent CVOD was prevented. Prolonged endogenous induction of iNOS seems to produce sufficient NO to reduce collagen synthesis, inhibit TGF-β1 expression and myofibroblast differentiation, and activate metalloproteinases that break down collagen I in Peyronie disease animal models, and may do similarly in corporal smooth muscle.[55]

Similar results to that obtained with chronic administration of vardenafil have been reported in other animal models of post-RP ED using long-term administration of sildenafil and tadalafil.[15,56–61] Additionally, Vignozzi and colleagues[52] found that chronic tadalafil administration (120 days) to rats was able to prevent the cavernosal smooth muscle fibrosis that occurred after bilateral cavernous neurotomy.

Moreover, PDE5i has been shown to have a protective effect against apoptosis. Das and colleagues[62,63] have shown that mouse cardiac myocyte cells exposed to hypoxia and reoxygenation showed less necrosis and apoptosis if they were treated with sildenafil compared with non-treated cells. These in vitro studies were confirmed in vivo, in a rabbit model of cardiac ischemia-reperfusion by Salloum colleagues[64–66] in which both sildenafil and vardenafil were shown to reduce the area of cardiac necrosis. Following these findings, Mulhall and colleagues[15] have shown that chronic administration of PDE5i was able to reduce the cavernosal apoptotic process after cavernous nerve injury. Lysiak and colleagues[17] demonstrated this effect was likely to be mediated by the phosphorylation of the survival associated kinases Akt and extracellular signal-regulated kinase.

Finally, PDE5i has also been shown to have a role in endothelial cell preservation. Behr-Roussel and colleagues[67] have shown that endothelium-dependent relaxations of cavernosal strips to acetylcholine of neurally intact rats were enhanced after subcutaneous chronic, 8-week treatment with sildenafil (60 mg/kg). Moreover, the same investigators showed the erectile responses to acute sildenafil were greater in chronically treated rats with sildenafil. They concluded that long-term sildenafil treatment might have long-lasting, physiologically significant erectile tissue benefits, probably mediated through the activation of Akt-dependent endothelial NOS (eNOS). This pathway was clearly highlighted in a subsequent study by Mulhall and colleagues,[51] where chronic administration of sildenafil given subcutaneously daily for three different durations (3, 10, 28 days) resulted in preservation of the smooth muscle to collagen ratio, and in the increased expression of Akt and eNOS. These conclusions have been confirmed by other investigators.[68–70]

However, it seems that PDE5i may as well induce endothelial cells preservation through another pathway. Recent studies have suggested a restoration of endothelial progenitor cells (EPCs) to normal levels in patients with ED treated chronically with PDE5i (either sildenafil, tadalafil, or vardenafil).[71–74] This may be due to the direct effect of PDE5i on the inhibition of PDE5 in the bone marrow where PDE5 messenger RNA have shown to be present.[75] Interestingly, it seems that the eNOS pathway itself directly interacts with EPCs. It has been demonstrated that a lack of eNOS induces defective hematopoietic recovery and EPC mobilization.[76]

Finally, the efficacy of PDE5i in tissue preservation is likely to be highly time-dependent. Indeed, the effect of sildenafil on all post-neural injury alterations (such as penile hypo-oxygenation and over-expression of the profibrotic ET-1 type B receptor) was more evident the earlier it was administered.[39] Furthermore, in the rat model, the highest rate of erectile function recovery occurred with higher doses and longer time of sildenafil administration.[15] In a study by Mulhall and colleagues,[15] rats with bilateral cavernous nerve crush receiving daily sildenafil had higher ICP to MAP ratios than the controls to which no sildenafil was given. Among the sildenafil daily-treatment group, the ICP to MAP ratios in animals that started sildenafil at a dose of 20 mg/kg for 3 days before cavernous nerve crush injury were higher than that in animals started on sildenafil 1 hour prior or 3 days after cavernous nerve crush.

HUMAN DATA SUPPORTING THE CONCEPT OF PENILE REHABILITATION

The human literature, albeit somewhat limited, is generally supportive of the concept of penile rehabilitation after RP. The first study to support the use of penile rehabilitation after RP was a randomized trial published in 1997 by Montorsi and colleagues.[77] A total of 30 patients with clinically localized prostate cancer was randomized after nerve-sparing RP to intracavernosal alprostadil (PGE1) injections 3 times per week for 12 weeks or observation without any treatment. Patients were assessed at the 6-month follow-up by sexual history, physical examination, color Doppler sonography of the cavernous arteries, and recording of nocturnal erections. Twelve of the 15 patients using injection therapy completed the trial, 8 of which (67%) reported the recovery of spontaneous erection sufficient for satisfactory sexual intercourse, compared with 3 out of 15 patients (20%) in the control group. All the patients in both groups that reported normal postoperative erections (except one) also showed normal erections on nocturnal testing, whereas color Doppler sonography demonstrated normal penile hemodynamics in all of them. In the control group, 53% of the patients with failure to recover functional erections had venous leak on Doppler penile ultrasound. Although limited by its small number, there is a signal from these data that early erections after RP are important to eventual erectile function recovery.

The actual histologic impact of sildenafil on corporal smooth muscle in men after RP was studied by Schwartz and colleagues[78] in 2004. In a randomized trial, 40 potent patients with prostate cancer underwent RP and were divided into two treatment groups. One group received 50 mg sildenafil and another 100 mg sildenafil every other night for 6 months beginning the day of catheter removal. Corporal biopsy was performed before RP and 6 months postoperatively. Twenty-one patients completed the study, 11 in 50 mg group and 10 in the 100 mg group. Histopathological analysis showed significant preservation of smooth muscle content with sildenafil use at both 50 and 100 mg levels (42.8% and 56.8%, respectively). These findings are in stark contrast to those of the aforementioned Iacono data. Furthermore, these data support the idea that PDE5i has a myoprotective and possibly even a myotrophic effect on the corporal smooth muscle.

In 2005, Mulhall and colleagues,[79] shed more light on potential benefits of early post-RP erections in both promoting the return of spontaneous erectile function, and improving the ability of patients to become a drug responder. They compared the erectile function outcomes at 18 months post-RP of a group of 58 patients undergoing penile rehabilitation (advised to obtain three erections per week using either sildenafil or intracavernosal injection therapy) and a group of 74 matched controls followed serially after RP who opted not to pursue a penile rehabilitation program. At 18 months post-RP, the patients opting for rehabilitation (R) had compared with the nonrehabilitation (NR) group significantly higher rates of medication-unassisted intercourse (R = 52% vs NR = 19%, $P<.001$); rates of sildenafil response (R = 64% vs NR = 24%, $P<.001$); and response to intracavernosal injection (R = 95% vs NR = 76%, $P<.01$).

The importance of the timing of penile rehabilitation after RP was confirmed in 2008 by Padma-Nathan and colleagues,[56] in publishing data from a Pfizer-sponsored trial, originally completed in 2002. In this study, 4 weeks after bilateral nerve-sparing radical retropubic prostatectomy, men with normal erectile function before surgery were randomized to double-blind sildenafil (50 or 100 mg) or placebo nightly for 36 weeks, followed by an 8-week drug-free period before assessment of erectile function. The 1-month delay to the commencement of the treatment was an arbitrary choice made because of the potential for sildenafil-induced erections in patients with an indwelling catheter. At 9 months after surgery, 27% of all patients using Viagra (there was no significant difference between 50 and 100 mg Viagra) had recovery of erections similar to their baseline erections compared with 4% of the patients in the placebo group. Whereas the erectile function recovery was shown to be higher in the Viagra group, the 25% response rate revealed by a mid-study blinded review of data, far lower than that reported in contemporary surgical series from centers of excellence, forced the investigators to cease the study accrual. Despite this, there was a sevenfold increase in the proportion of men having return of their erectile function back to baseline level when exposed to sildenafil after RP.

In a later study by Mulhall and colleagues,[80] compared the erectile function outcomes of two groups of patients with clinically organ-confined prostate cancer treated with bilateral nerve-sparing RP, matched for age, comorbidity status, and baseline EF. They were both instructed to obtain three erections per week using initially sildenafil and, if unsuccessful, intracavernous injections. The difference was that they were subdivided into those starting rehabilitation at less than 6 months after RP (early) and those starting at 6 months or more after RP (delayed). The mean duration after RP at the time of starting penile rehabilitation was 2 and 7 months in the early (48 patients) and delayed groups (36 patients), respectively ($P<.01$). At 2 years after surgery, there was a highly statistically significant difference in IIEF erectile function domain score between the early and delayed groups (22 vs 16, $P<.001$). There were also statistically significant differences between the groups in the percentage of men at 2 years after RP who had unassisted functional erections and sildenafil-assisted functional erections (58% vs 30%, $P<.01$; 86% vs 45%, $P<.01$, respectively).

These data suggest that delaying the start of penile rehabilitation after RP is associated with poorer outcomes for erectile function.

Additionally, in a nonrandomized study by Bannowsky and colleagues,[58] a strong benefit of penile rehabilitation was realized when it is started no later than the first day after RP. Indeed, in their study, 41 sexually active patients with preserved nocturnal erections (defined on nocturnal penile tumescence monitoring) were divided into a group of 23 patients who received sildenafil 25 mg/day at night and a control group of 18 patients followed but without the use of PDE5i (nonrandomized). A significant difference in IIEF-5 score and time to recovery of erectile function between the groups was observed ($P<.001$), with erectile function recovery rates of 86% versus 66% achieved in the respective groups. In addition to supporting the use of early postoperative low-dose sildenafil for erectile function recovery, this study demonstrated that a high proportion of men early after bilateral nerve-sparing surgery have good nocturnal erectile function.

Counter-balancing these encouraging data in favor of early penile rehabilitation, more recently, the Bayer-sponsored Recovery of Erections: Intervention with Vardenafil Early Nightly Therapy study has raised questions about the utility of penile rehabilitation.[81] The study was very complicated in its design. Within 14 days of bilateral nerve-sparing RP, patients were randomly assigned in a 1:1:1 ratio to receive either 9 months of treatment with vardenafil, 10 mg nightly (which could be decreased to 5 mg if required), plus on-demand placebo for sexual intercourse; 9 months of treatment with flexible-dose, on-demand vardenafil for sexual intercourse (starting at 10 mg with the option to titrate to 5 mg or 29 mg) plus nightly placebo; or 9 months of treatment with nightly placebo plus on-demand placebo for sexual intercourse. After this, a 2-month single-blind phase was conducted in which all patients received only placebo for sexual intercourse, this was, in turn, followed by a 2-month open-label phase in which all patients received vardenafil for sexual intercourse. The inclusion-exclusion criteria were standard for ED post-RP trials. This study, which has been criticized in detail elsewhere,[82] failed to demonstrate any difference in natural or vardenafil-assisted erectile function between men using vardenafil on-demand or daily, thus raising questions about rehabilitation as well as the design of the study. The implications of the difference in outcomes between the Pfizer- and Bayer-sponsored studies are unclear, but likely reside largely in the very different designs of the studies.

As a result, in the absence of definitive data to date, The International Consensus of Sexual Medicine (ICSM) 2009 committee on rehabilitation after RP could not define the optimal approach to rehabilitation at this time but recommended that clinicians should (1) discuss prevalence rates, (2) discuss the pathophysiology of ED after RP, (3) discuss the predictors of erectile function recovery, (4) use validated instruments respecting the published cut-offs for normalcy, (5) discuss rehabilitation outcomes with patients, and (6) discuss with patients the significant potential benefits that may be associated with rehabilitation.[83]

OTHER STRATEGIES

More recently, two other strategies have been explored for the purposes of penile rehabilitation post-prostatectomy: vacuum erectile device therapy and the use of transurethral prostaglandin.

Vacuum Devices

A number of centers have studied the role of vacuum devices (VDs) for the preservation of penile length post-prostatectomy and for rehabilitation. It has been well documented that the P_{O_2} and P_{CO_2} levels in the cavernosal sinusoids following the application of a vacuum device remain in the venous range.[84] Indeed, the oxygen saturation is approximately 80%. If one believes that cavernosal oxygenation is critical to erectile tissue health and penile rehabilitation outcomes, this finding would undermine the role of VD therapy as a rehabilitation strategy.

A study by Raina and colleagues[85] included 109 patients who were randomized to VD use daily for 9 months versus observation. Thirty-two percent of patients in the VD rehabilitation group versus 37% in the observation group had recovery of natural erections at 9 months after surgery. Seventy percent of the VD users were able to have sexual intercourse with the use of the VD at that time.

Dalkin and colleagues[86] studied 39 men with good preoperative erectile function who underwent nerve-sparing RP. Stretched flaccid penile length was evaluated preoperatively and at 3 months postoperatively by a single examiner. The VD was used daily starting the day after catheter removal and was continued for 90 days. In men using the VD on more than 50% of the possible days, only 3% had a decrease in stretched flaccid penile length of greater than 1cm. Of the three men with poor VD compliance, 67% had a penile length reduction of more than 1 cm.

Kohler and colleagues[87] analyzed 28 men after nerve-sparing RP who were randomly assigned to early VD use or a control group. The VD group had therapy commenced 1 month after RP, whereas the control group had VD therapy instituted 6 months after RP. Postoperative Sexual Health Inventory for Men (SHIM) scores (while using the VD) were higher in the treatment group at 6 months (12.4 vs 3.0). Furthermore, in the treatment group, no significant changes in stretched flaccid penile length were measured at 3 or 6 months postoperatively. In the control group, the mean penile length loss at 3 and 6 months was approximately 2 cm.

These data were recently supported by encouraging animal data from Yuan and colleagues[88] on the potential benefits of vacuum therapy in penile rehabilitation. In their study, three groups of rats were submitted to a bilateral cavernous nerve crush alone or crush plus VD therapy (5 minutes twice daily treatment with a 1 minute interval, Monday to Friday beginning at 2 weeks after crush surgery). After 4 weeks of treatment, the ICP to MAP ratio was measured as well as the duration (area under the curve) and for the structural analyses, the whole rat penes were harvested. The daily VD therapy in crush rats preserved the ICP to MAP ratios (0.53 ± 0.06 at 5 V and 0.65 ± 0.03 at 7.5 V), which was significantly higher compared with the sham group ($P<.01$). The structural analyses performed indicated that VD therapy in this model preserved erectile function through antihypoxic, antiapoptotic, and antifibrotic mechanisms.

Although not yet performed, there is a solid rationale for a large, multicenter analysis of VD therapy in a randomized controlled trial as a rehabilitation strategy to be conducted.

Intraurethral Prostaglandin Suppository

Recently there has also been resurgence in interest in the use of the intraurethral alprostadil suppository (MUSE; Vivus, Mountain View, CA) as a treatment strategy for ED as well as a penile rehabilitation strategy. Costabile and colleagues,[89] in a retrospective analysis of all alprostadil clinical trial data, analyzed 384 patients who were postprostatectomy. In this population, 40% had sexual intercourse on at least one occasion at home and 18% of patients had urethral pain and burning. The limiting factor in the use of alprostadil in the treatment of men postprostatectomy, particularly in the first year after surgery, is penile pain due to PGE1 hypersensitivity.

Raina and colleagues[90] studied 54 patients using alprostadil post-RP. Of these patients, 55% were capable of having sexual intercourse using alprostadil and 48% continued long-term therapy. The compliance with alprostadil was 63% at a mean follow-up of 2.3 years. Mean SHIM scores went from 19 preoperatively to 5 immediately postoperatively, and this increased to 16 with the use of alprostadil. A score of 16 on the SHIM questionnaire is not normal, although there appears to be a signal that there may be some benefit to alprostadil as a rehabilitation strategy. The same investigators studied 91 men who had undergone nerve-sparing RP with a mean follow-up of 6 months. Of these men, 56 were treated with alprostadil, 125 or 250 µg, three times per week for 6 months. Alprostadil was started 3 weeks after surgery. The control group was allowed to use erectogenic agents on-demand for sexual intercourse. Of the alprostadil rehabilitation patients, 50% had sexual intercourse without the use of any aides versus 37% of the untreated patients, 100% had penile pain, and 32% discontinued treatment.[91]

The first study to directly compare the ability of alprostadil and a PDE5i to enhance penile recovery subsequent to bilateral nerve-sparing RP was published by McCullough and colleagues[92] in 2010. In their prospective, randomized, open-label, multicenter trial, two groups of post-RP patients with clinically localized prostate cancer started nightly treatment within 1 month of surgery with intraurethral alprostadil (n = 139) and 50 mg oral sildenafil citrate (n = 73), respectively, for 9 months. Ninety-seven patients completed the trial in the alprostadil group and 59 in the sildenafil group. The benefit to return of erectile function of nightly sildenafil citrate versus intraurethral alprostadil was comparable within the first year of surgery with no statistical differences at any time-point between groups in the results of the sexual encounter profile, the Erectile Dysfunction Inventory of Treatment Satisfaction or measured stretched penile length.

THE MEMORIAL SLOAN KETTERING CANCER CENTER PENILE REHABILITATION ALGORITHM

It is the authors' preference that patients are sent to our Sexual Medicine Clinic before surgery so that we can discuss realistic expectations after surgery. We also encourage all patients to consider the use of low-dose PDE5i (typically sildenafil 25 mgs) on a nightly basis for the 2 weeks before the RP (**Fig. 1**). This strategy is based on the animal data discussed above that supports pretreatment. These patients are then told that with the catheter in place they should continue a low-dose PDE5i on a nightly basis. When they

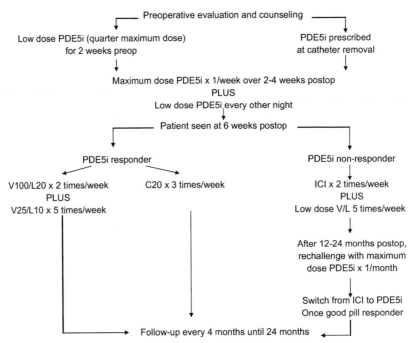

Fig. 1. The Memorial Sloan Kettering Cancer Center penile rehabilitation algorithm. C, Cialis (tadalafil); ICI, intracavernosal injections; L, Levitra (vardenafil); V, Viagra (sildenafil).

are given permission by their surgeon to resume attempts at obtaining erections, they switch to a low-dose PDE5i 6 nights a week and a maximum-dose pill 1 night per week with sexual stimulation. The patients are encouraged to return to the office 6 weeks after surgery, which will allow them approximately 4 weeks to try the maximum-dose medication (usually 3–4 attempts). For patients who have not been seen in the Sexual Medicine Clinic before surgery, the practice nurse writes a prescription for a PDE5i on the day the catheter is removed, and they are told to use a low-dose agent 6 nights a week and a maximum-dose medication 1 night a week with sexual stimulation from 2 weeks post-RP onwards.

Upon return to the office at 6 weeks after surgery, patients are asked about their response to the maximum-dose PDE5i. If the patient is a responder (defined as penetration hardness), they will use PDE5i alone for the purpose of penile rehabilitation: maximum-dose sildenafil or vardenafil 2 nights a week and a low dose on the other 5 nights. Alternatively, they can use tadalafil, 20 mg, three times a week. The patients are encouraged to get at least two erections per week. The major issue with this approach is cost, as a sildenafil responder will use 13 pills per month. The authors' have not yet explored the

tadalafil, 5 mg a day, strategy for this population because, after 5 days of continuous use of 5 mg daily, yield serum levels equivalent to a single 8 mg dose are achieved. This serum level is not likely sufficient for intercourse in the early stages after RP, so that supplementation using tadalafil 10 mgs 2 nights a week would be required translating into even greater cost.

Those patients who present at 6 weeks after surgery who have not responded to a PDE5i are driven directly to intracavernosal injection therapy. They are encouraged to undergo penile injection therapy training and to use injection therapy at least two times a week. On noninjection nights, they are told to use low-dose, a short-acting (sildenafil or vardenafil) PDE5i nightly as previously outlined. We discourage patients who are using regular injections from using tadalafil because of its long half-life. Toward the end of the first year after surgery, if patients are still using penile injection therapy they are encouraged to use a maximum-dose PDE5i at least once per month. This is performed in an effort to determine if the patient is responding to oral medication, as this will facilitate them ceasing injection therapy. It usually takes 10 to 14 months after surgery to start seeing some improvement in erectile function, but it is an 18 to 24 month time-frame before optimization of erectile function recovery is seen.

REFERENCES

1. Tal R, Alphs HH, Krebs P, et al. Erectile function recovery rate after radical prostatectomy: a meta-analysis. J Sex Med 2009;6:2538–46.
2. Quinlan DM, Epstein JI, Carter BS, et al. Sexual function following radical prostatectomy: influence of preservation of neurovascular bundles. J Urol 1991;145:998–1002.
3. Marien T, Sankin A, Lepor H. Factors predicting preservation of erectile function in men undergoing open radical retropubic prostatectomy. J Urol 2009;181:1817–22.
4. Catalona WJ, Carvalhal GF, Mager DE, et al. Potency, continence and complication rates in 1,870 consecutive radical retropubic prostatectomies. J Urol 1999;162:433–8.
5. Walsh PC, Partin AW, Epstein JI. Cancer control and quality of life following anatomical radical retropubic prostatectomy: results at 10 years. J Urol 1994;152:1831–6.
6. Zippe CD, Kedia AW, Kedia K, et al. Treatment of erectile dysfunction after radical prostatectomy with sildenafil citrate (Viagra). Urology 1998;52:963–6.
7. Moskovic DJ, Alphs H, Nelson CJ, et al. Subjective characterization of nerve sparing predicts recovery of erectile function after radical prostatectomy: defining the utility of a nerve sparing grading system. J Sex Med 2011;8(1):255–60.
8. Masterson TA, Serio AM, Mulhall JP, et al. Modified technique for neurovascular bundle preservation during radical prostatectomy: association between technique and recovery of erectile function. BJU Int 2008;101:1217–22.
9. Katz D, Bennett NE, Stasi J, et al. Chronology of erectile function in patients with early functional erections following radical prostatectomy. J Sex Med 2010;7:803–9.
10. Leungwattanakij S, Bivalacqua TJ, Usta MF, et al. Cavernous neurotomy causes hypoxia and fibrosis in rat corpus cavernosum. J Androl 2003;24:239–45.
11. User HM, Hairston JH, Zelner DJ, et al. Penile weight and cell subtype specific changes in a post-radical prostatectomy model of erectile dysfunction. J Urol 2003;169:1175–9.
12. Ferrini MG, Davila HH, Kovanecz I, et al. Vardenafil prevents fibrosis and loss of corporal smooth muscle that occurs after bilateral cavernosal nerve resection in the rat. Urology 2006;68:429–35.
13. Ferrini MG, Kovanecz I, Sanchez S, et al. Fibrosis and loss of smooth muscle in the corpora cavernosa precede corporal veno-occlusive dysfunction (CVOD) induced by experimental cavernosal nerve damage in the rat. J Sex Med 2009;6:415–28.
14. Kovanecz I, Rambhatla A, Ferrini MG, et al. Chronic daily tadalafil prevents the corporal fibrosis and veno-occlusive dysfunction that occurs after cavernosal nerve resection. BJU Int 2008;101:203–10.
15. Mulhall JP, Muller A, Donohue JF, et al. The functional and structural consequences of cavernous nerve injury are ameliorated by sildenafil citrate. J Sex Med 2008;5:1126–36.
16. Klein LT, Miller MI, Buttyan R, et al. Apoptosis in the rat penis after penile denervation. J Urol 1997;158:626–30.
17. Lysiak JJ, Yang SK, Klausner AP, et al. Tadalafil increases Akt and extracellular signal-regulated kinase 1/2 activation, and prevents apoptotic cell death in the penis following denervation. J Urol 2008;179:779–85.
18. Podlasek CA, Gonzalez CM, Zelner DJ, et al. Analysis of NOS isoform changes in a post radical prostatectomy model of erectile dysfunction. Int J Impot Res 2001;13(Suppl 5):S1–15.
19. Canguven O, Burnett A. Cavernous nerve injury using rodent animal models. J Sex Med 2008;5:1776–85.
20. Mullerad M, Donohue JF, Li PS, et al. Functional sequelae of cavernous nerve injury in the rat: is there model dependency. J Sex Med 2006;3:77–83.
21. Jin HR, Chung YG, Kim WJ, et al. A mouse model of cavernous nerve injury-induced erectile dysfunction: functional and morphological characterization of the corpus cavernosum. J Sex Med 2010;7(10):3351–64.
22. Iacono F, Giannella R, Somma P, et al. Histological alterations in cavernous tissue after radical prostatectomy. J Urol 2005;173:1673–6.
23. Rambhatla A, Kovanecz I, Ferrini M, et al. Rationale for phosphodiesterase 5 inhibitor use post-radical prostatectomy: experimental and clinical review. Int J Impot Res 2008;20:30–4.
24. Mulhall JP, Secin FP, Guillonneau B. Artery sparing radical prostatectomy—myth or reality? J Urol 2008;179:827–31.
25. Secin FP, Karanikolas N, Touijer AK, et al. Anatomy of accessory pudendal arteries in laparoscopic radical prostatectomy. J Urol 2005;174:523–6 [discussion: 526].
26. Secin FP, Karanikolas N, Kuroiwa K, et al. Positive surgical margins and accessory pudendal artery preservation during laparoscopic radical prostatectomy. Eur Urol 2005;48:786–92 [discussion: 793].
27. Polascik TJ, Walsh PC. Radical retropubic prostatectomy: the influence of accessory pudendal arteries on the recovery of sexual function. J Urol 1995;154:150–2.
28. Rogers CG, Trock BP, Walsh PC. Preservation of accessory pudendal arteries during radical retropubic prostatectomy: surgical technique and results. Urology 2004;64:148–51.
29. Droupy S, Hessel A, Benoit G, et al. Assessment of the functional role of accessory pudendal arteries in

erection by transrectal color Doppler ultrasound. J Urol 1999;162:1987–91.

30. Matin SF. Recognition and preservation of accessory pudendal arteries during laparoscopic radical prostatectomy. Urology 2006;67:1012–5.

31. Rosen MP, Greenfield AJ, Walker TG, et al. Arteriogenic impotence: findings in 195 impotent men examined with selective internal pudendal angiography. Young Investigator's Award. Radiology 1990;174:1043–8.

32. Gray RR, Keresteci AG, St Louis EL, et al. Investigation of impotence by internal pudendal angiography: experience with 73 cases. Radiology 1982;144:773–80.

33. Benoit G, Droupy S, Quillard J, et al. Supra and infralevator neurovascular pathways to the penile corpora cavernosa. J Anat 1999;195(Pt 4):605–15.

34. Breza J, Aboseif SR, Orvis BR, et al. Detailed anatomy of penile neurovascular structures: surgical significance. J Urol 1989;141:437–43.

35. Box GN, Kaplan AG, Rodriguez E Jr, et al. Sacrifice of accessory pudendal arteries in normally potent men during robot-assisted radical prostatectomy does not impact potency. J Sex Med 2010;7:298–303.

36. Moreland RB, Albadawi H, Bratton C, et al. O2-dependent prostanoid synthesis activates functional PGE receptors on corpus cavernosum smooth muscle. Am J Physiol Heart Circ Physiol 2001;281:H552–8.

37. Moreland RB, Gupta S, Goldstein I, et al. Cyclic AMP modulates TGF-beta 1-induced fibrillar collagen synthesis in cultured human corpus cavernosum smooth muscle cells. Int J Impot Res 1998;10:159–63.

38. Muller A, Tal R, Donohue JF, et al. The effect of hyperbaric oxygen therapy on erectile function recovery in a rat cavernous nerve injury model. J Sex Med 2008;5:562–70.

39. Vignozzi L, Morelli A, Filippi S, et al. Effect of sildenafil administration on penile hypoxia induced by cavernous neurotomy in the rat. Int J Impot Res 2008;20:60–7.

40. Kim N, Vardi Y, Padma-Nathan H, et al. Oxygen tension regulates the nitric oxide pathway. Physiological role in penile erection. J Clin Invest 1993;91:437–42.

41. Tal R, Mueller A, Mulhall JP. The correlation between intracavernosal pressure and cavernosal blood oxygenation. J Sex Med 2009;6:2722–7.

42. Lue TF, Takamura T, Schmidt RA, et al. Potential preservation of potency after radical prostatectomy. Urology 1983;22:165–7.

43. Knispel HH, Andresen R. Evaluation of vasculogenic impotence by monitoring of cavernous oxygen tension. J Urol 1993;149:1276–9.

44. Ghofrani HA, Voswinckel R, Reichenberger F, et al. Differences in hemodynamic and oxygenation responses to three different phosphodiesterase-5 inhibitors in patients with pulmonary arterial hypertension: a randomized prospective study. J Am Coll Cardiol 2004;44:1488–96.

45. Nehra A, Goldstein I, Pabby A, et al. Mechanisms of venous leakage: a prospective clinicopathological correlation of corporeal function and structure. J Urol 1996;156:1320–9.

46. Mulhall JP, Graydon RJ. The hemodynamics of erectile dysfunction following nerve-sparing radical retropubic prostatectomy. Int J Impot Res 1996;8:91–4.

47. Mulhall JP, Slovick R, Hotaling J, et al. Erectile dysfunction after radical prostatectomy: hemodynamic profiles and their correlation with the recovery of erectile function. J Urol 2002;167:1371–5.

48. Mulhall J, Barnas J, Aviv N, et al. Sildenafil citrate response correlates with the nature and the severity of penile vascular insufficiency. J Sex Med 2005;2:104–8.

49. Zhang R, Wang Y, Zhang L, et al. Sildenafil (Viagra) induces neurogenesis and promotes functional recovery after stroke in rats. Stroke 2002;33:2675–80.

50. Becher EF, Toblli JE, Castronuovo C, et al. Expression of caveolin-1 in penile cavernosal tissue in a denervated animal model after treatment with sildenafil citrate. J Sex Med 2009;6:1587–93.

51. Kovanecz I, Rambhatla A, Ferrini M, et al. Long-term continuous sildenafil treatment ameliorates corporal veno-occlusive dysfunction (CVOD) induced by cavernosal nerve resection in rats. Int J Impot Res 2008;20:202–12.

52. Vignozzi L, Filippi S, Morelli A, et al. Effect of chronic tadalafil administration on penile hypoxia induced by cavernous neurotomy in the rat. J Sex Med 2006;3:419–31.

53. Magee TR, Ferrini M, Garban HJ, et al. Gene therapy of erectile dysfunction in the rat with penile neuronal nitric oxide synthase. Biol Reprod 2002;67:1033–41.

54. Valente EG, Vernet D, Ferrini MG, et al. L-arginine and phosphodiesterase (PDE) inhibitors counteract fibrosis in the Peyronie's fibrotic plaque and related fibroblast cultures. Nitric Oxide 2003;9:229–44.

55. Gonzalez-Cadavid NF, Rajfer J. The pleiotropic effects of inducible nitric oxide synthase (iNOS) on the physiology and pathology of penile erection. Curr Pharm Des 2005;11:4041–6.

56. Padma-Nathan H, McCullough AR, Levine LA, et al. Randomized, double-blind, placebo-controlled study of postoperative nightly sildenafil citrate for the prevention of erectile dysfunction after bilateral nerve-sparing radical prostatectomy. Int J Impot Res 2008;20:479–86.

57. Parsons JK, Marschke P, Maples P, et al. Effect of methylprednisolone on return of sexual function after nerve-sparing radical retropubic prostatectomy. Urology 2004;64:987–90.

58. Bannowsky A, Schulze H, van der Horst C, et al. Recovery of erectile function after nerve-sparing radical prostatectomy: improvement with nightly low-dose sildenafil. BJU Int 2008;101:1279–83.

59. Penson DF, McLerran D, Feng Z, et al. 5-year urinary and sexual outcomes after radical prostatectomy: results from the prostate cancer outcomes study. J Urol 2005;173:1701–5.

60. Rozet F, Galiano M, Cathelineau X, et al. Extraperitoneal laparoscopic radical prostatectomy: a prospective evaluation of 600 cases. J Urol 2005;174:908–11.

61. Stanford JL, Feng Z, Hamilton AS, et al. Urinary and sexual function after radical prostatectomy for clinically localized prostate cancer: the Prostate Cancer Outcomes Study. JAMA 2000;283:354–60.

62. Das A, Xi L, Kukreja RC. Phosphodiesterase-5 inhibitor sildenafil preconditions adult cardiac myocytes against necrosis and apoptosis. Essential role of nitric oxide signaling. J Biol Chem 2005;280:12944–55.

63. Fisher PW, Salloum F, Das A, et al. Phosphodiesterase-5 inhibition with sildenafil attenuates cardiomyocyte apoptosis and left ventricular dysfunction in a chronic model of doxorubicin cardiotoxicity. Circulation 2005;111:1601–10.

64. Kukreja R, Salloum F, Xi L. Anti-ischemic effects of sildenafil, vardenafil and tadalafil in heart. Int J Impot Res 2007;19:226–7.

65. Salloum FN, Ockaili RA, Wittkamp M, et al. Vardenafil: a novel type 5 phosphodiesterase inhibitor reduces myocardial infarct size following ischemia/reperfusion injury via opening of mitochondrial K(ATP) channels in rabbits. J Mol Cell Cardiol 2006;40:405–11.

66. Salloum FN, Takenoshita Y, Ockaili RA, et al. Sildenafil and vardenafil but not nitroglycerin limit myocardial infarction through opening of mitochondrial K(ATP) channels when administered at reperfusion following ischemia in rabbits. J Mol Cell Cardiol 2007;42:453–8.

67. Behr-Roussel D, Gorny D, Mevel K, et al. Chronic sildenafil improves erectile function and endothelium-dependent cavernosal relaxations in rats: lack of tachyphylaxis. Eur Urol 2005;47:87–91.

68. Musicki B, Champion HC, Becker RE, et al. Erection capability is potentiated by long-term sildenafil treatment: role of blood flow-induced endothelial nitric-oxide synthase phosphorylation. Mol Pharmacol 2005;68:226–32.

69. Bivalacqua TJ, Liu T, Musicki B, et al. Endothelial nitric oxide synthase keeps erection regulatory function balance in the penis. Eur Urol 2007;51:1732–40.

70. De Young LX, Domes T, Lim K, et al. Endothelial rehabilitation: the impact of chronic PDE5 inhibitors on erectile function and protein alterations in cavernous tissue of diabetic rats. Eur Urol 2008;54:213–20.

71. Foresta C, De Toni L, Di Mambro A, et al. The PDE5 inhibitor sildenafil increases circulating endothelial progenitor cells and CXCR4 expression. J Sex Med 2009;6:369–72.

72. Foresta C, Di Mambro A, Caretta N, et al. Effect of vardenafil on endothelial progenitor cells in hypogonadotrophic hypogonadal patients: role of testosterone treatment. Clin Endocrinol 2009;71:412–6.

73. Foresta C, Ferlin A, De Toni L, et al. Circulating endothelial progenitor cells and endothelial function after chronic Tadalafil treatment in subjects with erectile dysfunction. Int J Impot Res 2006;18:484–8.

74. Foresta C, Lana A, Cabrelle A, et al. PDE-5 inhibitor, Vardenafil, increases circulating progenitor cells in humans. Int J Impot Res 2005;17:377–80.

75. Foresta C, Caretta N, Lana A, et al. Relationship between vascular damage degrees and endothelial progenitor cells in patients with erectile dysfunction: effect of vardenafil administration and PDE5 expression in the bone marrow. Eur Urol 2007;51:1411–7 [discussion: 1417–9].

76. Aicher A, Heeschen C, Mildner-Rihm C, et al. Essential role of endothelial nitric oxide synthase for mobilization of stem and progenitor cells. Nat Med 2003;9:1370–6.

77. Montorsi F, Guazzoni G, Strambi LF, et al. Recovery of spontaneous erectile function after nerve-sparing radical retropubic prostatectomy with and without early intracavernous injections of alprostadil: results of a prospective, randomized trial. J Urol 1997;158:1408–10.

78. Schwartz EJ, Wong P, Graydon RJ. Sildenafil preserves intracorporeal smooth muscle after radical retropubic prostatectomy. J Urol 2004;171:771–4.

79. Mulhall J, Land S, Parker M, et al. The use of an erectogenic pharmacotherapy regimen following radical prostatectomy improves recovery of spontaneous erectile function. J Sex Med 2005;2:532–40 [discussion: 540–2].

80. Mulhall JP, Parker M, Waters BW, et al. The timing of penile rehabilitation after bilateral nerve-sparing radical prostatectomy affects the recovery of erectile function. BJU Int 2010;105:37–41.

81. Montorsi F, Brock G, Lee J, et al. Effect of nightly versus on-demand vardenafil on recovery of erectile function in men following bilateral nerve-sparing radical prostatectomy. Eur Urol 2008;54:924–31.

82. Mulhall JP. Does on-demand vardenafil improve erectile function recovery after radical prostatectomy? Nat Clin Pract Urol 2009;6:14–5.

83. Mulhall JP, Bella AJ, Briganti A, et al. Erectile function rehabilitation in the radical prostatectomy patient. J Sex Med 2010;7:1687–98.

84. Bosshardt RJ, Farwerk R, Sikora R, et al. Objective measurement of the effectiveness, therapeutic success and dynamic mechanisms of the vacuum device. Br J Urol 1995;75:786–91.

85. Raina R, Agarwal A, Ausmundson S, et al. Early use of vacuum constriction device following radical prostatectomy facilitates early sexual activity and potentially earlier return of erectile function. Int J Impot Res 2006;18:77–81.

86. Dalkin BL, Christopher BA. Preservation of penile length after radical prostatectomy: early intervention with a vacuum erection device. Int J Impot Res 2007;19:501–4.

87. Kohler TS, Pedro R, Hendlin K, et al. A pilot study on the early use of the vacuum erection device after radical retropubic prostatectomy. BJU Int 2007;100:858–62.

88. Yuan J, Lin H, Li P, et al. Molecular mechanisms of vacuum therapy in penile rehabilitation: a novel animal study. Eur Urol 2010;58:773–80.

89. Costabile RA, Spevak M, Fishman IJ, et al. Efficacy and safety of transurethral alprostadil in patients with erectile dysfunction following radical prostatectomy. J Urol 1998;160:1325–8.

90. Raina R, Agarwal A, Zaramo CE, et al. Long-term efficacy and compliance of MUSE for erectile dysfunction following radical prostatectomy: SHIM (IIEF-5) analysis. Int J Impot Res 2005;17:86–90.

91. Raina R, Pahlajani G, Agarwal A, et al. The early use of transurethral alprostadil after radical prostatectomy potentially facilitates an earlier return of erectile function and successful sexual activity. BJU Int 2007;100:1317–21.

92. McCullough AR, Hellstrom WG, Wang R, et al. Recovery of erectile function after nerve sparing radical prostatectomy and penile rehabilitation with nightly intraurethral alprostadil versus sildenafil citrate. J Urol 2010;183:2451–6.

Testosterone and Prostate Cancer: What are the Risks for Middle-Aged Men?

Abraham Morgentaler, MD[a,b,*]

KEYWORDS

- Testosterone therapy • Prostate cancer • Testosterone
- Androgens • Testosterone deficiency

Over the last decade there has been a growing awareness of the health benefits of testosterone (T) therapy (TTh) for men with T deficiency, including improved sexual desire and performance, improved mood, increased muscle mass and strength, decreased fat mass, and improved bone mineral density.[1] These health benefits are of particular importance for middle-aged men, who generally are still in relatively good health and wish to live with a high quality of life. However, for approximately 70 years there has been a concern that higher serum T represents a risk for prostate cancer (PCa).[2] This concern regarding the relationship of T and PCa has been a major hurdle impeding more frequent use of TTh, because many physicians are reluctant to prescribe a beneficial treatment if there is a significant risk of precipitating cancer.

The basis for the historical fear regarding T and PCa stems from the experience that men with advanced PCa demonstrate rapid, dramatic regression of PCa based on serum markers such as prostate-specific antigen (PSA). This finding has led to the concept that PCa is androgen dependent, which in turn has led to the belief that ever-greater serum T would necessarily lead to ever-increasing PCa growth. If correct, then raising serum T with TTh might cause an occult quiescent prostate cancer to grow into an aggressive, clinically dangerous tumor.

However, over the last 10 to 15 years there has been a major reevaluation of the evidence regarding T and PCa. Whereas manipulation of serum T into and out of the castrate range clearly has a major impact on PCa growth, it now appears clear that variations in serum T within the naturally occurring range have minimal, if any effect on PCa.[2,3] This change in perspective has important implications for the safety of TTh in middle-aged men. In fact, emerging data suggest that low serum T may be a predictor of high-risk PCa, turning conventional wisdom regarding T and PCa on its head. In this article the author reviews the historical and current evidence regarding the relationship of T and PCa, and discusses implications for TTh for the middle-aged man.

ORIGIN OF THE CONCERN REGARDING TESTOSTERONE AND PROSTATE CANCER

In 1941 Charles Huggins and Clarence Hodges published the first report indicating that castration or treatment with estrogen in men with metastatic PCa caused a decline in the serum marker acid phosphatase.[4] Both treatments had the known effect of lowering serum T, and it was concluded that T caused an "enhanced rate of growth" of PCa. Androgen deprivation has been a mainstay of treatment for advanced PCa since that time. In addition, the investigators reported that T administration in these same men caused immediate PCa "activation" in all the individuals who received it.

In 1981 Fowler and Whitmore[5] reviewed the experience with T administration in men with

[a] Men's Health Boston, One Brookline Place, Suite 624, Brookline, MA 02445, USA
[b] Beth Israel Deaconess Medical Center, Harvard Medical School, Boston, MA, USA
* Men's Health Boston, One Brookline Place, Suite 624, Brookline, MA 02445.
E-mail address: amorgent@bidmc.harvard.edu

Urol Clin N Am 38 (2011) 119–124
doi:10.1016/j.ucl.2011.02.002

metastatic PCa at Memorial Sloan Kettering Cancer Center. Of 52 men who received T, 45 had an "unfavorable" response, most within 30 days. This study led to the widely repeated comment that offering T to a man with PCa was like "pouring gasoline on a fire," or "feeding a hungry tumor."

However, reexamination of these historical articles[2] revealed something quite different. In the article by Huggins and Hodges, 3 men were reported to receive T, yet results were only provided for 2 of these men, and 1 of these 2 had already been castrated.[4] Because we know today that an increase in serum T after androgen deprivation causes an increase in prostate markers such as PSA even in men without cancer, we can disqualify this individual from contributing to any general rule about T and PCa. In the end, the landmark article by Huggins and Hodges provides information on only a single man who received T administration without prior androgen deprivation. In this single case, the acid phosphatase results were erratic.[2]

The study by Fowler and Whitmore is even more instructive. Of the 52 men, only 4 were not yet androgen deprived by either castration or estrogen administration.[5] Of these 4 men, 1 had an early unfavorable result, and the other 3 continued to receive daily injections of T for 52, 55, and 310 days, without apparent negative effects. The investigators themselves were so surprised by these results that they postulated that naturally occurring serum T concentrations may be sufficient to produce maximal growth of PCa.[5]

What a reexamination of these and other articles from the pre-PSA era tell us is that T administration in men who were previously androgen deprived resulted in a rapid and near-universal growth in PCa manifestations, whereas T administration in hormonally intact men produced little or no effect.[2,3] This finding suggests that there is a limit to the ability of androgens to stimulate PCa growth.

LONGITUDINAL STUDIES

The relationship of T and other sex hormones to subsequent development of PCa has been extensively studied, in at least 21 population-based longitudinal studies.[6–12] In these studies a health history is obtained, and blood samples at baseline are then frozen for the duration of the study, in some cases up to 20 years or longer. At the end of the study men who have developed PCa are identified, and a matched set of men without PCa serve as controls.

Most of these studies surprisingly have shown no influence of serum T or other androgens on PCa risk. A small number have revealed weak associations with minor androgens, or ratios of one hormone to another, and in one case there was an association between quartile levels of free testosterone and PCa risk. However, these results have not been reproducible. It is worth noting that one large study of this type actually noted reduced PCa risk in men with higher T levels.[8]

In 2008 the investigators of 18 of these longitudinal studies pooled their data to form one large data set,[12] creating enough power to examine a variety of questions regarding serum sex hormones and PCa. In contrast to a meta-analysis, this was a single, actual study. With more than 3886 men with PCa and more than 6438 men as age-matched controls, this was one of the largest PCa studies published to date. The results showed no association between any androgens and PCa risk. Men with higher endogenous concentrations of serum T were at no greater risk of developing PCa than men with low levels of serum T.[12]

The importance of these studies is that they provide a sophisticated method of investigation to determine the long-term effects of endogenous hormone levels, especially testosterone, on the subsequent risk of development of PCa. Although such studies cannot entirely replace the value of a prospective long-term controlled study of TTh, they do address the question as to whether high levels of T (or other hormones) predispose men to a greater risk of later development of PCa. On this question, these prospective longitudinal studies provide two uniform and convincing answers: first, that men who develop PCa do not have higher baseline T levels, and second, men with higher T levels are at no greater risk of developing PCa than men with lower T concentrations.

TESTOSTERONE TRIALS

In the absence of any single large study on TTh, one must examine the results from smaller studies. One of these was a 12-month study of 371 men on T gel therapy.[13] Over the course of 1 year 3 cancers were detected, all due to an increase in PSA. One of these increases in PSA was transient and resolved; however, a biopsy was performed and revealed cancer. In this study the mean increase in PSA was 0.4 ng/mL. This increase was noted at 3 months, and PSA remained unchanged over the next 9 months.

Other studies have revealed a similar rate of cancer detection in TTh trials. In a review of 9 separate TTh trials involving 579 men and ranging from 3 to 36 months, 7 cancers were identified, representing a cancer detection rate of 1.2%.[14] Wang and colleagues[1] performed one of the longest TTh trials. In this study 163 men with a mean age of 51 years received T gel for 42 months. Over this time the mean PSA increased from 0.85 ng/mL at baseline to 1.1 ng/mL at 6 months, and then did not change significantly over the next 3 years of the study. Three men were diagnosed with prostate cancer, representing a cancer rate of less than 1% per year of treatment.

Prostate cancer rates were investigated among men with and without the prostatic precancerous lesion known as high-grade prostatic intraepithelial neoplasia (PIN). In this 12-month study 75 men with hypogonadism received TTh, including 55 men with benign pretreatment prostate biopsy, and 20 men with biopsy revealing PIN.[15] A similar 12-month increase in PSA of 0.3 ng/mL was seen in both groups, corresponding to a 15% rise. A single cancer was detected, in the PIN group, representing an overall cancer rate of 1.3%. The 5% cancer rate among men with PIN compares with a 25% risk over 3 years in this population, suggesting no significantly increased cancer risk.

One study that examined the effect of TTh on PSA found that the overall change was mild, and the individual response varied considerably. Among 58 men who underwent TTh for 1 year, the majority (32 men) demonstrated a mild PSA increase of 0.5 ng/mL or less.[14] There were also 14 men with a PSA increase greater than 0.5 ng/mL, but 12 men with a decline in PSA. No apparent differences in age, baseline T concentrations, or baseline PSA were noted between men with a PSA increase of greater than 0.5 ng/mL and men whose PSA declined. In 81 T-deficient men who received TTh, no increase was noted in PSA at 1-year intervals for up to 5 years.[16]

To put these studies and their results in perspective, it is important to be aware that the observed PSA changes in multiple studies of approximately 15% to 20% is not much greater than the 13% increase noted over 1 year in 50- to 60-year-old men participating in the placebo arm of an unrelated study.[17] In addition, the annual cancer rate of approximately 1% that shows up repeatedly in TTh trials compares favorably to cancer detection rates in men undergoing prostate cancer screening.[18]

A meta-analysis of 19 placebo-controlled TTh trials found that men who received T had no greater risk of PCa than men who received placebo.[19] There was also no greater risk of developing a PSA level of more than 4.0 ng/mL.

Remarkably, administration of supraphysiologic doses of T for 9 months in healthy men resulted in no increase in prostate volume or PSA.[20]

It is also worthwhile noting that two studies involving more than 400 men in total have shown that T-deficient men with PSA of 4.0 ng/mL or less have a biopsy-detectable cancer rate of 14% to 15%.[21,22] This result means that 1 in 7 men with normal PSA and low T has PCa. If raising T truly caused PCa to grow more rapidly, one would expect TTh trials to be associated with high rates of cancer. The fact that this does not occur argues strongly that PCa risk is unrelated to serum T concentration.

RESOLVING THE PARADOX

How is it possible that androgen deprivation and its discontinuation can have such a powerful effect on PCa growth, yet so much of the literature fails to demonstrate any effect of T on PCa?

The resolution of this paradox is the recognition that there is a finite ability of androgens to stimulate PCa. This concept has been formalized as the Saturation Model,[3] based on an accumulation of evidence from human trials, animal models, and PCa cell lines.

The key observation in all of these studies is that the prostate demonstrates exquisite sensitivity to changes in androgens at very low concentrations, but little or none at higher concentrations. Thus, a dose-response curve is easily shown in animals and PCa cell lines as androgens are increased; however, there then develops in all cases a plateau, beyond which even logarithmic increases in androgen concentrations elicit no further growth.[3]

One likely mechanism for the Saturation Model is via the androgen receptor (AR), which becomes maximally bound with androgen in human prostate at 4 nmol/L (approximately 120 ng/dL).[23] Because it is the androgen-AR complex that binds to genetic androgen response elements, once the AR has been maximally bound additional androgen is unable to influence cell activities via this mechanism, and serves merely as excess.

An additional mechanism is suggested by the work of Marks and colleagues,[24] in which hypogonadal men underwent prostate biopsy and comprehensive evaluation at baseline and after 6 months of injections of T or placebo every 2 weeks. Despite large changes in serum T concentrations, the intraprostatic concentrations of both T and dihydrotestosterone did not change significantly. Furthermore, no changes were noted in expression of androgen-related genes or genes associated with prostatic proliferation. These results indicate that substantial changes in serum androgen concentrations may occur without being reflected within the prostate, and do not appear to induce biologic changes within prostate tissue.

The Saturation Model explains why manipulating serum T into or out of the castrate range produces large changes in PCa, whereas variations in serum T within the naturally occurring range do not. Once the AR has been maximally bound (ie, saturated), one should expect minimal or no additional prostatic effect from higher serum androgens. Therefore, the one group at some increased risk of androgen-driven PCa stimulation includes men with severely depressed serum T, below the saturation point.

LOW TESTOSTERONE AND PROSTATE CANCER

As clinicians have begun to let go of the old belief that raising T would necessarily increase PCa risk, there has been a coincidental recognition that low T may itself represent a risk factor for PCa. There is now emerging data that testosterone deficiency is associated with greater risk of PCa, high Gleason scores, worse stage at presentation, and worse survival.[25]

A study of 345 men with hypogonadism and PSA levels of 4.0 ng/mL or less found that the group of men in the lowest tertile of total T had more than double the risk of cancer on biopsy compared with men in the highest tertile (odds ratio, 2.15; 95% confidence interval, 1.01–4.55).[21] In another study of 326 men who underwent radical prostatectomy, pretreatment T concentrations correlated with the likelihood of organ-confined disease.[26] In addition, there is now evidence correlating high Gleason scores with low T.[27]

Although not all studies have confirmed an association between low T and worrisome aspects of PCa, there is now an accumulation of studies that is certainly provocative. Whereas it was once believed that a long-term placebo-controlled study of TTh would almost certainly show an increase in the risk of PCa, now it must also be considered whether such a study might show a reduction in PCa, particularly high-risk PCa.

TESTOSTERONE THERAPY AFTER DIAGNOSIS OF PROSTATE CANCER

The growing number of men who appear to be cured from PCa after definitive therapy has created pressure to consider TTh in those men who are symptomatic for T deficiency. Although this has been a long-standing taboo, clinical experience with TTh together with the scientific evidence suggests this may be far less risky than had previously been assumed. Preliminary results from several small studies suggest that TTh may be used, with caution and in a carefully selected population, after PCa has been successfully treated.

The first of these was a small series of 7 cases in which TTh was provided to symptomatic hypogonadal men who had undergone radical prostatectomy and who had an undetectable postoperative PSA.[28] No recurrences were noted in these men despite 1 to 12 years of TTh in these individuals.

A second study reported similar reassuring results in 10 men who had also undergone radical prostatectomy with undetectable PSA.[29] Mean total T increased from 197 ng/dL to 591 ng/dL, and symptoms of hypogonadism improved. Most importantly, no PCa recurrences were noted with a median follow-up of 19 months.

A third study reported results in 31 men who received TTh after PCa treatment with brachytherapy.[30] In this group the median duration of treatment was 4.5 years with a range of 0.5 to 8.5 years. Total T concentrations rose from a median of 188 ng/dL to 498 ng/dL. No recurrences or PCa progression was noted, and all men remained with PSA less than 1.0 ng/mL at the end of the study.

There are now also reports of TTh in men with untreated PCa undergoing active surveillance. In one of these, an 84-year-old man with bilateral Gleason-6 PCa received 2 years of TTh with no increase in PSA.[31]

These various reports are consistent with the concept that PCa appears to be largely unaffected by variations in serum T within the naturally occurring range. Whereas not long ago any prior history of PCa was considered a lifelong contraindication to the use of TTh, the evidence no longer supports this notion. Although safety data are still lacking, it may now be reasonable to offer TTh to selected men with a history of PCa, as long as a discussion has taken place advising the patient that there is an unknown degree of risk of PCa progression or recurrence.

MONITORING FOR PROSTATE CANCER

Although there is little, if any, compelling evidence that TTh poses an increased risk of prostate cancer, it must also be recognized that there is great overlap between the population at risk for testosterone deficiency and the population at risk for prostate cancer, and it is thus highly recommended that men receiving TTh be monitored at regular intervals for prostate cancer. Monitoring should consist of PSA determination and digital rectal examination, with biopsy performed for development of an abnormal prostate examination, elevated PSA, or rapid increase in PSA.[18]

SUMMARY

In the absence of large, controlled prospective trials, it is impossible to definitively determine the safety of TTh in middle-aged men with T deficiency, especially with regard to the risk of PCa. However, there is now a large body of literature over several decades examining the relationship between androgens and PCa, providing a consistent picture that should provide a moderate degree of comfort to clinicians offering TTh.

Data from humans, animal models, and PCa cell lines indicate that while androgens are critical to the promotion of optimal PCa growth, there is a finite degree of androgen-dependent growth. These data show that the limit to maximal androgen-mediated PCa growth is reached at serum T levels that are well below most naturally occurring serum T concentrations (approximately 120 ng/dL), and that therefore the raising of serum T via TTh is unlikely to affect PCa growth. The single, important exception is the man with severe T deficiency, in whom there remains unmet androgen-driven capacity to stimulate PCa growth.

The field has changed so rapidly that it is no longer unusual to offer TTh to men with a history of treated PCa, and there are even reports of TTh in men undergoing active surveillance with untreated PCa, without evidence of clinical PCa progression. A new consideration is that low T may predispose to a greater risk of PCa, especially high-risk PCa.

The field of androgens and PCa has been turned upside down. With the new perspectives offered by science over the last decade or more, clinicians must balance the proven benefits of TTh against the historical fears regarding PCa that have failed to find evidentiary support.

REFERENCES

1. Wang C, Cunningham G, Dobs A, et al. Long-term testosterone gel (AndroGel) treatment maintains beneficial effects on sexual function and mood, lean and fat mass, and bone density in hypogonadal men. J Clin Endocrinol Metab 2004;89:2085–98.
2. Morgentaler A. Testosterone and prostate cancer: an historical perspective on a modern myth. Eur Urol 2006;50:935–9.
3. Morgentaler A, Traish AM. Shifting the paradigm of testosterone and prostate cancer: the Saturation Model and the limits of androgen-dependent growth. Eur Urol 2009;55:310–21.
4. Huggins C, Hodges CV. Studies on prostatic cancer: I. The effect of castration, of estrogen and of androgen injection on serum phosphatases in metastatic carcinoma of the prostate. Cancer Res 1941;1:293–7.
5. Fowler JE, Whitmore WF Jr. The response of metastatic adenocarcinoma of the prostate to exogenous testosterone. J Urol 1981;126:372–5.
6. Hsing AW. Hormones and prostate cancer: what's next? Epidemiol Rev 2001;23:42–58.
7. Eaton NE, Reeves GK, Appleby PN, et al. Endogenous sex hormones and prostate cancer: a quantitative review of prospective studies. Br J Cancer 1999; 80:930–4.
8. Stattin P, Lumme S, Tenkanen L, et al. High levels of circulating testosterone are not associated with increased prostate cancer risk: a pooled prospective study. Int J Cancer 2004;108:418–24.
9. Barrett-Connor E, Garland C, McPhillips JB, et al. A prospective, population-based study of androstenedione, estrogens, and prostatic cancer. Cancer Res 1990;50:169–73.
10. Parsons JK, Carter HB, Platz EA, et al. Serum testosterone and the risk of prostate cancer: potential implications for testosterone therapy. Cancer Epidemiol Biomarkers Prev 2005;14:2257–60.
11. Gann PH, Hennekens CH, Ma J, et al. Prospective study of sex hormone levels and risk of prostate cancer. J Natl Cancer Inst 1996;88:1118–26.
12. Endogenous Hormones Prostate Cancer Collaborative Group, Roddam AW, Allen NE, et al. Endogenous sex hormones and prostate cancer: a collaborative analysis of 18 prospective studies. J Natl Cancer Inst 2008;100:170.
13. Dean JD, Carnegie C, Rodzvilla J, et al. Long-term effects of Testim 1% testosterone gel in hypogonadal men. Rev Urol 2004;6:S22–9.
14. Rhoden EL, Morgentaler A. Influence of demographic factors and biochemical characteristics on the prostate-specific antigen (PSA) response to testosterone replacement therapy. Int J Impot Res 2006;18:201–5.
15. Rhoden EL, Morgentaler A. Testosterone replacement therapy in hypogonadal men at high risk for prostate cancer: results of 1 year of treatment in men with prostatic intraepithelial neoplasia. J Urol 2003;170:2348–51.
16. Coward RM, Simhan J, Carson CC 3rd. Prostate-specific antigen changes and prostate cancer in hypogonadal men treated with testosterone replacement therapy. Br J Urol 2009;103:1179–83.
17. D'Amico AV, Roehrborn CG. Effect of 1 mg/day finasteride on concentrations of serum prostate-specific antigen in men with androgenic alopecia: a randomised controlled trial. Lancet Oncology 2007;8:21–5.

18. Rhoden EL, Morgentaler A. Risks of testosterone-replacement therapy and recommendations for monitoring. N Engl J Med 2004;350:482–92.

19. Calof OM, Singh AB, Lee ML, et al. Adverse events associated with testosterone replacement in middle-aged and older men: a meta-analysis of randomized, placebo-controlled trials. J Gerontol A Biol Sci Med Sci 2005;60:1451.

20. Cooper CS, Perry PJ, Sparks AE, et al. Effect of exogenous testosterone on prostate volume, serum and semen prostate specific antigen levels in healthy young men. J Urol 1998;159:441.

21. Morgentaler A, Bruning CO III, DeWolf WC. Incidence of occult prostate cancer among men with low total or free serum testosterone. JAMA 1996;276:1904–6.

22. Morgentaler A, Rhoden EL. Prevalence of prostate cancer among hypogonadal men with prostate-specific antigen of 4.0 ng/ml or less. Urology 2006;68:1263–7.

23. Traish AM, Williams DF, Hoffman ND, et al. Validation of the exchange assay for the measurement of androgen receptors in human and dog prostates. Prog Clin Biol Res 1988;262:145.

24. Marks LS, Mazer NA, Mostaghel E, et al. Effect of testosterone replacement therapy on prostate tissue in men with late-onset hypogonadism: a randomized controlled trial. JAMA 2006;296:2351–61.

25. Morgentaler A. Testosterone deficiency and prostate cancer: emerging recognition of an important and troubling relationship. Eur Urol 2007;52:623–5.

26. Isom-Batz G, Bianco FJ Jr, Kattan MW, et al. Testosterone as a predictor of pathological stage in clinically localized prostate cancer. J Urol 2005;173:1935–7.

27. Hoffman MA, DeWolf WC, Morgentaler A. Is low serum free testosterone a marker for high grade prostate cancer? J Urol 2000;163:824–7.

28. Kaufman JM, Graydon RJ. Androgen replacement after curative radical prostatectomy for prostate cancer in hypogonadal men. J Urol 2004;172:920–2.

29. Agarwal PK, Oefelein MG. Testosterone replacement therapy after primary treatment for prostate cancer. J Urol 2005;173:533–6.

30. Sarosdy MF. Testosterone replacement for hypogonadism after treatment of early prostate cancer with brachytherapy. Cancer 2007;109:536–41.

31. Morgentaler A. Two years of testosterone therapy associated with decline in prostate-specific antigen in a man with untreated prostate cancer. J Sex Med 2009;6:574–7.

Erectile Dysfunction and Depression: Screening and Treatment

Michael A. Perelman, PhD[a,b],*

KEYWORDS
- Depression • Erectile dysfunction • Sexual dysfunction
- Metabolic syndrome • Combination treatment

The comorbid conditions erectile dysfunction (ED) and depression are both highly prevalent in men. The National Comorbidity Survey found a lifetime prevalence of major depression of 12.7% for men in a representative sample of the US population, with minor depression affecting an estimated 10% of the population aged 15 to 54 years.[1] In the Massachusetts Male Aging Study, high depression scores were associated with frequent reports of moderate ED (for men aged 40–70 years), with the prevalence of severe, or complete, ED estimated at 10%.[2] Multiple regression analysis to control for all other predictors of ED still found that men with high depression scores were nearly twice as likely to report ED than nondepressed men.[3] Depression continues to be among the most common comorbid problems seen in men with ED, both in the community and in clinical samples.[2–5]

There is a very low rate of recognition of depression by urologists and other nonpsychiatric physicians. Lee and colleagues[6] determined that 33% of the 120 men presenting to a sexuality clinic had a major current psychiatric disorder. Of these 40 men, only one-third had been identified as having a mental disorder by the study urologist. Major depression was present in 15 (12.5%) of those men and was the second most common category of mental illness (chemical dependence was first). This failure to properly diagnose has 2 obvious negative consequences. First, the mental disorders detected were hardly trivial: 2 of the men required psychiatric hospitalization, 1 made a suicide attempt, and 1 required electroconvulsive therapy (ECT). Failure to properly diagnose is in itself serious and could have extremely deleterious consequences. Second, there is a growing body of evidence that underdiagnosed and untreated psychosocial-cultural factors contribute significantly to ED treatment discontinuation and failure.[7,8] In fact, Mallis and colleagues[9] determined that more than 50% of their study participants reported a lifetime history of psychiatric difficulties, concluding that obtaining a patient's psychosocial history is essential when evaluating and treating ED.

The effect of depression on the course of ED is multifaceted because of systemic pathophysiologic implications as well as psychological and behavioral ramifications. Although the relative contributions of organic and psychosocial-cultural causes to depression is open to discussion, there is little debate that depression can have a deleterious effect on the treatment of ED. Confounding this problem is the reality that a proper psychiatric diagnosis usually requires a 45- to 90-minute interview by a trained psychiatrist, whereas a urologist's time is often limited to

Disclosures: Bayer Schering Pharma AG, Consultant, Speaker; Eli Lilly, Consultant, Lecturer/Speakers Bureau; Glaxo Smith Kline, Investigator, Consultant; Johnson & Johnson, Investigator, Consultant; Palatin Technologies, Consultant; Shionogi, Consultant.
a Human Sexuality Program, Payne Whitney Clinic, The New York Presbyterian Hospital, New York, NY, USA
b New York Weill Medical College of Cornell University, New York, NY, USA
* 70 East 77th Street, Suite 1C, New York, NY 10075.
E-mail address: perelman@earthlink.net

Urol Clin N Am 38 (2011) 125–139
doi:10.1016/j.ucl.2011.03.004

15 to 30 minutes, almost all of it occupied with acquiring medical information. This article reviews the current knowledge about the relationship between ED and depression, the effect of treatments for depression on ED, ways to improve screening for depression, and treatment of ED in patients experiencing this common comorbidity.

Every patient who seeks treatment of ED should be screened for a major mood disorder (MMD) or depression. Depression in the medically ill is generally underdiagnosed and undertreated.[10] Patients with ED have an increased likelihood of depression and vice versa. In patients with ED, it is of course normal to have a distressed response to this condition. Indeed, distress or bother is generally a part of the diagnostic criteria for ED. Whereas many of these symptoms resolve themselves with the effective treatment of the ED, for those individuals who have significant depressive disorder (associated with ED rather than caused by ED), this is not the case. Failure to screen for MMD can result in significant risk to the patient in terms of both morbidity and mortality.

WHAT IS DEPRESSION?

ED has been extensively characterized elsewhere. However, before proceeding further, it would be useful to define and characterize depression. It is a significant error to view depression as "only" a psychosocial-cultural phenomenon. A severe major depression is frequently organic in derivation and some think that depression is a systemic disease with distinct subtypes, each with unique organic pathophysiology.[10] Yet, it is clear that behavioral, psychosocial, and cultural factors also play a role in the cause of depression in much the same way they do in sexual dysfunction (SD) generally and ED specifically. Like ED, there are omnipresent psychogenic components existing in most depressed patients regardless of the degree of organicity. The degree of manifest dysfunction frequently exceeds the degree of organic impairment even in men who are "organically" depressed. In other words, like ED, despite the existence of organic pathogenesis, depression always has a psychogenic component, even if the depression was initially the result of constitution, illness, surgery, or other treatments.[11]

Depressed mood is common in everyday life and may be a normal and expectable reaction to adverse events. However, when depressed mood lasts for 2 weeks or more, is associated with certain other symptoms, such as insomnia and agitation, and causes serious distress or impairment in functioning, a diagnosis of a mood disorder should be considered. The algorithm required and the multiple terms used to diagnose specific mood disorders in the current the American Psychiatric Association's *Diagnostic and Statistical Manual of Mental Disorders* (Fourth Edition Text Revision) (DSM-IV-TR)[12] can be confusing for the uninitiated. **Box 1** provides the nomenclature used in DSM-IV-TR to categorize the various mood disorders.

Major depressive episode and major depressive disorder sound similar but are conceptually distinct. Major depressive episode denotes a period of at least 2 weeks marked by the presence of at least 5 of 7 specific symptoms, 1 of which must be either depressed mood or markedly diminished interest or pleasure. The term major depressive episode is not applied when the patient also meets the following criteria: (1) if the symptoms do not cause clinically significant distress or impairment for a manic episode, (2) if the symptoms are directly attributable to substance or medical condition, or (3) if the symptoms are because of bereavement (this last item is controversial). Many patients with a major depressive episode qualify for a diagnosis of major depressive disorder, either single episode or recurrent. But a diagnosis of major depressive disorder is only made if certain other disorders are ruled out (such as schizophrenia) and if the patient has never had a manic episode. The DSM-IV-TR recommends the diagnosis of major depressive disorder only for those patients who do not have a bipolar disorder, or what used to be called manic-depressive disorder. If there is a past history of a manic episode, the diagnosis is bipolar I disorder. If only milder manic-range episodes, called hypomanic episodes, have been present, the diagnosis is bipolar II disorder. Bipolar disorders are less common than major depressive disorders. However, the inadvertent prescription of an antidepressant to patients with bipolar disorder can destabilize them and is a major iatrogenic risk associated with primary care physicians (PCPs) or urologists prescribing antidepressants. Bottom line, the clinician initially consulted should screen every patient with ED for major mood disorders. However, once screened and identified as potentially having a major mental disorder, the patient should be referred to a mental health professional (MHP), typically a psychiatrist for sophisticated diagnostic typing.

Depression, like ED, occurs more frequently in the medically ill. Rates of depression have been shown to increase with the increasing number and acuity of medical illnesses.[13] For example, studies have found increased risk for major depression in patients with cardiovascular, endocrine, and inflammatory diseases at rates triple

Box 1
The current mood disorder nomenclature

Mood episodes

    Major depressive episode

    Manic episode

    Mixed episode

    Hypomanic episode

Depressive disorders

    Major depressive disorder

    Dysthymic disorder

    Depressive disorder not otherwise specified

Bipolar disorders

    Bipolar I disorder

    Bipolar II disorder (recurrent major depressive episodes with hypomanic episodes)

    Cyclothymic disorder

    Bipolar disorder not otherwise specified

Other mood disorders

    Mood disorders due to a general medical condition

    Substance-induced mood disorder

    Mood disorder not otherwise specified

Specifiers, describing current or most recent episode

    Severity/psychotic/remission specifiers for major depressive episode

    Severity/psychotic/remission specifiers for manic episode

    Severity/psychotic/remission specifiers for mixed episode

    Chronic specifier for a major depressive episode

    Catatonic features specifier

    Melancholic features specifier

    Atypical features specifier

    Postpartum onset specifier

Specifiers, describing course of recurrent episodes

    Longitudinal course specifiers (with and without full interepisode recovery)

    Seasonal pattern specifier

    Rapid cycling specifier

Adapted from Diagnostic and statistical manual of mental disorders, 4th edition, Text Revision (DSM-IV-TR). Washington, DC: American Psychiatric Association; 2000; with permission.

those of usual populations.[14–20] Furthermore, depression is an independent risk factor for those diseases including greater risk of mortality after acute myocardial infarction.[21,22]

ETIOLOGY: THE BIDIRECTIONAL RELATIONSHIP BETWEEN ED AND DEPRESSION

Correlations have been noted between depression and aspects of sexual function, including erectile function. Experiencing ED can of course be a cause or precipitator of a depression of greater magnitude. History taking is critical in determining whether depression is a consequence of the ED, or if ED is more determined by the depression and its treatments. Most cases of reactive depression resolve upon improvement of sexual function.[23,24] In fact, for a select subpopulation of depressed men with ED, the use of phosphodiesterase 5 (PDE5) inhibitors alone is adequate in resolving the depression.[25,26]

Shabsigh and colleagues[27] concluded that ED is associated with a high incidence of depressive symptoms independent of age, marital status, or comorbid conditions and that depressed patients with ED had a lower libido than patients who did not exhibit depression. These patients were also less likely than others to continue a treatment of ED. There is a link between depression and nocturnal penile tumescence (NPT). In an early case report, 2 severely depressed men with ED were noted to have virtually absent NPT, which normalized, with successful antidepressant treatment.[28] A subsequent series measuring NPT found that, compared with nondepressed controls, men with depression showed decreased total sleep tumescence time and were more likely to have absence of rigid nocturnal erections.[29–31]

The relationship between depression and ED is complex, and it can be difficult to distinguish which occurred first. Depression can be a major consequence of ED, yet inversely, depression and its treatments can both cause ED.[32,33] Finally, although factors such as stress, alcohol, or hypogonadism can contribute to both depression and ED, it is quite plausible that a mechanism, as yet unknown, may lead to both ED and depression. Such an interaction can be understood in terms of several theoretical models that discuss how the mind and body both inhibit and excite sexual response, creating a unique dynamic balance.[34–38]

Bancroft[39] and Kaplan[40] both described a delicate balance between central excitatory and inhibiting mechanisms, adding greater understanding of the role of anxiety and other psychogenic factors in ED. Subsequently, Perelman[35–38] postulated The Sexual Tipping Point (STP) model, which expanded this dual control concept to include all aspects of sexual functioning and dysfunction. This useful heuristic model defined a characteristic threshold for the expression of a sexual response for any individual, which could vary dynamically within and between individuals and for any given sexual experience (**Fig. 1**).[38]

Although the exact nature of a biological predisposition is not known, it is reasonable to conclude that the threshold for onset of either erectile difficulty and/or depression may have a distribution curve like that of numerous other human variables, such as height.[8,41,42] The specific threshold for any specific function is determined by multiple factors for any given moment or circumstance. One or another factor dominates, whereas the others recede in importance.[41–43] Determining whether the exact physiologic mechanisms of such thresholds are central, peripheral, and/or some combination requires further research.

These biological set points for erectile latency and depression (as well as other comorbid disease thresholds) are affected by multiple organic and psychogenic factors in varying combinations over the course of a man's life cycle. However, this pattern of biological susceptibility presumably interacts with a variety of circumstances and intrapersonal and interpersonal dynamics, in addition to environmental and medical risk factors, resulting in manifest disorders. These concepts can help us understand both ED and depression, as well as lead to identification of both the types and severity of factors that underlie both disorders. Clinicians can understand both ED and depression by recognizing how these predisposing, precipitating, and maintaining psychosocial-cultural causes, organic causes, and risk factors are all interrelated. Yet, ED and depression can both be elicited by a purely organic factor at one time and a completely cultural/environmental in another instance. There is a subsequent typical cascade of secondary

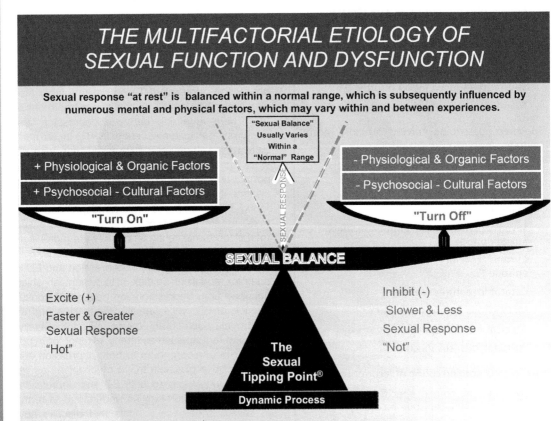

Fig. 1. The Sexual Tipping Point is the characteristic threshold for the expression of a sexual response for any person that may vary within and between sexual experiences. This model demonstrates both the mental and physical contributors to sexual function and dysfunction. At rest, the range of sexual response is normally balanced around neutral by these same dynamically opposing inhibitory and excitatory forces. At rest, a given individual is usually neither "turned on" nor "turned off"; "sexual balance" usually varies within a "normal range." (*Adapted from* Perelman MA. The Sexual Tipping Point: a mind/body model for sexual medicine. J Sex Med 2009;6:630; with permission.)

physiologic and psychosocial consequences that exacerbate the end points of the depressed mood, energy level, appetites, and sexual function. To further explore the cause of comorbid ED and depression, the next section focuses on some of the key factors. Although there is a spurious risk of oversimplifying a multidimensional nuanced cause, clarity of presentation requires such an organizational structure.

Depression, ED, and the Metabolic Syndrome

Clinicians have often observed that men with depression and hypogonadism often report a similar set of symptoms: fatigue, lack of sexual energy, depressed mood, and a sense of diminished psychological well-being. It may be difficult to determine the correct diagnosis, and the 2 conditions may also coexist in the same patient. Some evidence suggests that testosterone supplementation may benefit at least some men who are depressed, particularly those with low serum testosterone levels. Studies by Kupelian and colleagues[44] and Pope and colleagues[45] have successfully documented the potential role for testosterone augmentation therapy in depressed men with testosterone levels in the low-normal range.

The multiple biological mechanisms that can be involved causing ED (including type 2 diabetes, insulin resistance, abdominal obesity, hypertension, and dyslipidemia) characterize the metabolic syndrome. Recent advances in understanding the systemic effects of depression have suggested that depression can exacerbate, can contribute to, and is highly associated with this syndrome. In particular, older men may develop a major depressive episode along with ED, sometimes in association this metabolic syndrome.[46,47] There are of course other endocrine concerns, which are discussed by Guay elsewhere in this issue.

Psychogenic

Psychological issues often involve personality disorders, loss, and stresses of life, such as financial pressures. Relationship problems and other psychosocial events/stresses frequently contribute to, result from, or sometimes cause both ED and depression. The relevance of psychogenic factors should especially be considered for men with acquired and/or situational ED. Alterations in perceptual and attention processes (negative cognitions) can directly result in both mood and erectile variations.[48,49] In addition, performance anxiety may lead a man to engage in behaviors such as "spectatoring" during intercourse, which focuses attention away from arousing stimulus and instead on negative cognitions and consequently has a dampening effect on both erectile capacity and mood.[50] Thought affects the body biologically, not just psychologically. "In the anxious individual, there can be over-activity of the sympathetic system leading to increased smooth muscle tone. Alternatively, signals from the brain of an individual with a psychogenic issue can override the erotogenic parasympathetic output from the sacral spinal cord."[4]

Treatments for Depression Resulting in ED

Drugs, whether prescribed or taken recreationally, are perhaps one of the most common causes of diminished sexual capacity. Commonly prescribed medications are known to affect erectile function. For a detailed discussion of pharmacology and sex, the reader is recommended to the International Society for Sexual Medicine (ISSM) Consultation texts on Sexual Medicine.[51] Some of the most important groups of pharmacologic agents to consider are antidepressants, centrally acting antihypertensive drugs, central nervous system depressants, β-adrenoceptor antagonists, and any drug that has an anticholinergic action.[4] It is ironic that antidepressants seem to be independently associated with male sexual disorders.[23] It is difficult to separate the ED risk of antidepressants from ED associated with depression. In individual cases, a thorough baseline history of erectile function before antidepressant treatment usually helps in clarifying the cause of the ED.

The chronic nature of depression in many cases and the subsequent need for long-term administration of antidepressants has enriched our knowledge of the sexual side effects of these medications. Estimates of the percentage of patients affected in later studies are likely to be more accurate than the estimates in earlier studies that relied on spontaneous reporting, which is known to underestimate the true incidence.[52–56] Side effects of antidepressant treatment on sexual function are a serious issue for patients and their partners. Semipermanent interruption of sexual function by these medications is a significant barrier to medication adherence.

Clinicians should be aware that the sexual side effects of antidepressant medications are quite variable.[57,58] The mechanisms by which selective serotonin reuptake inhibitor (SSRI) antidepressants impair sexual function is the focus of ongoing research, but it is presumed to be caused by differential action of the relevant neurotransmitters. For instance, serotonin is known to act as an inhibitor of sexual response, so that drugs such as SSRIs, which increase serotonin levels, probably inhibit sexual function.[59] In addition, there is speculation that some SSRI antidepressants by centrally inhibiting nitric oxide synthetase may be involved in SSRI-related ED.[60] However, the primary sexual side effect associated with SSRIs is their effect on ejaculation and orgasm, with libido being second. Although SSRIs may also have a secondary effect on the erectile capacity, ED is the least common of the sexual negative effects with approximately 10% occurrence rate; however, in some cases, it has been reported to be irreversible.[58,61]

DIAGNOSIS AND SCREENING

The history obtained by PCPs and urologists is frequently limited to an end-organ focus and fails to reveal significant psychosocial barriers to successful restoration of sexual health. These obstacles or resistances represent an important cause of nonresponse and treatment discontinuation.[62] These barriers manifest themselves in varying levels of complexity, which individually and/or collectively must be understood and managed for the pharmaceutical treatment to be optimized.[63–65] Only recently have clinicians begun incorporating sex therapy concepts and have recognized that resistance to lovemaking is often emotional. Most of these barriers to success can be managed as part of the treatment, yet too few clinicians are trained to do so.[64,66]

Screening

Although the patient is initially evaluated for ED, there is a secondary goal of evaluating the management algorithm for any other significant disease or disorder. When depression is suspected, the physician must explore the mental status of the patient with an emphasis on assessing this mood disorder. This assessment can be done by the examining clinician alone or by working within a multidisciplinary team. The primary goal of the evaluation visit is to obtain the necessary information to assess the nature of the ED and to begin developing a treatment plan. Guidance for brief screening or a "sex status" examination of the patient with ED has been well described elsewhere.[8,67] Therefore, it is only briefly summarized in the following section, whereas specific screening techniques and questionnaires for depression are highlighted.

The Sexual Status Examination or Sex Status Exam

The sex status focuses on finding potential physical and specific psychosocial factors relating to

the disorder.[68] It is also important to ascertain why the patient is seeking assistance at that particular time. The clinician should first obtain a clear and detailed description of the patient's sexual symptoms, as well as information about the onset and progression of symptoms. The details of the physical and emotional circumstances surrounding the onset of a difficulty are important for the assessment of both physical and psychological causes. The ideal history is an integrated, fluid assessment, in which the patient's response is continuously reevaluated during follow-up. The successful treatment of ED requires answers to 3 key questions regarding diagnosis, cause, and treatment: (1) Does the patient really have a sexual disorder and what is the differential diagnosis? (2) What are the underlying organic and/or psychosocial factors? (3) Should the patient be treated or not? Do the underlying organic and psychosocial factors require priority treatment, or can the treatment of these factors be bypassed or concurrent? These decisions are dynamic and should be consistently reevaluated as the treatment proceeds.[67]

The methodology used to answer these questions is a focused history. Obviously, the clinician must determine whether the patient has an illness or is taking a drug that could be causing the symptom. However, this article presumes that the necessary assessment steps and procedures, including physical examination, as well as laboratory tests have been conducted in a manner consistent with the parameters recommended by Broderick elsewhere in this issue. By the end of the evaluation visit, the physician should have already ascertained or identified the necessary next steps to determine the extent to which there is an endocrine (eg, diabetes, androgens), neurogenic, vascular, psychogenic, and/or drug-related basis to the patient's ED. However, the clinician should not arbitrarily separate the psychosocial/sexual history from the medical history. An integrated medical and sexual history yields a significant amount of information regarding all aspects of a man's sexual health and relationships.

It is not necessary to do an exhaustive sexual and family history for most evaluations. The investigation of these issues should be selective so that the interview does not become unnecessarily lengthy. The clinician should briefly screen all patients for obvious psychopathology that would significantly interfere with the initiation of treatment of ED. Yet, the clinician will also want to know whether psychiatric symptoms, if present, are the cause and/or the consequence of the sexual disorder. If the patient is depressed, the severity of his depression must be clarified. Any patient who experiences major depression should be queried about suicide risk.

For all men, clinicians should assess the living and marital/dating status. Contextual factors, including difficulties with the current interpersonal relationship and whether the partner has an SD, should be clarified. The clinician may grasp the couple's interactions from the first interview's sex status. Numerous partner-related nonsexual issues may adversely affect the outcome. The degree of acrimony should be monitored when the patient describes his complaints, including is the anger, resentment, hurt, or sadness a maintaining or precipitating factor, or are the emotions more mild manifestations of the frustrations of daily life. Severe marital strife will inevitably require a referral to an MHP, albeit it may not be successfully accepted.[35,64,65] The single patient with ED must be assessed in the same manner as if the patient was in a relationship. The patient's sexual symptom may or may not relate to difficulties in his relationships. Needless to say, sexual orientation issues, for both single and coupled men, require the same, if not even greater sensitivity on the clinician's part.

Questionnaires

Chochinov and colleagues[10] were able to demonstrate that the mere asking of a single question, "Are you depressed?" was at least as effective as questionnaires in detecting depression. Yet, some clinicians may choose to use current or future instruments to facilitate the history-taking process. Two such instruments are briefly described below, but such instruments must be incorporated in a manner that does not interfere with rapport. The Patient Health Questionnaire-9 (PHQ-9) rating scale, developed specifically for the medical office practice,[69,70] is a convenient way to screen medical office patients for major depressive episode. It can be completed either by the patient himself or by the practitioner interviewing the patient. The PHQ-9 scale is easily scored to provide a measure of depression severity, and includes an item asking specifically about suicidal thoughts. In addition, the Depression in the Medically Ill Scale is a 10-item questionnaire that is 85% effective in detecting depression without the necessity of a psychiatric evaluation, which can be used by busy clinicians as a screening device.[10]

WHEN TO REFER?

When a patient with a variety of psychopathologic states (eg, stress, phobias, personality disorders) is evaluated for sexual complaints, the clinician must consider whether that patient's emotional conflicts are too severe for a focused treatment of the sexual problem and whether such treatment should either be safely postponed for another time or occur concurrently with treatment of the emotional distress. With more severe situations, the modal choice is likely to be a simultaneous initiation of the SD treatment along with a referral to an MHP to facilitate patient management. Yet, a person who is currently addicted to drugs and/or alcohol is not a suitable candidate for treatment until he has been detoxified and is off the drug. However, it is usually not necessary to postpone treatment of ED.[40,67]

Combination Therapy: Who and When?

Typically, PCPs and urologists integrate counseling with their sexual pharmaceutical armamentarium to treat ED. If an antidepressant is needed, they might consider initially prescribing themselves depending on the presenting symptoms, their own expertise, and level of interest. However, in the presence of an MMD, a referral to a psychiatrist is strongly recommended. What follows is a general algorithm for evaluating the referral necessity for any comorbidity.

Whether or not a clinician works alone or in combination with a psychiatrist or other health care specialists is determined by the complexity of the case.[51,63,65] The treating clinician would diagnose the patients as having mild, moderate, or severe treatment obstacles (TOs) to the successful restoration of sexual function and satisfaction. TOs could either be organic, pharmaceutical, and/or psychosocial-cultural in any combination. However, the TO categories would be segmented as follows: (1) mild TOs, no significant or mild obstacles to successful medical treatment of ED; (2) moderate TOs, some significant obstacles to successful medical treatment of ED; and (3) severe TOs, substantial to overwhelming obstacles to successful medical treatment of ED[65]; Althof, 2003, #9076.[63] This characterization would be based on an assessment of all the available information obtained during the evaluation. The physician would continue treatment and/or make referrals based on the progress obtained. The matrix determining who might treat is presented in **Table 1**.

Clearly, a multidisciplinary team including multiple medical specialists and a sex therapist could attempt to treat almost every case. However, treatment by a team is a labor-intensive approach and frequently unrealistic, both economically and geographically in terms of available expertise and manpower. However, in a common clinical practice

Table 1
ED management guidelines based on treatment obstacles

	Mild TOs	Moderate TOs	Severe TOs
Solo Physician	Frequently	Sometimes	Rarely
Multidisciplinary Team	Frequently	Frequently	Frequently

Data from Perelman M. Combination therapy for sexual dysfunction: integrating sex therapy and pharmacotherapy. In: Balon R, Segraves RT, editors. Handbook of Sexual Dysfunction. Boca Raton (FL): Taylor & Francis; 2005. p. 13–41.

scenario, the physician who first evaluates a patient with ED (this would of course be true for all SDs) could integrate counseling with the needed medical treatment, often resulting in a successful outcome.[71] Presumably, in such a scenario, a PDE5 would probably be chosen. Indeed, for some patients this prescription might adequately treat a mild depression effectively as well.[26]

Again, all does not have to be accomplished in the first visit, when using a case management approach based on Perelman's combination treatment STP model.[71] Such an approach always includes: (1) a thorough evaluation including a focused sex history or sex status exam; (2) integration of sexual pharmaceuticals with counseling for psychosocial-cultural factors while recognizing that the prescribed pharmaceuticals are both potentially restorative, as well as therapeutic probes (illuminators of failure or nonresponse; (3) integration of weaning and/or relapse prevention when possible; and (4) continued follow-up and referral as needed. ED is recognized as a progressive disease in terms of the underlying organic abnormality, which may play a role in altering the threshold for response and potential reemergence of dysfunction. Perelman recommended that the clinician schedule booster or follow-up sessions to help the patient stay the course and provide opportunity for additional treatment when necessary[64,65,72]; Perelman, 2005, #102132.[8] Generally speaking, treatment of ED should be started as soon as possible, with reevaluations of the patient's responses occurring as treatment proceeds. Retaking a quick current and mental health sex status provides a convenient model for managing follow-up.

Returning specifically to the issue of comorbid depression and ED, most patients seeking treatment of ED will not be manifesting such severe symptoms that a referral would be required. Many PCPs who more and more are the first ones a man with ED seeks treatment from are themselves willing and able to treat mild to moderate depression as well as the ED concurrently. In addition, there are numerous organically

determined reasons for making referral to a multiplicity of medical specialists (gynecologists, neurologists, endocrinologists, etc) when necessary and appropriate.[65] However, the next section highlights what to expect when the severity of the patient's depression requires referral to a psychiatrist for adjunctive treatment. In fact, the value of working with a board-certified psychiatrist when diagnosing and treating a severe depression could not be overemphasized.

WHAT TO EXPECT AFTER MAKING A REFERRAL?

Generally, the psychiatrist works with the referring physician to optimize the treatment of both the depression and the ED while also helping with the management of any other comorbid medical conditions. The psychiatrist typically provides pharmacotherapy for depression, and like any qualified mental health specialist, may also provide psychotherapy for both depression and ED. It is hoped that all the practitioners caring for the patient have special training and experience in the treatment of men with sexual issues.

If a patient with ED fulfills the criteria for major depression, the recommendation to the patient and referring physician should be to treat the depression. A referring physician should expect that if the patient is indeed diagnosed as having an MMD, treatment options (depending on severity) are likely to include psychopharmacology, psychotherapy, more rarely ECT, and when necessary, psychiatric hospitalization. The side-effect burden of these treatments, once the depression has lifted, requires collegial consultation to determine the best balance of treatment for the patient seeking improvement in sexual functioning. Discussion with the patient, his partner, when possible and appropriate, and the psychiatrist can help guide the decision whether or not concurrent treatment of the ED should be attempted or postponed. Both the referring physician and the psychiatrist should be aware of the particular risk of drug treatments and maintain the following cautionary viewpoint. Because many antidepressants carry the risk of erectile toxicity, there is a theoretical concern that depressed men may be at a particular risk of ED from long-term antidepressant treatment. Therefore antidepressants with the lowest risk of sexual side effects should be selected. Once treatment of ED is initiated, men on antidepressants should be asked regularly and specifically about the quality of their erections (with partner, with self-stimulation, and on awakening). If at all possible, the antidepressant treatment should be discontinued if ED recurs or worsens (Stephen Snyder, MD, New York, NY, USA, personal communication, January 2011).

There are several strategies for minimizing harm to erections, particularly during antidepressant treatment. These strategies may be summarized under the following general headings: (1) wait for spontaneous remission, (2) drug holiday, (3) decrease dosage (4) antidepressant selection and switching agents, and (5) antidotes.[53,73] These strategies are all discussed later, but only choices 4 and 5 represent truly valid approaches. Several reviews of this topic provide tables summarizing the advantages of one drug or method over the others.[4,23,53,74] However, the research underlying such studies frequently uses different methodologies and different thresholds for diagnosing SD, thus limiting the value of such comparison tables (Taylor Segraves, MD, Cleveland, OH, USA, personal communication, February 2011). Instead, in this article, the drugs mentioned are identified in **Box 2** with the relevant research summarized within the text.

Like urology, the concept of watchful waiting has its adherents, however, meta-analysis suggests that less than 10% of patients experience spontaneous improvement from the initially developed antidepressant sexual side effects.[57,75] A drug holiday may make a difference for a small percentage of patients, but the risk of depression reoccurrence makes this an imprudent strategy because skipping medicine can certainly lead to relapse.[76] Although reducing dose has a theoretical appeal, there is no indication that the antidepressant affect can be maintained at a level in which no sexual side effects occur. Finally, sudden discontinuation can cause a serotonin discontinuation syndrome with symptoms including light-headedness, nausea, vomiting, irritability, electric shock paresthesias, and sudden depression, among others.[53]

Switching medications in combination with altering dosage and using multiple medications to achieve an individualized optimized response is a common strategy. The basis for this popularity

---

Box 2
Names of medicines mentioned in this article and their customary dosages

SSRIs

 Fluoxetine (Prozac), 20 to 80 mg

 Sertraline (Zoloft), 50 to 200 mg

 Paroxetine (Paxil), 20 to 60 mg

 Fluvoxamine (Luvox), 150 to 300 mg

 Citalopram (Celexa) 20 to 60 mg

 Escitalopram (Lexapro), 10 to 20 mg

Norepinephrine and dopamine reuptake inhibitors

 Venlafaxine (Effexor), 75 to 375 mg

 Duloxetine (Cymbalta), 30 to 120 mg

 Desvenlafaxine (Pristiq), 50 to 100 mg

 Trazodone extended release (Oleptro), 150 to 375 mg

Tricyclic antidepressants

 Clomipramine (Anafranil), 75 to 225 mg

Other antidepressants

 Bupropion (Wellbutrin), 225 to 450 mg

 Nefazodone (Serzone), 300 to 600 mg

 Mirtazapine (Remeron), 15 to 45 mg

Antidotes

 Amantadine (Symmetrel), 100 to 200 mg

 Buspirone (BuSpar), 20 to 60 mg

 Cyproheptadine (Periactin), 4 to 12 mg

 Gingko biloba, 120 to 240 mg

 Granisetron (Kytril), 2 mg

 Yohimbine (Yocon, Aphrodyne), 5.4 to 32.4 mg

PDE5 inhibitors

 Sildenafil (Viagra), 50 to 100 mg

 Tadalafil (Cialis for use as needed), 10 to 20 mg, (Cialis for daily use), 2.5 mg and 5 mg

 Vardenafil (Levitra), 10 to 20 mg

Stimulants

 Methylphenidate (Ritalin, Concerta, Focalin, and others), 15 to 60 mg

 Mixed amphetamine salts (Adderall), 15 to 60 mg

 Dextroamphetamine (Dexedrine), 10 to 60 mg

Courtesy of Adam Ashton, MD; with permission.

is determined by the numerous studies demonstrating variability of side effects noted both between and within given individuals in response to different antidepressants.[56,58,77–96] The methodological limitations independent of the popularity of these studies and the ubiquity of this strategy among psychiatrists should be remembered. For instance, Segraves[58] in a multicenter trial compared sustained-release bupropion with the SSRI sertraline. It was determined that the 2 drugs were similarly effective in treating depression but the side-effect profiles varied, with the sertraline patients having more sexual disorders than those assigned to the bupropion SR group. Similarly Modell and colleagues[82] compared the sexual side effects associated with bupropion and the SSRIs fluoxetine, paroxetine, and sertraline. Patients using SSRIs experienced significant decreases in libido, arousal, and duration and intensity of orgasm. In contrast, patients treated with bupropion reported significant improvements in libido, arousal, and orgasm intensity and duration. Only 27% of patients treated with SSRIs reported no adverse sexual side effects, compared with 86% of bupropion-treated patients who reported no sexual problems, with some reporting improvement in some aspect of their sexual functioning. Generally speaking, clinicians agree that the incidence of SD with bupropion, mirtazapine, moclobemide, nefazodone, and, maybe, reboxetine is lower than with other drugs. Norepinephrine and dopamine reuptake inhibitors, such as duloxetine, are also being used regularly now by psychiatrists. Segraves and colleagues[52,61] recommend duloxetine for depressed patients with sexual problem who need a selective and nonselective serotonin reuptake inhibitors.

Some noted psychiatrists think that the drugs with the most frequent sexual side effects are the tricyclic antidepressants.[52,97–99] Among the SSRIs, paroxetine has the worst reputation for side effects, which may ironically be related to why it is frequently used as an off-label treatment of premature ejaculation.[57,82,100,101] Of related concern, antipsychotics are somewhat notorious for having persistent sexual side effects after discontinuing medication.[102] However, the second-generation antipsychotics (eg, aripiprazole) can sometimes be used without adding significant burden to the sexual side effect profile beyond that existing for the antidepressant being augmented (Adam Ashton, MD, Amherst, NY, USA, personal communication, February 2011).

Although some might question whether to use an SSRI at all in a patient with depression and ED, the answer depends on considering the whole array of sexual symptoms. The SSRIs can affect all 4 components of sexual function, including desire, arousal/erection, orgasm, and resolution. In this situation, a careful sexual history can help determine whether a trial of an SSRI antidepressant is reasonable. For instance, a depressed man with psychogenic ED who is a rapid ejaculator and has good sexual desire would be a good candidate for an SSRI. Yet conversely, a man with organic ED who has difficulty ejaculating and lacks sexual desire would be a poor candidate for an SSRI, and for such a patient, it may be preferable to prescribe a non-SSRI such as bupropion. However, it is worth remembering that some men find improved sexual function in all 4 phases in response to successful treatment of their depression whether by drugs, cognitive-behavioral psychotherapy, and/or both. As mood improves there is less anhedonia, and a happier person is more likely to have sex.

Augmenting the primary antidepressant with antidotes is a very commonly used approach. Regrettably, the results are often less than totally satisfactory, and like "switching," usually require a considerable trial and error process to find the correct dosage and/or the most effective dosing schedule.[53] A number of these antidotes are only briefly discussed below because none of them met with the success originally predicted for them. The 5-hydroxytryptamine receptor 1A (5-HT$_{1A}$) agonist buspirone has been reported to improve sexual functioning in patients treated for generalized anxiety disorder[103] and to assist in reversing SSRI-induced SD.[104] However, buspirone is not frequently used in the United States for either purpose. While frequently discussed in the nutraceutical literature, Gingko biloba probably has only exceedingly modest effect in treating SSRI-induced SD.[105–107] A few case studies have suggested benefit from cyproheptadine in reversing SSRI-induced SD.[108–111] Recently, urologists have discussed using midodrine to treat anejaculation in men with spinal cord injuries, as well as those with SSRI side effects. Most found it ineffective, with proponents acknowledging noticeable variability in response from patient to patient.[112] A variety of psychostimulants (dopamine-releasing agents with enhancing noradrenergic benefits) have been reported, again with mixed and minimal success.[113] The centrally acting presynaptic α_2-antagonist yohimbine that is approved to treat male erectile disorder[114] has been described in studies dating back to more than 25 years.[53,115–117] The results of these studies on reversing SSRI-induced SD are both conflicting and generally poor.[53,111,118–120] However, the most important work to date in the pharmacologic management of ED and depression was after the release of the PDE5 inhibitors.[53]

An important use of sildenafil in cases of depression is to counteract the effect of antidepressants.[4,121,122] Fava and colleagues[123] also assessed the safety and efficacy of sildenafil with ED caused by SSRI antidepressants, with those randomized to receive sildenafil reporting significant improvement in the number of successful sexual intercourse attempts per week. For ED in particular, the likely use of any of the PDE5 inhibitors by the initially consulting physician will work well with the drugs used by most psychiatrists for treating men with comorbid ED and depression. Although it is clear that additional research is needed, until more is known, the strategies outlined earlier can be used to assist many of the patients experiencing a comorbid ED and depression.[53]

Generally, in addition to pharmacotherapy, the psychiatrist also provides psychotherapy for both the depression and the ED. Psychotherapeutic treatment by MHP adds benefit, improves the chance of long-term success, and specifically can improve patients' adherence to medical treatments for ED and depression. Although there are a wide variety of psychotherapeutic techniques, a combination treatment using cognitive-behavioral approach, integrated with the use of as-needed antidepressant medication is recommended.[26,124–128]

SUMMARY

Sexuality is a complex interaction of biology, culture, intrapersonal and interpersonal psychology. A biopsychosocial model of SD provides a compelling argument for a combination treatment, which integrates counseling and pharmaceuticals. It is certainly a primary goal of pharmaceutical companies to develop new drugs for the treatment of depression, which do not have negative sexual side effects. While more research is needed, it seems probable that combination therapy will be the treatment of choice for all SDs, as new pharmaceuticals are developed for desire, arousal, and orgasm problems in both men and women.[64,65,67,101]

Obtaining a sex status or focused sex history and continuous reassessment based on follow-up are the foundations of this approach. Restoration of lasting and satisfying sexual function requires a multidimensional understanding of all the forces that created the problem, whether a solo clinician or multidisciplinary team approach is used. All clinicians need to carefully evaluate their own competence and interest when considering the treatment of a man's ED so that the patient receives optimized care regardless of the modalities used.

The initially consulted physician for a man with ED must screen for a MMD, given the high incidence of comorbidity. The consulting psychiatrist is expected to suggest both pharmacologic and psychotherapeutic strategies because psychosocial issues always arise when medicating a man's mood and sexuality.

ACKNOWLEDGMENTS

The author gratefully acknowledges Stephen Snyder, MD, for his contributions to the manuscript and many useful suggestions. The author also thanks Adam Ashton, MD, Anita Clayton, and Taylor Segraves for their support and personal communications.

REFERENCES

1. Kessler RC, Zhao S, Blazer DG, et al. Prevalence, correlates, and course of minor depression and major depression in the National Comorbidity Survey. J Affect Disord 1997;45:19–30.
2. Feldman HA, Goldstein I, Hatzichristou DG, et al. Impotence and its medical and psychosocial correlates: results of the Massachusetts Male Aging Study. J Urol 1994;151:54–61.
3. Araujo AB, Durante R, Feldman HA, et al. The relationship between depressive symptoms and male erectile dysfunction: cross-sectional results from the Massachusetts Male Aging Study. Psychosom Med 1998;60:458–65.
4. Wylie K, MacInnes I. Erectile dysfunction. In: Balon R, Segraves RT, editors. Handbook of sexual dysfunction. London: Taylor and Francis; 2005. p. 155–91.
5. Blazer DG, Kessler RC, McGonagle KA, et al. The prevalence and distribution of major depression in a national community sample: the National Comorbidity Survey. Am J Psychiatry 1994;151:979–86.
6. Lee IC, Surridge D, Morales A, et al. The prevalence and influence of significant psychiatric abnormalities in men undergoing comprehensive management of organic erectile dysfunction. Int J Impot Res 2000;12:47–51.
7. Althof SE. Sexual therapy in the age of pharmacotherapy. Annu Rev Sex Res 2006;17:116–31.
8. Perelman MA. Psychosocial evaluation and combination treatment of men with erectile dysfunction. Urol Clin North Am 2005;32:431–45, vi.
9. Mallis D, Moysidis K, Nakopoulou E, et al. Psychiatric morbidity is frequently undetected in patients with erectile dysfunction. J Urol 2005;174:1913–6.
10. Chochinov H, Wilson K, Enns M, et al. "Are you depressed?" Screening for depression in the terminally ill. Am J Psychiatry 1997;154(5):674–6.
11. Perelman MA. Rehabilitative sex therapy for organic impotence. In: Segraves T, Haeberle E,

editors. Emerging dimensions of sexology. New York: Praeger Publications; 1984. p. 181–8.

12. Association AP. Diagnostic and statistical manual of mental disorders. Text Revision (DSM-IV-TR). 4th edition. Washington, DC: American Psychiatric Association; 2000.

13. Sutor B, Rummans TA, Jowsey SG, et al. Major depression in medically ill patients. Mayo Clin Proc 1998;73:329–37.

14. Rudisch B, Nemeroff CB. Epidemiology of comorbid coronary artery disease and depression. Biol Psychiatry 2003;54:227–40.

15. Flores BH, Musselman DL, DeBattista C, et al. Biology of mood disorders. In: Nemeroff CB, Schatzberg AF, editors. The American psychiatric publishing textbook of psychopharmacology. Arlington (VA): American Psychiatric Publishing; 2004. p. 717–63.

16. Nemeroff CB, Musselman DL. Are platelets the link between depression and ischemic heart disease? Am Heart J 2000;140:57–62.

17. Hughes JW, Stoney CM. Depressed mood is related to high-frequency heart rate variability during stressors. Psychosom Med 2000;62:796–803.

18. Miller GE, Stetler CA, Carney RM, et al. Clinical depression and inflammatory risk markers for coronary heart disease. Am J Cardiol 2002;90:1279–83.

19. Otte C, Marmar CR, Pipkin SS, et al. Depression and 24-hour urinary cortisol in medical outpatients with coronary heart disease: the Heart and Soul Study. Biol Psychiatry 2004;56:241–7.

20. Musselman DL, Nemeroff CB. Depression really does hurt your heart: stress, depression, and cardiovascular disease. Prog Brain Res 2000;122: 43–59.

21. Frasure-Smith N, Lesperance F, Talajic M. Depression following myocardial infarction. Impact on 6-month survival. JAMA 1993;270:1819–25.

22. Burg MM, Abrams D. Depression in chronic medical illness: the case of coronary heart disease. J Clin Psychol 2001;57:1323–37.

23. Althof S. Depression and erectile dysfunction. Men's Sexual Health Consultation Collections November 2006;29–34.

24. Montorsi F, Adaikan G, Becher E, et al. Summary of the recommendations on sexual dysfunctions in men. J Sex Med 2010;7:3572–88.

25. Rosen R, Shabsigh R, Berber M, et al. Efficacy and tolerability of vardenafil in men with mild depression and erectile dysfunction: the depression-related improvement with vardenafil for erectile response study. Am J Psychiatry 2006;163:79–87.

26. Seidman SN, Roose SP, Menza MA, et al. Treatment of erectile dysfunction in men with depressive symptoms: results of a placebo-controlled trial with sildenafil citrate. Am J Psychiatry 2001; 158:1623–30.

27. Shabsigh R, Klein LT, Seidman S, et al. Increased incidence of depressive symptoms in men with erectile dysfunction. Urology 1998;52:848–52.

28. Roose SP, Glassman AH, Walsh BT, et al. Reversible loss of nocturnal penile tumescence during depression: a preliminary report. Neuropsychobiology 1982;8:284.

29. Thase ME, Reynolds CF, Glanz LM, et al. Nocturnal penile tumescence in depressed men. Am J Psychiatry 1987;144:89–92.

30. Thase ME, Reynolds CF, Jennings JR, et al. Diminished nocturnal penile tumescence in depression: a replication study. Biol Psychiatry 1992;31:1136–42.

31. Nofzinger EA, Thase ME, Reynolds CF III, et al. Sexual function in depressed men: assessment by self-report, behavioral, and nocturnal penile tumescence measures before and after treatment with cognitive behavior therapy. Arch Gen Psychiatry 1993;50:24.

32. Strand J, Wise TN, Fagan PJ, et al. Erectile dysfunction and depression: category or dimension? J Sex Marital Ther 2002;28:175–81.

33. Seidman SN, Roose SP. The relationship between depression and erectile dysfunction. Curr Psychiatry Rep 2000;2:201–5.

34. Bancroft J, Janssen E. The dual control model of male sexual response: a theoretical approach to centrally mediated erectile dysfunction. Neurosci Biobehav Rev 2000;24:571–9.

35. Perelman M, editor. Integration of sex therapy and pharmacological therapy in FSD Female Sexual Dysfunction 2005: a multidisciplinary update on female sexual dysfunction. New York (NY): Columbia University College of Physicians and Surgeons; 2005. p. 153–78.

36. Perelman M, editor. Prevalence, definition, etiology and diagnosis of premature ejaculation: D. o. U. Columbia University College of Physicians and Surgeons, Trans. In: Male Sexual Dysfunction. New York: Columbia University College of Physicians and Surgeons, Department of Urology; 2005. p. 75–9.

37. Perelman M. Idiosyncratic masturbation patterns: a key unexplored variable in the treatment of retarded ejaculation by the practicing urologist. J Urol 2005;173(4):340 [abstract: 1254].

38. Perelman MA. The sexual tipping point: a mind/body model for sexual medicine. J Sex Med 2009;6:629–32.

39. Bancroft J. Central inhibition of sexual response in the male: a theoretical perspective. Neurosci Biobehav Rev 1999;23:763–84.

40. Kaplan HS. The evaluation of sexual disorders: psychologic and medical aspects. New York: Brunner/Mazel; 1995.

41. Perelman MA. Integrating sildenafil and sex therapy: unconsummated marriage secondary to ED and RE. J Sex Educ Ther 2001;26:13–21.

42. Waldinger MD. The neurobiological approach to premature ejaculation. J Urol 2002;168:2359–67.

43. Waldinger MD, Zwinderman AH, Olivier B, et al. Proposal for a definition of lifelong premature ejaculation based on epidemiological stopwatch data. J Sex Med 2005;2:498–507.

44. Kupelian V, Shabsigh R, Araujo AB, et al. Erectile dysfunction as a predictor of the metabolic syndrome in aging men: results from the Massachusetts Male Aging Study. J Urol 2006;176:222–6.

45. Pope HG, Cohane GH, Kanayama G, et al. Testosterone gel supplementation for men with refractory depression: a randomized, placebo-controlled trial. Am J Psychiatry 2003;160:105–11.

46. Seidman SN. Exploring the relationship between depression and erectile dysfunction in aging men. J Clin Psychiatry 2002;63(Suppl 5):5–12 [discussion: 23–5].

47. Traish AM, Feeley RJ, Guay A. Mechanisms of obesity and related pathologies: androgen deficiency and endothelial dysfunction may be the link between obesity and erectile dysfunction. FEBS J 2009;276:5755–67.

48. Rosen RC. Psychogenic erectile dysfunction. Classification and management. Urol Clin North Am 2001;28:269–78.

49. Zilbergeld B. The new male sexuality. Revised edition. New York: Bantam Books; 1999.

50. Masters WH, Johnson VE. Human sexual inadequacy. Boston: Little, Brown & Co; 1970.

51. Lue TF, Basson R, Rosen R, et al, editors. Sexual medicine: sexual dysfunctions in men and women. Paris: Health Publications; 2004.

52. Segraves RT, Balon R. Sexual pharmacology fast facts. New York: W.W. Norton & Company; 2003.

53. Ashton AK. The new sexual pharmacology - a guide for the clinician. In: Leiblum S, editor. Principles and practice of sex therapy. New York: The Guilford Press; 2007. p. 509–41.

54. Frank E, Kupfer DJ, Perel JM, et al. Three-year outcomes for maintenance therapies in recurrent depression. Arch Gen Psychiatry 1990;47:1093–9.

55. Mueller TI, Leon AC, Keller MB, et al. Recurrence after recovery from major depressive disorder during 15 years of observational follow-up. Am J Psychiatry 1999;156:1000–6.

56. Clayton AH, Pradko JF, Croft HA, et al. Prevalence of sexual dysfunction among newer antidepressants. J Clin Psychiatry 2002;63:357–66.

57. Montejo-Gonzalez AL, Llorca G, Izquierdo JA, et al. SSRI-induced sexual dysfunction: fluoxetine, paroxetine, sertraline, and fluvoxamine in a prospective, multicenter, and descriptive clinical study of 344 patients. J Sex Marital Ther 1997;23:176–94.

58. Segraves RT. Sexual dysfunction associated with antidepressant therapy. Urol Clin North Am 2007; 34:575–9, vii.

59. Halaris A. Neurochemical aspects of the sexual response cycle. CNS Spectr 2003;8:211–6.

60. Finkel MS, Laghrissi-Thode F, Pollock BG, et al. Paroxetine is a novel nitric oxide synthase inhibitor. Psychopharmacol Bull 1996;32:653–8.

61. Segraves RT, Lee J, Stevenson R, et al. Tadalafil for treatment of erectile dysfunction in men on antidepressants. J Clin Psychopharmacol 2007;27:62–6.

62. Kaplan HS. The new sex therapy. New York: Brunner/Mazel; 1974.

63. Althof SE. Therapeutic weaving: the integration of treatment techniques. In: Levine SB, editor. Handbook of clinical sexuality for mental health professionals. New York: Brunner-Routledge; 2003. p. 359–76.

64. Perelman MA. Sex coaching for physicians: combination treatment for patient and partner. Int J Impot Res 2003;15(Suppl 5):S67–74.

65. Perelman MA. Combination therapy for sexual dysfunction: integrating sex therapy and pharmacotherapy. In: Balon R, Segraves RT, editors. Handbook of sexual dysfunction. Boca Raton (FL): Taylor & Francis; 2005. p. 13–41.

66. Althof SE. When an erection alone is not enough: biopsychosocial obstacles to lovemaking. Int J Impot Res 2002;14(Suppl 1):S99–104.

67. Perelman MA. Psychosocial history. In: Goldstein I, Meston CM, Davis SR, et al, editors. Women's sexual function and dysfunction: study, diagnosis and treatment. London: Taylor and Francis; 2006. p. 336–42.

68. Perelman MA. Commentary: pharmacological agents for erectile dysfunction and the human sexual response cycle. J Sex Marital Ther 1998;24:309–12.

69. Kroenke K, Spitzer RL, Williams JB. The PHQ-9: validity of a brief depression severity measure. J Gen Intern Med 2001;16:606–13.

70. Williams JWJ, Noel PH, Cordes JA, et al. Is this patient clinically depressed? JAMA 2002;287: 1160–70.

71. Perelman MA. Integrated sex therapy: a psychosocial-cultural perspective integrating behavioral, cognitive, and medical approaches. In: Carson CC, Kirby RS, Goldstein I, et al, editors. Textbook of erectile dysfunction. London: Informa Healthcare; 2008. p. 298–305.

72. McCarthy BW. Relapse prevention strategies and techniques with erectile dysfunction. J Sex Marital Ther 2001;27:1–8.

73. Balon R. The effects of antidepressants on human sexuality: diagnosis and management. Prim Psychiatr 1995;2:2–10.

74. Rosen RC, Marin H. Prevalence of antidepressant-associated erectile dysfunction. J Clin Psychiatry 2003;64(Suppl 10):5–10.

75. Ashton AK, Rosen RC. Accommodation to serotonin reuptake inhibitor-induced sexual dysfunction. J Sex Marital Ther 1998;24:191–2.

76. Rothschild AJ. Selective serotonin reuptake inhibitor-induced sexual dysfunction: efficacy of a drug holiday. Am J Psychiatry 1995;152:1514–6.

77. Croft H, Settle EJ, Houser T, et al. A placebo-controlled comparison of the antidepressant efficacy and effects on sexual functioning of sustained-release bupropion and sertraline. Clin Ther 1999;21:643–58.

78. Coleman CC, King BR, Bolden-Watson C, et al. A placebo-controlled comparison of the effects on sexual functioning of bupropion sustained release and fluoxetine. Clin Ther 2001;23:1040–58.

79. Coleman CC, Cunningham LA, Foster VJ, et al. Sexual dysfunction associated with the treatment of depression: a placebo-controlled comparison of bupropion sustained release and sertraline treatment. Ann Clin Psychiatry 1999;11:205–15.

80. Segraves RT, Kavoussi R, Hughes AR, et al. Evaluation of sexual functioning in depressed outpatients: a double-blind comparison of sustained-release bupropion and sertraline treatment. J Clin Psychopharmacol 2000;20:122–8.

81. Walker PW, Cole JO, Gardner EA, et al. Improvement in fluoxetine-associated sexual dysfunction in patients switched to bupropion. J Clin Psychiatry 1993;54:459–65.

82. Modell JG, Katholi CR, Modell JD, et al. Comparative sexual side effects of bupropion, fluoxetine, paroxetine, and sertraline. Clin Pharmacol Ther 1997;61:476–87.

83. Labbate LA, Brodrick PS, Nelson RP, et al. Effects of bupropion sustained-release on sexual functioning and nocturnal erections in healthy men. J Clin Psychopharmacol 2001;21:99–103.

84. Clayton AH, McGarvey EL, Abouesh AI, et al. Substitution of an SSRI with bupropion sustained release following SSRI-induced sexual dysfunction. J Clin Psychiatry 2001;62:185–90.

85. Feiger A, Kiev A, Shrivastava RK, et al. Nefazodone versus sertraline in outpatients with major depression: focus on efficacy, tolerability, and effects on sexual function and satisfaction. J Clin Psychiatry 1996;57(Suppl 2):53–62.

86. Ferguson JM, Shrivastava RK, Stahl SM, et al. Re-emergence of sexual dysfunction in patients with major depressive disorder: double-blind comparison of nefazodone and sertraline. J Clin Psychiatry 2001;62:24–9.

87. Kennedy SH, Eisfeld BS, Dickens SE, et al. Antidepressant-induced sexual dysfunction during treatment with moclobemide, paroxetine, sertraline, and venlafaxine. J Clin Psychiatry 2000;61:276–81.

88. Delgado PL, Brannan SK, Mallinckrodt CH, et al. Sexual functioning assessed in 4 double-blind placebo- and paroxetine-controlled trials of duloxetine for major depressive disorder. J Clin Psychiatry 2005;66:686–92.

89. Ashton AK. Reversal of SSRI-induced sexual dysfunction by switching to escitalopram. J Sex Marital Ther 2005;31(3):257–62.

90. Nafziger AN, Bertino JSJ, Goss-Bley AI, et al. Incidence of sexual dysfunction in healthy volunteers on fluvoxamine therapy. J Clin Psychiatry 1999; 60:187–90.

91. Nemeroff CB, Ninan PT, Ballenger J, et al. Double-blind multicenter comparison of fluvoxamine versus sertraline in the treatment of depressed outpatients. Depression 1995;3:163–9.

92. Gardner EA, Johnston JA. Bupropion–an antidepressant without sexual pathophysiological action. J Clin Psychopharmacol 1985;5:24–9.

93. Gelenberg AJ, McGahuey C, Laukes C, et al. Mirtazapine substitution in SSRI-induced sexual dysfunction. J Clin Psychiatry 2000;61:356–60.

94. Guelfi JD, Ansseau M, Timmerman L, et al. Mirtazapine versus venlafaxine in hospitalized severely depressed patients with melancholic features. J Clin Psychopharmacol 2001;21:425–31.

95. Clayton AH. Epidemiology and neurobiology of female sexual dysfunction. J Sex Med 2007; 4(Suppl 4):260–8.

96. Knegtering H, Bruggeman R, Castelein S, et al. Antipsychotics and sexual functioning in persons with psychoses. Tijdschr Psychiatr 2007;49: 733–42 [in Dutch].

97. Couper-Smartt JD, Rodham R. A technique for surveying side-effects of tricyclic drugs with reference to reported sexual effects. J Int Med Res 1973;1:473–6.

98. Karp JF, Frank E, Ritenour A, et al. Imipramine and sexual dysfunction during the long-term treatment of recurrent depression. Neuropsychopharmacology 1994;11:21–7.

99. Mavissakalian M, Perel J, Guo S. Specific side effects of long-term imipramine management of panic disorder. J Clin Psychopharmacol 2002;22: 155–61.

100. Kiev A, Feiger A. A double-blind comparison of fluvoxamine and paroxetine in the treatment of depressed outpatients. J Clin Psychiatry 1997;58: 146–52.

101. Perelman MA, McMahon C, Barada J. Evaluation and treatment of the ejaculatory disorders. In: Lue T, editor. Atlas of male sexual dysfunction. Philadelphia: Current Medicine, Inc; 2004. p. 127–57.

102. Csoka AB, Shipko S. Persistent sexual side effects after SSRI discontinuation. Psychother Psychosom 2006;75:187–8.

103. Othmer E, Othmer SC. Effect of buspirone on sexual dysfunction in patients with generalized anxiety disorder. J Clin Psychiatry 1987;48:201–3.

104. Norden MJ. Buspirone treatment of sexual dysfunction associated with selective serotonin re-uptake inhibitors. Depression 1994;2:109–12.

105. Ashton AK, Ahrens K, Gupta S, et al. Ginkgo biloba: Efficacy in SSRI-induced sexual dysfunction. Am J Psychiatry 2000;157:836–7.

106. Cohen AJ, Bartlik B. Ginkgo biloba for antidepressant-induced sexual dysfunction. J Sex Marital Ther 1998; 24:139–43.

107. Levine SB. Caution recommended. J Sex Marital Ther 1999;25:2–5.

108. McCormick S, Olin J, Brotman AW. Reversal of fluoxetine-induced anorgasmia by cyproheptadine in two patients. J Clin Psychiatry 1990;51:383–4.

109. Feder R. Reversal of antidepressant activity of fluoxetine by cyproheptadine in three patients. J Clin Psychiatry 1991;52:163–4.

110. Lauerma H. Successful treatment of citalopram-induced anorgasmia by cyproheptadine. Acta Psychiatr Scand 1996;93:69–70.

111. Keller Ashton A, Hamer R, Rosen RC. Serotonin reuptake inhibitor-induced sexual dysfunction and its treatment: a large-scale retrospective study of 596 psychiatric outpatients. J Sex Marital Ther 1997;23: 165–75.

112. Courtois F, Charvier K. [ISSMList] International Society for Sexual Medicine listserv. Available at: ISSMLIST@ist.issm.info. Accessed February 9, 2011.

113. Bartlik BD, Kaplan P, Kaplan HS. Psychostimulants apparently reverse sexual dysfunction secondary to selective serotonin re-uptake inhibitors. J Sex Marital Ther 1995;21:264–71.

114. PDR Staff. Physicians desk reference. Montvale (NJ): Thomson; 2005.

115. Morales A. Yohimbine in erectile dysfunction: the facts. Int J Impot Res 2000;12(Suppl 1):S70–4.

116. Margolis R, Prieto P, Stein L, et al. Statistical summary of 10,000 male cases using Afrodex in treatment of impotence. Curr Ther Res Clin Exp 1971;13:616–22.

117. Susset JG, Tessier CD, Wincze J, et al. Effect of yohimbine hydrochloride on erectile impotence: a double-blind study. J Urol 1989;141:1360–3.

118. Jacobsen FM. Fluoxetine-induced sexual dysfunction and an open trial of yohimbine. J Clin Psychiatry 1992;53:119–22.

119. Hollander E, McCarley A. Yohimbine treatment of sexual side effects induced by serotonin reuptake blockers. J Clin Psychiatry 1992;53:207–9.

120. Michelson D, Kociban K, Tamura R, et al. Mirtazapine, yohimbine or olanzapine augmentation therapy for serotonin reuptake-associated female sexual dysfunction: a randomized, placebo controlled trial. J Psychiatr Res 2002;36:147–52.

121. Nurnberg HG, Seidman SN, Gelenberg AJ, et al. Depression, antidepressant therapies, and erectile dysfunction: clinical trials of sildenafil citrate (Viagra) in treated and untreated patients with depression. Urology 2002;60:58–66.

122. Nurnberg HG, Gelenberg A, Hargreave TB, et al. Efficacy of sildenafil citrate for the treatment of erectile dysfunction in men taking serotonin reuptake inhibitors. Am J Psychiatry 2001;158: 1926–8.

123. Fava M, Nurnberg HG, Seidman SN, et al. Efficacy and safety of sildenafil in men with serotonergic antidepressant-associated erectile dysfunction: results from a randomized, double-blind, placebo-controlled trial. J Clin Psychiatry 2006; 67:240–6.

124. Perelman MA. Treatment of premature ejaculation. In: Leiblum S, Pervin L, editors. Principles and practice of sex therapy. New York: Guilford Press; 1980. p. 199–233.

125. Barlow DH. Causes of sexual dysfunction: the role of anxiety and cognitive interference. J Consult Clin Psychol 1986;54:140–8.

126. Pampallona S, Bollini P, Tibaldi G, et al. Combined pharmacotherapy and psychological treatment for depression: a systematic review. Arch Gen Psychiatry 2004;61:714–9.

127. Cuijpers P, van Straten A, van Oppen P, et al. Are psychological and pharmacologic interventions equally effective in the treatment of adult depressive disorders? A meta-analysis of comparative studies. J Clin Psychiatry 2008;69:1675–85 [quiz: 1839–41].

128. Melnik T, Soares BG, Nasselo AG. Psychosocial interventions for erectile dysfunction. Cochrane Database Syst Rev 2007;3:CD004825.

Psychological Factors Associated with Male Sexual Dysfunction: Screening and Treatment for the Urologist

Stanley E. Althof, PhD[a,b,*], Rachel B. Needle, PsyD[a,c,d,e]

KEYWORDS

- Erectile dysfunction • Hypoactive sexual desire disorder
- Premature ejaculation • Delayed ejaculation

Male sexual dysfunctions, including erectile dysfunction (ED), hypoactive sexual desire disorder (HSDD), premature ejaculation (PE), and delayed ejaculation (DE), are a complex amalgam of interrelated biological, psychological, and contextual variables that can combine to produce distressing symptoms both for the male diagnosed with the dysfunction and for his partner. In some instances psychological factors may precipitate a man's sexual dysfunction or further worsen and complicate the sexual dysfunction.[1,2]

This article describes the assessment process for identifying the psychological concerns associated with a man's sexual complaint and presents a stepwise algorithm for treating them. Physicians' awareness of the psychological and interpersonal issues will help them better manage patients' ongoing medical treatment and limit discontinuation of efficacious therapies. Other articles in this issue address the medical aspects of the evaluation and treatment of male sexual dysfunction. The authors recommend that clinicians use a biopsychosocial model, which allows the provider to capture the ever-changing blend of biological, psychological, relational, and contextual factors that interact to precipitate and maintain the dysfunction. Biological influences include illness, medication, surgery, and lifestyle factors (eg, obesity). The psychological/interpersonal aspects include the preexisting psychological life of the man, the psychological impact the dysfunction has on the man independent of his sexual life,

Dr Stanley Althof's disclosures of commercial interests: Boehringer-Ingelheim: receives honorarium for roles as Principal Investigator, Advisory Board, Speaker; Johnson & Johnson: receives honorarium for roles of Principal Investigator, Consultant; Eli Lilly: receives honorarium for role of Consultant; Neurohealing: unpaid role on Advisory Board; Palitan: receives honorarium for role of Consultant; Pfizer: unpaid role of Consultant; Shionogi: receives honorarium for roles of Consultant, Advisory Board, Speaker.
Dr Rachel Needle's disclosures of commercial interest: Boehringer-Ingelheim: receives salary for role of Sub-Investigator; Johnson & Johnson: receives salary for role of Sub-Investigator.

[a] Center for Marital and Sexual Health of South Florida, 1515 North Flagler Drive, Suite 540, West Palm Beach, FL, USA
[b] Case Western Reserve University School of Medicine, Cleveland, OH, USA
[c] South University, West Palm Beach, FL, USA
[d] Nova Southeastern University, 1111 West Broward Boulevard, Fort Lauderdale, FL, USA
[e] Positive Friends, USA
* Corresponding author. Center for Marital and Sexual Health of South Florida, 1515 North Flagler Drive, Suite 540, West Palm Beach, FL.
E-mail address: stanley.althof@case.edu

Urol Clin N Am 38 (2011) 141–146
doi:10.1016/j.ucl.2011.02.003

and the impact the dysfunction has on the couple's sexual and nonsexual life. A careful assessment will delineate all the factors—medical, psychological, interpersonal, and contextual—that contribute to the onset and maintenance of the sexual dysfunction.

EVALUATION

Psychosexual evaluation goes beyond traditional psychological assessment to examine the patient's or couple's sexual history, current sexual practices, relationship quality and history, emotional health, and contextual factors (eg, young children, chronic illness, financial concerns, cultural beliefs, and so forth) currently influencing their lives. The patient's developmental history is examined for influences on current functioning (eg, sexual or physical abuse) or the impact of a serious medical illness. Assessment of all the relevant medical and biological factors is necessary to understand the genesis and maintenance of the current difficulty.[3]

The manner in which questions are presented is especially significant because patients usually have an unsophisticated view of their dysfunction and the impact it has on their lives. Patients are also often unaware of the relationship between this symptom and multiple disease processes and/or the relationship to their psychological and interpersonal issues.[4] However, by following this method of logical and empathic questioning, the patient often gains a fresh perspective on the multiple issues that may be related to his dysfunction.

Although the partner does not often participate in the initial assessment meeting, clinicians should be aware that partner perspectives are frequently illuminating. When present, partners can provide important insight about the sexual and psychological dynamics of the relationship, and can become an important ally for both patient and clinician in a successful treatment intervention.[5]

The assessment outline that follows is meant to guide the clinician from a first-person standpoint. The outline is not meant to impede on or supplant an individual clinician's personal style or technique.

Begin by asking the patient, "What brought you in to see me?" Or, if the clinician is aware that the patient's visit concerns a sexual problem, ask him to clarify the nature of the problem.

Clarify the Sexual Problem

Even though the patient has self-diagnosed the sexual problem, determine whether he is experiencing ED, HSDD, PE, DE, or more than one dysfunction. Patients may mislabel their sexual conditions; for instance, some men describe PE as ED. If the patient acknowledges multiple sexual issues, take a separate history for each dysfunction.

Ascertain the Onset and Course of the Sexual Dysfunction

Once the type of sexual problem has been clarified, use the following questions to distinguish between lifelong or acquired type, and what factors precipitate and maintain the dysfunction:

- When did the patient first notice the symptoms of the specific sexual dysfunction?
- Was the onset sudden or gradual?
  If the onset was sudden, look for temporally related precipitants (eg, starting a new medication or being laid off from a job)
- What has the course of the sexual dysfunction been? In other words, has it gotten better or worse over time?
  Delineate what led to improvement
  Delineate what led to worsening.

Current Experience

At this point, attempt to further clarify the dysfunction by asking the patient (and partner if applicable) to recount, in as much detail as possible, a recent sexual experience. During the patient's recollections, probe him for what he was thinking and feeling at the time. For example, did he wish to avoid lovemaking so that he would not embarrass himself? Did he have little confidence in his ability to achieve an erection? Did he feel angry toward his partner? Was he afraid of his partner's possible contempt? How did his partner respond if the patient lost his erection during lovemaking?

Use this kind of questioning to identify the degree of performance anxiety, lack of confidence, distractibility, and attraction to the partner.

Treatment Avoidance

Before moving on to any intervention, assess the patient's risk for early discontinuation of treatment. In other words, if you find that the sexual dysfunction has been present for more than 6 months prior to the current evaluation, ask the patient why he did not come in sooner. The answer(s) to this question may be predictive of issues related to early discontinuation of treatment. For example, patients may have avoided treatment if such avoidance helped maintain the quality of a relationship with a depressed or sexually unwilling partner.[4,6]

In addition to ascertaining the reasons for possible delayed evaluation, it is equally important to find out what has motivated the patient to come in now. Again, some patients are motivated by partner pressure or concern.

Previous Treatment for Sexual Dysfunction

Determine if the patient has previously sought treatment for any sexual dysfunction. If this is the case, ascertain what type of treatment the patient received. For example, previous treatments may have focused solely on a psychological treatment while neglecting biomedical factors. In addition, by reviewing the patient's previous treatment experience, the clinician may gain insight about treatment avoidance not covered by the previous section. In other words, such additional questioning may reveal barriers that could inhibit, or completely disrupt, the current treatment. Such barriers may include unrealistic treatment expectations or genital pain in partners.[4,7]

Partner Response

A partner's response to the patient's sexual dysfunction can greatly affect the success of treatment. Clinicians should determine the following:

- Does the partner miss sexual intimacy?
- Is the partner angry or frustrated over the patient's avoidance of treatment?
- Is the partner pleased that sexual intercourse is no longer a part of the relationship?
- Is the partner a willing and supportive partner in the patient's treatment?
- Does the partner suffer from low desire?
- Does the partner suffer from genital pain?

Clinicians may need to discuss the use of lubrication, noncoital sexual behavior, or hormone replacement therapy as an adjunct to intercourse.[6]

Lifestyle Factors

Assessment of lifestyle factors is also an important part of the evaluation of sexual dysfunction. Factors such as cigarette smoking, excessive consumption of alcohol, and substance abuse have all been associated with diminished ED. In addition, the sexual willingness of partners may be diminished in the face of a patient's obesity, smoking, or alcohol consumption.

Nonsexual Relationships with a Partner

To restore intimacy between a patient and his partner, obstacles that may have arisen during the asexual months or years prior to evaluation must be overcome. On average, patients wait until 3 to 6 years after the sexual dysfunction symptoms appear before seeking treatment. The majority of men with sexual problems tend not to seek evaluation or treatment. During this protracted period of asexuality, both the frequency of sexual activity and other expressions of intimacy (like hand-holding, touching, and so forth) are greatly diminished. This situation occurs because men wish to avoid embarrassment and tend to withdraw emotionally. Some partners misinterpret the man's avoidance to mean that he is involved with another partner or no longer finds her attractive, which may cause her to withdraw as well. Research has identified issues of trust, infidelity, sex-role demands, and power struggles as interpersonal problems in partner relationships of those with ED.[4,7–10] For clinicians to help patients and partners overcome these issues, they must ascertain the dynamics and solidarity of the partner relationship. Regardless of the partner's presence at the evaluation, clinicians should determine:

- The patient's satisfaction with his current partner relationship(s)
- The patient's sexual function in previous relationships
- The impact of the sexual dysfunction on the current relationship
- If any struggles over power, control, intimacy, or finances exist between the patient and his partner
- The partner's level of sexual desire and overall sexual function
- The partner's mental health
- If there are any other current stressors on the relationship (children, finances, and so forth).

Vocational Life/Patient Occupation

A patient's work-related stress or concern about financial well-being may contribute to or maintain the sexual dysfunction. Clinicians should be aware that patients are often intuitive about the impact of work-related stress on physical symptoms such as a headache or stomachache. However, they are often psychologically naïve about the impact of work-related stress on sexual function.

Major Stress and/or Stress Management

Exposure to acute and chronic stress can also contribute to the sexual dysfunction.[11] Common examples of life stressors include bankruptcy, children with addiction, ill parents or other family members, and diagnosis of a serious health problem in the patient or his partner.

Mental Health History

Mental health disorders, like depression, have been associated with ED and HSDD as both a precipitating and maintaining factor. Mental health disorders have also been identified as an inhibitor of successful psychological treatment.[10,12–14] In addition, other psychological concerns such as performance anxiety, distractibility, and negative expectations can exacerbate sexual dysfunction. Clinicians can assess a patient's mental health by asking about:

- Performance Anxiety
  Distractibility
- Depression
  Mood
  Sleep
  Appetite
  Decreases in energy
  Outlook on the future
  Suicidal ideation
  Libido
  Prior or family history of depression
- Generalized Anxiety Disorder
  Shortness of breath
  Racing heart
  Decreased concentration
  Nervousness or agitation
  Sleep disturbance
  Excessive or unrealistic fears
- Obsessional Traits
  Excessive focus or preoccupation with sexual function.

TREATMENT

Clinicians are fortunate to have a wide range of effective biological and psychological therapies available for men who suffer from ED. Unfortunately, in the United States there are no approved medications for PE (although dapoxetine has been approved in 25 countries), DE, or HSDD. To clarify one point, HSDD is not synonymous with hypogonadism, as men can complain of low sexual interest although their testosterone levels are well within the normal range.

The medical therapies for male sexual dysfunctions are covered in other articles in this issue. Making the proper choice is sometimes more intuitive than evidenced based. In addition, there have been several recent studies that combining medical and psychological therapies are more efficacious than simply giving the drug alone.[12–17] At present, combination therapy is more of an ideal than a reality but it holds great promise as a treatment intervention.

This article is not intended to train urologists in sex therapy or psychotherapy. The goal is to help interested urologists broaden their treatment of male sexual dysfunction.

The major psychological factors that precipitate sexual dysfunction or worsen sexual dysfunction arising from medical factors are depression, anxiety, sexual confidence concerns, and relational issues. In addition, contextual factors such as partners working different shifts, illness in the partner, financial concerns, and death of a close family relative or friend may also affect sexual function. The article by Perelman addresses the issue of depression; this article focuses on all of the other psychosocial issues.

When the patient presents with severe psychopathology, referral to a mental health specialist is the appropriate course of action. However, the mild and moderate psychological concerns can often be helpfully addressed by the urologist. This article presents a treatment algorithm called PLISSIT, a model that guides the urologist in a stepwise fashion to address the psychological concerns of the patient and his partner.[18]

The PLISSIT Model

Introduced by Jack Annon,[18] the PLISSIT model is a stepwise algorithm for treating sexual problems. PLISSIT consists of 4 escalating levels of intervention beginning with P for permission giving, LI for providing limited information, SS for offering specific suggestions, and IT for intensive therapy. Annon believed that the degree of psychosocial complexity determined the level of intervention and that every patient did not require intensive psychotherapy. Depending on the man or couples' needs, some will do well with only permission and limited information. Those with a greater degree of psychosocial complexity (eg, significant performance anxiety) may need specific suggestions, and those with serious psychological and interpersonal problems will likely require referral for intensive psychotherapy.

Permission

For some men sex has become boring, predictable, mechanical, and devoid of mental or physical excitement. These men might present with HSDD. Moreover, without sufficient mental or physical excitement the patient will not achieve a firm, long-lasting erection even with a phosphodiesterase type 5 inhibitor (PDE5i). It is not uncommon for these men to ask the clinician if a certain behavior is normal. These individuals are looking to modify or expand the repertoire of their sexual behavior, and are seeking advice and permission.

By utilizing his or her mantle of authority the clinician grants "permission" to the patient to experiment with different sexual behaviors that are likely to increase his level of sexual excitement. Some men were taught that sex is dirty, sinful, only for procreation, and can only be conducted in a rigidly prescribed manner (eg, in the dark in the missionary position). It is not surprising that these individuals may have difficulty achieving or maintaining erections, as over time their excitement dwindles. In general, people outgrow or learn to modify rigid learning patterns, and do not require permission to experiment sexually. However, some may turn to us for permission to engage in oral sex or different positions, or to share fantasies with their partner. The aim is not to push individuals into behaviors that are abhorrent to them or fundamentally against their values. Permission giving seeks to facilitate the patient's passion and excitement within the bounds of their value system. Sometimes doing something slightly different, which for them may border on taboo, can be extremely exciting and can help to reinvigorate their sexual life and restore function.

Limited information

Limited information is the next level of the algorithm, which refers to making specific suggestions to the man or couple with the aim of improving the efficacy of an intervention or easing the anxiety associated with the sexual problem. For example, the urologist might suggest reading materials or videos to help men with specific problems. The book by Metz and McCarthy[19] is an excellent resource to suggest to men who suffer from rapid ejaculation.

Other forms of limited information might include the window of opportunity for the different PDE5i drugs and the need for some sexual excitement in conjunction with using these drugs. Too often men return to us saying, "it didn't work," when a careful inquiry would reveal that they expected the drug to induce an erection prior to any sexual excitement.

Sometimes men present with a self-diagnosed sexual problem. These men assert that they suffer from PE but their intravaginal ejaculatory latency time is 8 minutes. Providing patients with information on what is normal or what is expected may prove helpful to some. For others, who insist that they have the condition and who are unable or unwilling to process what is normal, a referral is required.

Specific suggestions

Offering "specific suggestions" is aimed at men with uncomplicated psychosocial issues that can be addressed with targeted behavioral interventions. Examples of specific suggestions include the prescription of sensate focus to men with significant performance anxiety thought to interfere with achieving or maintaining erection, or the stop/start technique or squeeze technique for men with PE.[11,20]

Another example of limited information might include suggesting that the man with PE focus on his level of arousal so that he can learn to modulate his excitement.[21] Awareness of his level of excitement allows the man to slow his thrusting, or even possibly stop movement. Men tend to avoid focusing on their level of excitement, fearing that it will cause them to ejaculate even more rapidly. However, distraction is unsuccessful and leads to continued early ejaculations. The urologist might also suggest the stop/start or squeeze technique to improve ejaculatory control.

To overcome performance anxiety associated with ED, the urologist might suggest that the man use a PDE5i to help regain his confidence. He or she might then suggest that he begin to wean himself away from the PDE5i and try intercourse without any medication. Simply knowing that the medication is available provides "insurance" to help the man feel more confident about his sexual performance.

The urologist might also recommend some commonsense solutions to simple marital issues. More complex marital concerns will require a referral for therapy. Mothers of young children often feel that there is no break in their routine, and after having been touched all day by children do not desire further touching by their male partner. The clinician may help the man understand some of the burdens of motherhood and suggest that he find ways for her to have time alone, or have an "adult night" away from the kids.

Intensive therapy

"IT" refers to intensive therapy, which is generally conducted by a mental health clinician. Psychotherapy refers to more global treatment of psychological problems (eg, anxiety, depression, couples therapy). Sex therapy is a specialized form of psychotherapy that draws on an array of technical interventions known to effectively treat male and female sexual dysfunctions. Treatment may be conducted in individual, couples or group format, depending on the initial problem, the judgment of the therapist, the motivation of the patient(s), and practical considerations of both patient(s) and therapist.[22]

Sexual therapy techniques comprise behavioral/cognitive interventions as well as psychodynamic, systems, relationship, and educational interventions (eg, reading, videotapes, illustrations, anatomic models). While employing traditional psychotherapeutic techniques—support, interpretation, confrontation, cognitive reframing, and homework, to name a few—sex therapy incorporates specific technical interventions such as sensate focus to diminish performance anxiety. Effective comprehensive treatment often involves collaboration with other specialists such as urologists, gynecologists, endocrinologists, family practice physicians, internists, cardiologists, neurologists, nurse practitioners, physician assistants, or physical therapists.

By following the PLISSIT model, the urologist can offer stepwise practical interventions that are likely to prove helpful to the man and/or couple. If the patient does not respond to permission giving, limited information, or specific suggestions, the urologist can offer a referral to a mental health specialist. The patient is likely to appreciate the urologist's interest and logical stepwise approach, and may be more receptive to a referral than when a referral is made at the initial consultation.

SUMMARY

This article presents a model for both the evaluation and treatment of the psychological concerns of men with sexual problems. By following the PLISSIT algorithm, the urologist can skillfully and empathically treat their patient's medical and mild to moderate psychological concerns. Psychosocial intervention need not be a time-consuming, seemingly endless process. Rather, in many instances these psychosocial concerns will improve. Patients are grateful that the clinician understands them and is able to treat them in a more holistic manner.

REFERENCES

1. Althof S. Psychogenic impotence: treatment of men and couples. In: Leiblum S, Rosen R, editors. Principles and practice of sex therapy. New York: Guilford Press; 1989. p. 237–68.
2. Althof S. Treatment of rapid ejaculation: psychotherapy, pharmacotherapy, and combined therapy. In: Leiblum S, editor. Principles and practice of sex therapy. 4th Edition. New York: Guilford Press; 2007.
3. McCabe M, Althof SE, Assalian P, et al. Psychological and interpersonal dimensions of sexual function and dysfunction. J Sex Med 2010;7(1 Pt 2):327–36.
4. LoPiccolo J. Psychological assessment of erectile dysfunction. In: Carson C, Kirby R, Goldstein I, editors. Textbook of erectile dysfunction. Oxford (UK): Isis Medical Media Ltd; 1999. p. 183–94.
5. Pollets D, Ducharme S, Pauporte J. Psychological considerations in the assessment of erectile dysfunction. Sex Disabil 1999;17(2):129–45.
6. Althof S. When an erection alone is not enough; biopsychosocial obstacles to lovemaking. Int J Impot Res 2002;14(Suppl 1):S99–104.
7. Ackerman M, Carey M. Psychology's role in the assessment of erectile dysfunction: historical precedents, current knowledge, and methods. J Consult Clin Psychol 1995;63(6):862–76.
8. Melman A, Levine S, Sachs B, et al. Psychological issues in diagnosis and treatment. In: Jardin A, Wagner G, Khoury S, et al, editors. Erectile dysfunction. Paris: International Society for Impotence Research; 1999. p. 407–24.
9. Wincze J, Carey M. Sexual dysfunction: a guide for assessment and treatment. 2nd edition. New York: Guilford Press; 2001.
10. McCabe M. Satisfaction in marriage and committed heterosexual relationships: past present and future. Annu Rev Sex Res 2006;XVII:39–58.
11. Semans J. Premature ejaculation. South Med J 1956;49:352–8.
12. Aubin S, Heiman J, Berger R, et al. Comparing sildenafil alone vs. sildenafil plus brief couple sex therapy on erectile dysfunction and couples' sexual and marital quality of life: a pilot study. J Sex Marital Ther 2009;35:122–43.
13. Melnik T, Abdo CH. Psychogenic erectile dysfunction: comparative study of three therapeutic approaches. J Sex Marital Ther 2005;31(3):243–55.
14. Perelman M. A new combination treatment for premature ejaculation. A sex therapist's perspective. J Sex Med 2006;3:1004–12.
15. Abdo CH, Afif-Abdo J, Otani F, et al. Sexual satisfaction among patients with erectile dysfunction treated with counseling, sildenafil, or both. J Sex Med 2008; 5(7):1720–6.
16. Althof S. Sex therapy in the age of pharmacotherapy. Annu Rev Sex Res 2006;17:116–32.
17. Perelman M. Sex coaching for physicians: combination treatment for patient and partner. Int J Impot Res 2003;15:S67–74.
18. Annon J. Behavioral treatment of sexual problems: brief therapy. Hagerstown (MD): Harper & Row; 1976.
19. Metz M, McCarthy B. Coping with premature ejaculation: how to overcome PE, please your partner & have great sex. Oakland (CA): New Harbinger Publications; 2003.
20. Masters W, Johnson V. Human sexual inadequacy. Boston: Little, Brown; 1970.
21. Althof S. Psychological treatment strategies for rapid ejaculation: Rationale, practical aspects and outcome. World J Urol 2005;23(2):89–92.
22. Althof SE. What's new in sex therapy (CME). J Sex Med 2010;7(1 Pt 1):5–13 [quiz: 14–15].

Doppler Blood Flow Analysis of Erectile Function: Who, When, and How

Timothy J. LeRoy, MD, Gregory A. Broderick, MD*

KEYWORDS

- Erectile dysfunction • Penile Doppler sonography
- Ultrasonography • Peyronie's disease

OVERVIEW

Since the introduction of several effective oral treatments for erectile dysfunction (ED), primary care physicians and midlevel providers manage most patients wishing treatment of male sexual dysfunction. ED is defined as the consistent or recurrent inability to attain and/or maintain penile erection sufficient for sexual performance.[1] ED constitutes an evolving public health concern. Studies from the 1990s estimated that half of men older than 40 years had ED.[2] Public awareness, pharmaceutical marketing, and new areas of research, such as cancer survivorship, are also increasing. In aggregate, this research and awareness is increasing the demand for treatment to the primary provider. Failure or poor efficacy of first-line treatments often leads to specialty referral. Other reasons for specialty referral may be trauma, uncertainty of diagnoses, or simply, the wish of the patient or provider.

Broadly categorized, there are 3 types of ED: neurogenic, psychogenic, and vasculogenic. Neurogenic and psychogenic causes are discussed by Altof and Needle elsewhere in this issue. Vasculogenic causes can be arterial, venoocclusive, or some combination of the two. Vasculogenic ED may account for up to 60% to 80% of all cases reported.[3]

There has been considerable research into diagnostic techniques over the past few decades. Without invasive testing, the urologist was limited to inferences made from physical examination and patient-based questionnaires. More data were often required to make solid clinical and surgical decisions. This requirement of data prompted several different types of investigations. The first-line diagnostic test for vasculogenic ED has been combined intracavernous injection and stimulation (CIS) and direct assessment by an observer.[4] This test is used to bypass both neurologic and hormonal influences and allow the provider to directly evaluate the vascular status of the penis. A normal response from CIS is associated with appropriate venous occlusion. False-negative results are found in as many as 20% of patients with intermediate arterial inflow. False-positive result could also commonly occur.

If more testing is thought to be needed or an operative intervention is being considered, such as for Peyronie's disease or for pelvic trauma, a second-line study is warranted. The pharmacopenile Doppler ultrasonography (PDDU) is a diagnostic modality useful in determining the subtype of vasculogenic ED as well as the magnitude of its severity. PDDU involves injecting a vasoactive penile stimulant followed by genital self-stimulation, audiovisual stimulation, or in some cases, repeat injection during which blood flow is assessed by color duplex Doppler ultrasonography. This procedure allows for both a direct and a quantifiable evaluation of ED. Ultrasonography is also able to provide information on the

Disclosure statement: The authors have nothing to disclose.
Department of Urology, Mayo Clinic Florida, 4500 San Pablo Road, Jacksonville, FL 32224, USA
* Corresponding author.
E-mail address: Broderick.gregory@mayo.edu

Urol Clin N Am 38 (2011) 147–154
doi:10.1016/j.ucl.2011.03.003

underlying soft tissue abnormalities such as a Peyronie's plaque.

PENILE ANATOMY

Three cylindrical structures, the corpus spongiosum, ventrally containing the urethra, and the paired corpora cavernosa, form the penis. The corpora cavernosa are covered by a 2-layer tunica with outer longitudinal fibers and inner circular fibers. There are also fibrous struts that help add support to the erect penis. The intracavernosal septum incompletely divides the 2 cylinders. Clinically, this anatomy is advantageous because only a single injection to the corporal body is required. The medication will circulate to the contralateral side. The tunica albuginea itself is also covered with a more superficial Buck fascia and a loose connective tissue and skin (**Fig. 1**). On ultrasonography, the corpora cavernosa appears hypoechoic and encased in a hyperechoic tunica.

Arterial supply to the penis is from the branches of the common penile artery, which is the direct continuation of the internal pudendal artery bilaterally. This artery branches into 3 named arteries. The cavernosal artery pierces the corporal body and travels in the center of the erectile tissue. These arteries are evaluated during the ultrasonographic study as discussed later. The bulbourethral artery enters the spongiosum superiorly and supplies the urethra, the spongiosum, and the glans penis. The third artery is the dorsal artery of the penis that courses between the dorsal vein and penile nerves. It gives off branches to the cavernous bodies and circumferential branches to the spongiosum. As with much of the pelvic vasculature, considerable variations have been found in the arterial supply to the penis.[5,6] On ultrasonography, the arteries can be found in several imaging planes and are easily seen as bright parallel lines because the arterial walls are hyperechoic (**Fig. 2**). The venous drainage of the corpora begin with the intersinusoidal and subtunical venous plexuses. This venous drainage continues to the emissary veins and then to larger channels such as the dorsal vein of the penis. The venous function in ED is described later.

PHYSIOLOGY OF ERECTION

In a flaccid state, the subtunical and intersinusoidal veins freely flow to the emissary veins. The arterioles and sinusoids maintain a high resting tone, which limits the inflow into the corpora. When combined, these yield a flaccid penis. After appropriate neural stimulation, a cascade of neurotransmitters, such as nitric oxide, affect the vascular supply to the penis. This starts with relaxation of the smooth muscle in the cavernosal arteries and then proceeds to the sinusoids. This

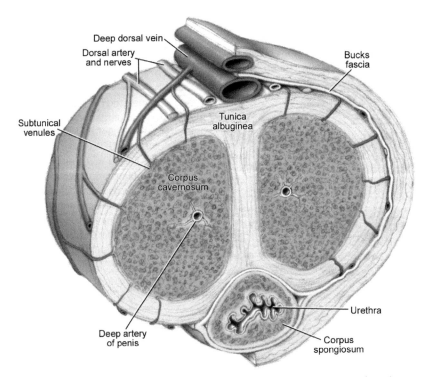

Fig. 1. Cross section of the penis demonstrating the visual anatomy noted on a typical study.

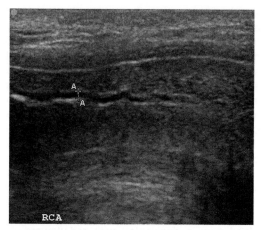

Fig. 2. A cavernous artery is seen in this sagittal ultrasonography. The appearance of the arterial walls is consistent with arthrosclerosis and/or calcification. RCA, right cavernous artery.

relaxation promotes a high inflow to the corporal bodies. Tumescence continues as the sinusoids fill with blood and begin to engorge. As the tunica elongates and expands, it begins to occlude the emissary veins between the inner circular and outer longitudinal layers described earlier. **(Fig. 3)** The occlusion propagates the erection because inflow is high and vascular outflow is at a minimum. Eventually, the intracorporal pressure increases to systemic levels and the inflow becomes reduced as well. Initially, the glans penis and corpora spongiosum react similarly in regard to flow. The major difference is the lack of tunical coverings and thus minimal venous occlusion. These structures continue to have high arterial inflow and function similar to an arteriovenous shunt. Just as tumescence proceeds step-wise, detumescence does so as well, with several separate stages proceeding according to penile pressure as the penis returns to its normal state.

PATIENT SELECTION

As with most diagnostic interventions, the patient selection process begins only after a satisfactory evaluation has been performed. A full patient history should be obtained, including a medical, surgical, sexual, and psychosocial history. The use of a patient self-assessment such as the International Index of Erectile Function or the Sexual Health Inventory for Men is also helpful in the

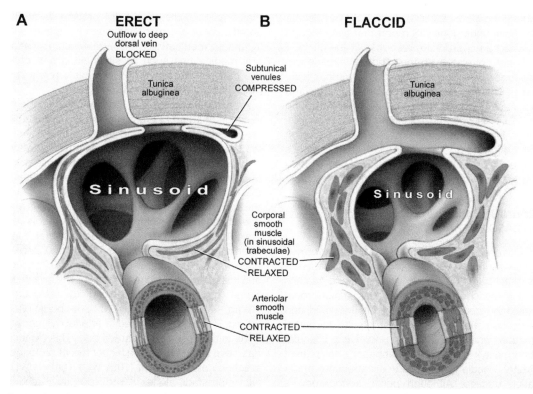

Fig. 3. Physiology of erection revealing the changes in the corporal smooth muscle and the accompanying vasculature. (*A*) The normal anatomy and physiology in the erect phallus, (*B*) the normal anatomy and physiology in the flaccid phallus.

standard evaluation. Given the considerable patient, and potentially even physician awkwardness of this type of interaction, the authors recommend an attitude of comfort and adaptability throughout the evaluation process.[7] Physical examination should include a broad screening for medical comorbid conditions relevant to ED, such as body habitus and blood pressure measurements. Urologic evaluation may reveal physical findings such as Peyronie's plaques, and neurologic evaluation may yield clues to neurogenic causes including presence of the bulbocavernosus reflex or peripheral neuropathy suggesting diabetes. Laboratory studies to identify or confirm a specific cause, such as hypogonadism, may be used as appropriate.

Many patients have an obvious and often severe cause of ED, such as Peyronie's disease, pelvic surgery, or metabolic syndrome. Another large subset of patients would have tried and failed oral treatments with phosphodiesterase 5 inhibitors. Further testing to confirm the cause is not mandatory for the urologist. First and foremost, the provider should review the medications tried and their doses to ensure that first-line trials have been appropriate. The provider may then pursue other empirical treatments such as intracavernosal injections, but the patient should have an option of undergoing more definitive studies. Some patients who have undergone CIS report that even though they had an appropriate response in the clinic, it does not correlate with their "home" experience. This report might be an indication of venous leak, and PDDU may be helpful to better understand the cause of the patient's ED.[4] Another indication for PDDU is operative planning. If, for example, the urologist is deciding between plaque excision and grafting and a penile implant for Peyronie's disease, a quantifiable examination of penile blood flow may provide the data needed for the decision.

TECHNIQUE OF PENILE DOPPLER ULTRASONOGRAPHY

As with any invasive procedure, a proper informed consent should be undertaken with the patient outlining the purpose, alternatives, risks, and benefits of the testing process. The examination room should be comfortable, safe from intrusion and distraction. False-positive test results (a partial erection when there is no underlying vascular abnormality) may ensue secondary to patient anxiety, needle phobia, and/or inadequate medication dosage. Although penile sonography is noninvasive to the patient, intracavernous injections (ICI) have morbidity that both the examiner and patient should be informed of. It is reported

that 1 in 5 neurologically intact men complain of an ache in the penis after prostaglandin E_1 injections. Prolonged erection is another well-known risk and must be pharmacologically reversed with subsequent injections to avoid priapism and its subsequent morbidity. Equipment needed includes a 5/8-in needle (27–29 gauge) and syringe for injection and the vasoactive medication chosen by the examiner for the study. A high-resolution ultrasonographic probe (7–10 MHz) is able to perform real-time ultrasonography and color pulsed Doppler. This technique allows the examiner to evaluate penile blood flow changes throughout the various phases of erection. In color-coded duplex sonography, the direction of blood flow is designated with red (toward the probe) or blue (away from the probe), making the identification of the small cavernous vessels and recording of blood flow easier.[8,9]

Attempts have been made to lessen the invasiveness of PDDU by substituting an oral medication such as sildenafil for injectable medications. These studies did show an increase in the peak flow velocities that were comparable to those seen with ICI, but the time frame was considerably longer. Testing may begin in 1 to 20 minutes with injectables versus in 30 to 90 minutes after an oral medication.[10] Other similar studies found that oral medications did not provide as strong an efficacy or any response when compared with injectable medications.[11,12] Further complicating oral medications such as sildenafil is that often the patient selected for PDDU has already had poor efficacy with that treatment type.

An example protocol of study would include an injection of 10 μg of prostaglandin E_1 (alprostadil). Direct pressure may be applied to the injection site for 2 to 3 minutes to prevent hematoma formation. If the examiner suspects a robust response given the patient's history and physical examination, this dose may be decreased by half. If necessary, the dose may be escalated up to 20 μg. This is only one of several possible medication protocols that have been described. Other agents that have been used include papaverine (7.5–60 mg), papaverine with the addition of phentolamine (0.1–1 mg), and papaverine + phentolamine + alprostadil. Some protocols use redosing of alprostadil, 10 μg, + phentolamine, 1 mg, + papaverine, 30 mg, (Trimix) to help predict arterial dysfunction if the initial dose of alprostadil fails. This protocol has been shown to have a higher risk of prolonged erections and priapism (10% with Trimix vs 1% with alprostadil alone).[13] The initial flows should be measured 5 to 10 minutes after injection. Some investigators recommend measurements every 5 minutes for the first 20 to 30 minutes, but this is often not practical in a busy practice. It is not unusual for the initial response time to be changed based on the patient's mental state and medical conditions. For example, a delayed response can be found in the hypertensive patient as well as the anxious patient. A rapid and robust response can be expected in the young man with psychogenic ED and patients with a neurogenic cause (including after prostatectomy and colorectal surgery). The examiner should record the erection hardness and correlate this with the PDDU measurements. A recent validated scale, the Erection Hardness Score (scale 1–4) can be used to standardize responses.[14] As first described by Donatucci and Lue,[4] the combination of injection plus manual self-stimulation leads to higher rates of rigid erections compared with injection alone. As such, the patient should be reexamined after self-stimulation. Other investigators suggest repeat pharmacostimulation as an adjuvant if self-stimulation is not preformed.[15] When there is full tumescence (or best achieved rigidity), grayscale imaging for the presence of nonvascular abnormalities such as plaques and fibrosis should be performed and noted. Doppler evaluations should include samples at the penoscrotal junction for the evaluation of blood flow at intervals described earlier and any physical deformity noted (such as a Peyronie's plaque). Evaluating the blood flow at the base of the penis limits the effect of penile pressure on arterial inflow.[15] Both arteries should be evaluated in a typical study.

At then end of the testing period, it is important to ensure a complete detumescence. The patient should not leave the office until the penis returns to a normally flaccid state. This will sometimes require injecting a diluted phenylephrine (an α-adrenergic agonist) solution of 200 μg /mL, given 1 mL every 3 to 5 minutes until detumescence. The patient should be monitored for symptoms such as acute hypertension, tachycardia, arrhythmias, and palpitations. Some providers choose to use a cardiac monitor during this process.

NORMAL STUDY

The PDDU should be preformed as described earlier. Measurements and rigidity should be recorded. **Fig. 4** demonstrates the normal Doppler waveform of a PDDU over time. Initially, the penile flow is elevated, both systolic and diastolic, because of smooth muscle relaxation. As the penile pressure increases the diastolic flow decreases and eventually reverses direction. At peak pressures, the arterial flow is dampened and no diastolic flow is noted. There are several possible parameters that might be measured, but the most common ones are peak systolic velocity (PSV), arterial diameter, end-diastolic velocity (EDV), and resistive index (RI). These variables are described in context with the pathologic condition they best elucidate. Performing an evaluation as described earlier should allow the examiner to understand the cause of a vasculogenic ED, if present in the patient.

ARTERIAL INSUFFICIENCY

Sufficient arterial inflow is of paramount importance to the study because without it, adequate

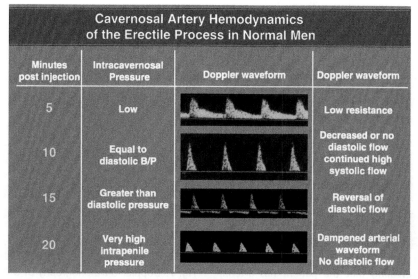

Minutes post injection	Intracavernosal Pressure	Doppler waveform	Doppler waveform
5	Low		Low resistance
10	Equal to diastolic B/P		Decreased or no diastolic flow continued high systolic flow
15	Greater than diastolic pressure		Reversal of diastolic flow
20	Very high intrapenile pressure		Dampened arterial waveform No diastolic flow

Cavernosal Artery Hemodynamics of the Erectile Process in Normal Men

Fig. 4. The normal Doppler waveform changes over time in the normal subject. As the penile pressure increases the waveform initially shows a diastolic flow. This then stops and even reverses direction. B/P, blood pressure.

erectile rigidity is unlikely to be obtained. Inflow is directly related to both arterial diameter as well as blood flow velocity. Whereas diameter can be useful, it is many variables such as location of examination (distal vs proximal), compression with the probe, and normal anatomic differences that make it difficult to use arterial inflow as the sole standard. The finding typically used is the PSV. PSV represents the highest recoded blood flow in the artery during systole. In the historical literature, in patients with abnormal pudendal arteriography, PSV less than 25 cm/s has a sensitivity of 100% and a specificity of 95%.[16] Severe unilateral cavernous arterial insufficiencies (AIs) are manifested by an asymmetry of PSV greater than 10 cm/s from the contralateral side. Many investigators conclude that a normal PSV should be greater than 35 cm/s. An example of a Doppler waveform of AI is shown in **Fig. 5**.

VENOOCCLUSIVE DYSFUNCTION OR VENOUS LEAKAGE

The trapping of blood within the corpora cavernous limits the venous outflow and is necessary for tumescence to occur. Cavernous venous occlusive disease (CVOD) is defined as the inability to achieve and maintain adequate erections despite appropriate arterial inflow. On PDDU, if the Doppler waveform continues to manifest high systolic flows and persistent EDV greater than 5 to 7 cm/s, the patient is considered to have CVOD. As seen in **Fig. 4**, the only time one expects to see elevated diastolic flow is at the beginning of tumescence. A continually high EDV is typically evident in CVOD. EDV alone looses specificity for venous leakage if it is associated with AI.[17] As such,

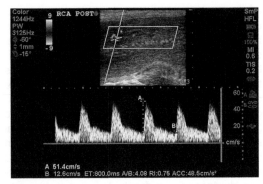

Fig. 6. This PDDU shows sufficient arterial inflow at 51.4 cm/s poststimulation but an RI consistent with CVOD. A/B, points A & B; ACC, acceleration index; ET, elapsed time; RCA, right cavernous artery.

many investigators include another value that takes PSV into account. This value is the RI. The formula for RI is as follows:

$$RI = (PSV - EDV)/PSV$$

As the penile pressure equals or exceeds the diastolic pressure, the diastolic flow in the corpora approaches zero and the value for RI approaches 1. During tumescence as well as in partial erections, the diastolic flow remains and the RI value is less than 1.0. Naroda and colleagues[18] concluded that an RI of less than 0.75 predicts CVOD in nearly 95% of patients and that an RI greater than 0.9 to 1 is normal. RI is typically recorded at the 20-minute mark of the study. **Fig. 6** shows the typical waveform noted in CVOD.

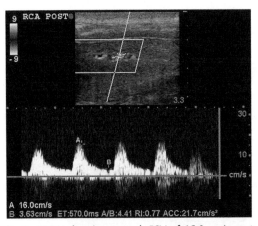

Fig. 5. PDDU showing a peak PSV of 16.0 cm/s poststimulation revealing that the patient has arterial insufficiency. A/B, points A & B; ACC, acceleration index; ET, elapsed time; RCA, right cavernous artery.

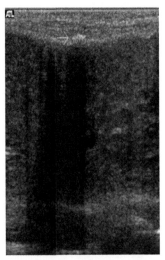

Fig. 7. Doppler ultrasonography of a Peyronie's plaque. The plaque often manifests as a hyperechoic to isoechoic finding with through shadowing.

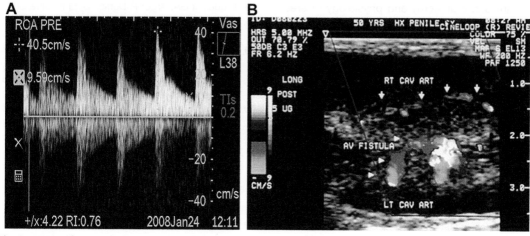

Fig. 8. PDDU of an arteriolar-sinusoidal fistula as is seen in nonischemic priapism. (*A*) PDDU waveform, note the elements of both a high PSV (in this study 40 cm/s) and elevated diastolic flow. (*B*) Color Doppler view over the fistula showing high flows of the left cavernous artery (LT CAV ART). RT CAV ART, right cavernous artery.

COMBINED DISEASE

As expected, combined disease manifests features of both AI and CVOD. The extent of each component may not be as severe when present in combination. The typical findings include a lower PSV, greater than 25 cm/s but not higher than 35 cm/s. In addition to this finding, there will be evidence of CVOD. As discussed earlier, the specificity of EDV is blunted in the presence of low arterial inflow. Therefore, the authors use RI and expect to see a value less than 0.9 in a combined disease picture.

PEYRONIE'S DISEASE

Peyronie's disease is a male sexual disorder that may be associated with ED and pain on erection. It is a condition of the tunica albuginea characterized by the formation of plaques of fibrous tissue that results in various severities of penile curvature. The authors do not recommend PDDU as a first-line evaluation of Peyronie's disease. A significant proportion of patients with this condition never require medical or surgical intervention. The discussion of the cause and medical/surgical interventions in Peyronie's disease is outside the scope of this discussion. However, if there is significant ED or severe curvature precluding sexual intercourse, the PDDU can be invaluable for surgical planning and patient counseling. Plaque length and characteristics can be readily demonstrated on Doppler ultrasonography. The PDDU is performed as described for the normal study. The pharmacologically produced erection also gives the examiner an idea of the severity and direction of penile curvature during tumescence. These

plaques often manifest as hyperechoic or isoechoic lesions with through shadowing (**Fig. 7**). A careful examination of the patient's erectile quality is also paramount because it can determine if the patient is ultimately a candidate for a penile implant or one of the various incision/plication/grafting techniques available.

PRIAPISM

Priapism is defined as a full or partial erection that continues more that 4 hours beyond sexual stimulation or is unrelated to sexual stimulation. The 2 broad categories are ischemic (low flow, venoocclusive) and nonischemic (high flow, arterial) priapism. The dysregulated arterial inflows with or without a fistula can best be distinguished from a persistent ischemic priapism with PDDU. In the setting of priapism, no injectable medications should be used as part of the study. Doppler examination should include the cavernosal arteries from the base of the corpora (ie, below the penoscrotal junction) proceeding distally in an attempt to find a potential fistula. On PDDU, an ischemic priapism simply shows no or very minimal arterial flow through the corpora. In high flow priapism, the examiner often finds a high PSV consistent with increased arterial inflow. There is often a high diastolic flow accompanying this observation if examining the arteriolar-sinusoidal fistula (**Fig. 8**).

SUMMARY

In the appropriately selected patient, PDDU can be extremely valuable to the urology practitioner. Use of PDDU does require an understanding of the relevant penile anatomy and physiology of erection as well as their clinical correlations to ED. It also requires that the practitioner have access to the Doppler equipment and pharmacotherapy for injection. Following the steps outlined in this article to perform the study, and by applying the basic understanding of the main vascular causes of ED, PDDU can be used to diagnose and guide the patient and practitioner to the best treatment options.

REFERENCES

1. Jardin A, Wagner G, Khoury S, et al. Erectile dysfunction: first international consultation on erectile dysfunction. Plymouth (England): Health Publications; 2000. p. 711–23.
2. Feldman HA, Goldstein I, Hatzichristou DG, et al. Impotence and its medical and psychosocial correlates: results of the Massachusetts Male Aging Study. J Urol 1994;151(1):54–61.
3. Altinkilic B, Hauck EW, Weidner W. Evaluation of penile perfusion by color-coded duplex sonography in the management of erectile dysfunction. World J Urol 2004;22:361–4.
4. Donatucci CF, Lue TF. The combined intracavernous injection and stimulation test: diagnostic accuracy. J Urol 1992;148:61–2.
5. Bare RL, DeFranzo A, Jarow JP. Intraoperative arteriography facilitates penile revascularization. J Urol 1994;151:1019–21.
6. Bahren W, Gall H, Scherb W, et al. Arterial anatomy and arteriographic diagnosis of arteriogenic impotence. Cardiovasc Intervent Radiol 1988;11(4):195–210.
7. Rosen RC, Hatzichristou D, Broderick G, et al. Clinical evaluation and symptom scales: sexual dysfunction assessment in men. In: Lue TF, Basson R, Rosen R, et al, editors. Sexual medicine: sexual dysfunctions in men and women. Paris: Health Publications; 2004. p. 173–220.
8. Broderick GA, Arger P. Duplex Doppler ultrasonography: noninvasive assessment of penile anatomy and function. Semin Roentgenol 1993;28:43–56.
9. Landwehr P. Penile vessels: erectile dysfunction. In: Wolf KJ, Fobbe F, editors. Color duplex sonography: principles and clinical application. Stuttgart (Germany): Thieme Medical; 1995. p. 204–15.
10. Arslan D, Esen AA, Secil M, et al. A new method for the evaluation of erectile dysfunction: slidenafil plus Doppler ultrasonography. J Urol 2001;66(1):181–4.
11. Copel L, Katz R, Blachar A, et al. Clinical and duplex US assessment of effects of sildenafil on cavernosal arteries of the penis: comparison with intracavernosal injection of vasoactive agent- initial experience. Radiology 2005;237(3):986–91.
12. Erdogru T, Usta MF, Ceken K, et al. Is sildenafil citrate an alternative agent in the evaluation of penile vascular system with color Doppler ultrasound. Urol Int 2002;68(4):255–60.
13. Seyam R, Mohamed K, Akhras AA, et al. A prospective randomized study to optimize the dosage of trimix ingredients and compare its efficacy and safety with prostaglandin E1. Int J Impot Res 2005;17:346–53.
14. Cappelleri JC, Bushmakin AG, Symods T, et al. Scoring correspondence in outcomes related to erectile dysfunction treatment on a 4-point scale (SCORE-4). J Sex Med 2009;6(3):809–19.
15. Halls J, Bydawell G, Patel U. Erectile dysfunction: the role of penile Doppler ultrasound in diagnosis. Abdom Imaging 2009;34:712–25.
16. Lewis RW, King BF. Dynamic color Doppler sonography in the evaluation of penile erectile disorders [abstract]. Int J Impot Res 1994;6:A30.
17. Wilkins CJ, Sriprasad S, Sidhu PS. Color Doppler ultrasound of the penis. Clin Radiol 2003;58(7):514–23.
18. Naroda T, Yamanaka M, Matsushita K, et al. Clinical studies for venogenic impotence with color Doppler ultrasonography- evaluation of resistance index of the cavernous artery. Nippon Hinyokika Gakkai Zasshi 1996;87(11):1231–5 [in Japanese].

Newer Phosphodiesterase Inhibitors: Comparison with Established Agents

Erin R. McNamara, MD, Craig F. Donatucci, MD*

KEYWORDS

- Erectile dysfunction • Phosphodiesterase 5
- Phosphodiesterase 5 inhibitors • Oral therapy

KEY POINTS

- Neurologic and vascular contribution to erectile physiology
- The role of nitric oxide in smooth muscle relaxation
- First-line therapy for erectile dysfunction: phosphodiesterase 5 inhibitors
- Newer phosphodiesterase 5 inhibitors
- Safety; efficacy; and use of sildenafil, vardenafil, and tadalafil
- Future of oral therapy.

Erectile dysfunction (ED) is defined as the consistent or recurrent inability to attain or maintain penile erection sufficient for sexual performance.[1] Self-reported ED has increased significantly as men seek effective therapy, such as oral phosphodiesterase inhibitors (PDE5i). It is estimated that 15 to 30 million men report sexual dysfunction.[2] Although the search for the causes of ED has extended over centuries, it is only recently that we have gained an understanding of the neurovascular physiology of erection. As a result of these efforts therapeutic agents targeted at specific underlying pathology are now available. The dawn of effective pharmacologic treatment occurred in the 1980s with the introduction of vasoactive agents for self-injection.

Intracavernosal therapy was the primary and most efficacious treatment at that time and remained so until the discovery of nitric oxide (NO) and its role in erection physiology in the next decade.

Twelve years ago the Food and Drug Administration (FDA) approved sildenafil as the first oral phosphodiesterase inhibitor, and there is a new algorithm of treatment that is centered on patients' goals and motivations and evidence-based principles.[3] More than 70% of erectile dysfunction can now be treated with oral medications. Oral pharmacotherapy is the first-line treatment without question for almost all types of erectile dysfunction according to the American Urological Association and European Urological Association guidelines and the World Health Organization-sponsored International Consultation on treatment for erectile dysfunction.[4–6]

With the availability of effective oral medications, the point of care for men suffering from ED moved from urologists to primary care physicians; these health care providers now perform the majority of evaluation and management of men with erectile dysfunction. By 2002, the majority of sildenafil prescriptions were written by primary care physicians (69%) as compared with urologists (13%).[2] With this transition, it is important

Consultant: Pfizer, Lilly; Coinvestigator: Vivus.
The authors have nothing to disclose.
Division of Urology, Department of Surgery, Duke University Medical Center, Box 2374, Durham, NC 27710, USA
* Corresponding author.
E-mail address: donat001@mc.duke.edu

Urol Clin N Am 38 (2011) 155–163
doi:10.1016/j.ucl.2011.03.005

Consultant: Pfizer, Lilly; Coinvestigator: Vivus.
The authors have nothing to disclose.
Division of Urology, Department of Surgery, Duke University Medical Center, Box 2374, Durham, NC 27710, USA
* Corresponding author.
E-mail address: donat001@mc.duke.edu

Urol Clin N Am 38 (2011) 155–163
doi:10.1016/j.ucl.2011.03.005

for urologists to stress to the primary care community the need to be thoughtful in the treatment of erectile dysfunction. Recent evidence has demonstrated that ED may be a precursor to coronary artery disease and is associated with other chronic illnesses, such as diabetes mellitus, hyperlipidemia, obesity, hypertension, and depression; thus health care providers should discuss possible causes and all treatment options with patients.[7] PDE5i are now the drugs of choice in the initial therapy of ED. This review compares the currently available PDE5i with the second-generation PDE5i, which are soon to be available.

MECHANISM OF ERECTION

Erections are initiated, maintained, and terminated because of a complex interaction between the neural and vascular components. Both central and peripheral factors are responsible for successful erections. The main physiologic event is the release of nitric oxide both from the autonomic nerve endings and the endothelial cells in the corpora cavernosum. After release NO rapidly enters the smooth muscle cells leading to smooth muscle relaxation and tumescence followed by passive veno-occlusion as the subtunical venule plexus is compressed against the rigid tunica albuginea. Nitric oxide facilitates vasodilatation and relaxation by activating guanylate cyclase. This enzyme converts guanosine triphosphate to cyclic guanosine monophosphate (cGMP), which is directly responsible for smooth muscle relaxation by its effect on intracellular calcium levels. Hyperpolarization occurs at the cell membrane. There is a decrease in cytoplasmic calcium and the smooth muscle cell relaxes (**Fig. 1**). Levels of cGMP in the smooth muscle cells of the penis are regulated by the enzyme phosphodiesterase type 5 (PDE-5).[8–10] Detumescence occurs with sympathetic nerve firing. Adrenergic nerves release norepinephrine that binds to $\alpha1$ or $\alpha2$ receptors on the smooth muscle cell. This neurotransmitter is responsible for the activation of a G-protein and an influx of calcium into the smooth muscle cell. As PDE-5 continues to breakdown cGMP to guanosine monophosphate, the smooth muscle cells and endothelial cells contract. This condition is the chronic state of the flaccid penis (**Fig. 2**).

ORAL PHOSPHODIESTERASE INHIBITORS

Phosphodiesterase is found in multiple tissues throughout the body and has been categorized into 11 families. Phosphodiesterase type 5 is the predominant subtype in corpora cavernosal tissue as well as vascular smooth muscle. Thus, drugs were targeted to inhibit this enzyme and increase the NO in corporal smooth muscle cells, which resulted in improved erectile function.

PDE5i were first marketed in 1998 with the introduction of sildenafil. This introduction was followed in 2003 by vardenafil and tadalafil. When choosing a PDE5i for patients with ED, considerations include the onset of action, efficacy, and duration of effect of the individual agent. Pharmacokinetic serum levels have defined the maximal plasma concentration, time to reach this plasma concentration (Tmax), and the plasma half-life (t½) for each agent and are included in the product label of the 3 current agents. How well these laboratory findings correlate to clinical results is sometimes difficult to determine and the measuring tool most commonly used to evaluate efficacy is the International Index of Erectile Function (IIEF) erectile function (EF) domain score.

Sildenafil Citrate

The first and most extensively investigated of these agents is sildenafil citrate. The registration trial for sildenafil, published in 1998, demonstrated a clinically and statistically significant improvement in IIEF erectile function domain scores for men suffering from ED for greater than 5 years.[11] Sildenafil is absorbed in the small bowel after gastric emptying, with onset of action of sildenafil in approximately 20 minutes, a reported t½ of 3 to 5 hours, and duration of action as long as 12 hours.[12] Sildenafil undergoes first pass metabolism in the liver by the P-450 enzymes CYP3A4 and CYP2C9 and metabolism within the gut wall. This metabolism allows only 38% to 41% of the drug available to elicit a drug effect.[13] Further experience with sildenafil revealed that it should not be taken with high-fat meals because the delay in gastric emptying results in decreased absorption, reduced peak serum concentrations, and decreased efficacy.[9,14]

Vardenafil

The FDA approved vardenafil in 2003 after a study of 805 men with ED demonstrated a clinically and statistically significant improvement in IIEF scores when compared with placebo. In this pivotal trial, 3 therapeutic doses were evaluated (5, 10, and 20 mg) and men were classified with mild, moderate, and severe ED based upon baseline IIEF EF domain scores. Approximately 40% of men with moderate or severe ED had improvement with the highest dose and more than 79% of men with mild ED had improvement.[15,16] Vardenafil is quickly absorbed with a Tmax of 45 minutes and a reported t½ of 4 to 5 hours. Onset of action

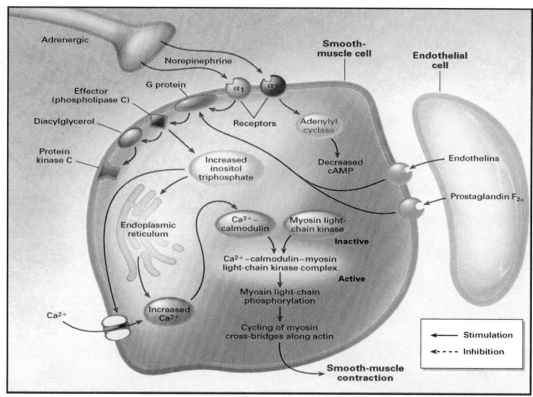

Fig. 1. Mechanism of smooth muscle contraction. (*From* Lue TF. Erectile dysfunction. N Engl J Med 2000; 342(24):1802–13; with permission. Copyright © 2000, Massachusetts Medical Society.)

has been recorded as early as 10 minutes.[17] Vardenafil is also metabolized by the liver; however, the degree of hepatic metabolism for vardenafil is less than that of sildenafil resulting in greater bioavailability of this agent. Just as with sildenafil, it is recommended that high-fat meals are avoided.[18]

Tadalafil

Tadalafil was also approved in 2003 and is the most selective of the 3 PDE5i medications. Tadalafil has a completely different structure than the other 3 marketed PDE5i (**Fig. 3**). The onset of action has been recorded at 20 minutes, whereas the Tmax of tadalafil is closer to 2 hours and the t½ is 17.5 hours with a clinical efficacy reported of 12 to 36 hours.[19] The registration trial for tadalafil involved 1112 men with a mean duration of ED greater than 1 year. After ingestion more than 80% of the men taking tadalafil had improved erections with duration of efficacy up to 36 hours after administration of the drug.[20] Because of slower uptake in the small bowel tadalafil does not seem to be as affected by high dietary fat intake, thus there are no dietary restrictions with the use of this agent.[21,22]

Since the introduction of the last of the currently marketed PDE5i in 2003 several novel PDE5i that have been investigated, with the hope that different pharmacokinetic parameters may lead to a decrease in adverse effects while or increasing efficacy. To this date, most of the newer PDE5i have exhibited pharmacokinetic profiles similar to the older PDE5i, and although the newer agents show more promise in vitro, true clinical evidence is still lacking. At the time of this article, none of these have been approved in the United States.

Avanafil

Avanafil (TA-1790, Vivus, Inc) has a much shorter onset of action and half-life than currently approved PDE5i; after ingestion the Tmax has been measured at 35 minutes with a half-life of less than 1.5 hours.[22] Preliminary trials examined doses of 50 mg, 100 mg, and 200 mg; all 3 doses significantly improved IIEF EF domain scores versus placebo. Phase I and II trials looking at safety and efficacy of the drug for ED have been completed and currently phase III trials are underway in the United States. The adverse event

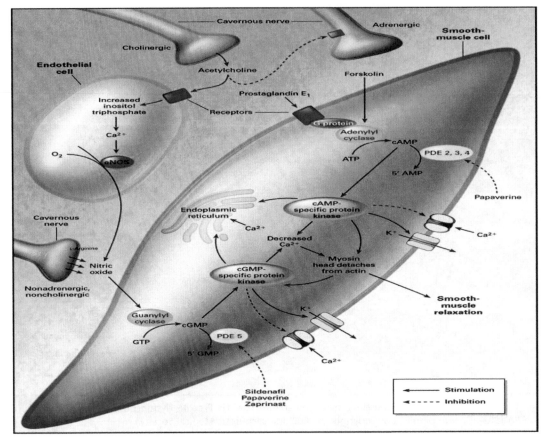

Fig. 2. Mechanism of smooth muscle relaxation and role of PDE5 and nitric oxide. (*Data from* Lue TF. Erectile dysfunction. N Engl J Med 2000;342(24):1802–13.)

profile is similar to that of the other known PDE5i.[23,24]

Udenafil

Udenafil is the only other PDE5i marketed and is available in South Korea and approved for distribution in the Russian Federation. The structure of udenafil is similar to that of sildenafil and vardenafil. The pharmacokinetic profile of udenafil demonstrates a Tmax of 60 minutes and a t½ of 11 to 13 hours; thus the duration of action of udenafil falls in between those of sildenafil/vardenafil and tadalafil.[25] Animal studies showed improved erectile function with the use of udenafil versus placebo in diabetic rats and in rats with cavernosal nerve injury.[26,27] In human studies, improvement in IIEF EF domain scores has been shown in both healthy men and men after prostatectomy ED.[28] Other studies have looked at the effect of udenafil in a diabetic population with reports that improvement in IIEF scores from baseline were unaffected by initial glycosylated hemoglobin levels, which

could be promising for this group of patients who can be refractory to oral medications.

Lodenafil

Lodenafil carbonate is a PDE5i developed in Brazil and has completed phase II and III trials that show safety and efficacy in treating ED. Lodenafil has a unique chemical structure; a carbonate bridge unites 2 molecules of lodenafil, after ingestion the carbonate bridge is broken freeing each molecule of lodenafil for biologic effect (**Fig. 4**). Lodenafil has a Tmax of 80 minutes and a t½ of 2.4 hours.[29,30]

In a phase III prospective, randomized, double-blind, placebo-controlled clinical trial of 350 men with ED, 2 doses of lodenafil carbonate (40 mg and 60 mg) were tested over a 4-week period. Efficacy was determined using the IIEF EF domain scores and Sexual Encounter Profile (SEP) questions 2 and 3. After 4 weeks of therapy subjects using 80 mg of lodenafil achieved clinically meaningful and statistically significant changes in all parameters of IIEF EF domain and SEP.[30] Adverse

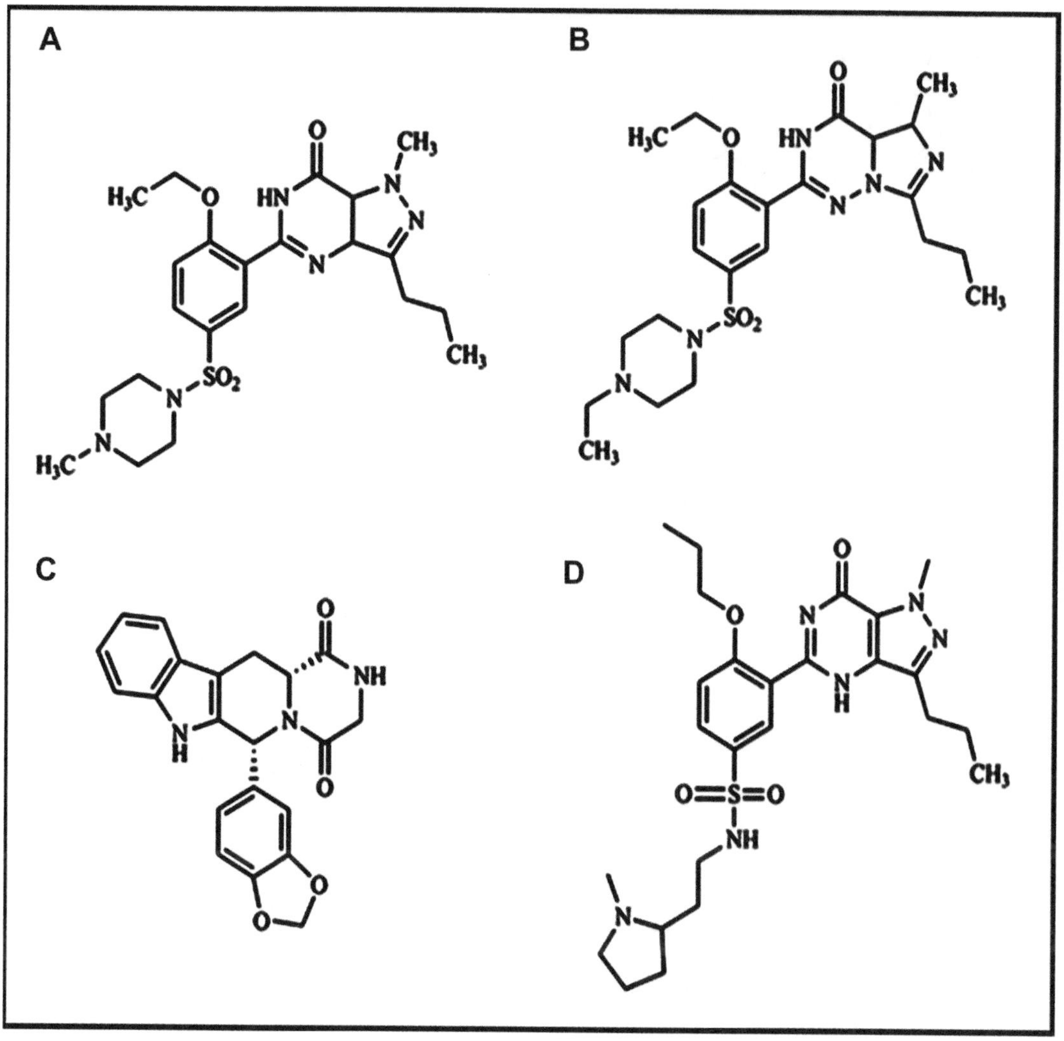

Fig. 3. Molecular structure of marketed PDE5i: (*A*) sildenafil, (*B*) vardenafil, (*C*) tadalafil, (*D*) udenafil. (*Data from* Kouvelas D, Goulas A, Papazisis G, et al. PDE5 inhibitors: in vitro and in vivo pharmacologic profile. Curr Pharm Des 2009;15(30):3464–75.)

events noted during this phase III trial were typical for class (headache, rhinitis, flushing, color, visual disturbance, and dyspepsia). A full 12-week trial is necessary to further establish the efficacy and safety of this agent.

Mirodenafil

Mirodenafil is another PDE5i available in South Korea. Animal studies have been promising in that the maximum concentration of mirodenafil is much higher than sildenafil in the plasma and corpus cavernosum tissue; however, the Tmax and t½ were similar between the two drugs.[31,32] Mirodenafil has also been studied in humans and the Tmax is reported to be 90 minutes, whereas the t½ was 2.4 hours. In a prospective, randomized, double-blind, placebo-controlled trial, doses of

50 and 100 mg were tested in 223 men with erectile dysfunction over 12 weeks; 215 men completed the trial.[33] In this study efficacy was also determined using the IIEF EF domain scores and SEP questions 2 and 3. Subjects using active therapy at both dose levels demonstrated improved erectile function (clinically meaningful and statistically significant improvement in IIEF and SEP scores). In addition, a strong positive response was noted in both the Global Assessment and the Life Satisfaction Checklist. Adverse events were typical of class; no novel adverse events emerged in the study.

SLx-2101

The last new agent, SLx-2101, is different from the others because it has an active metabolite,

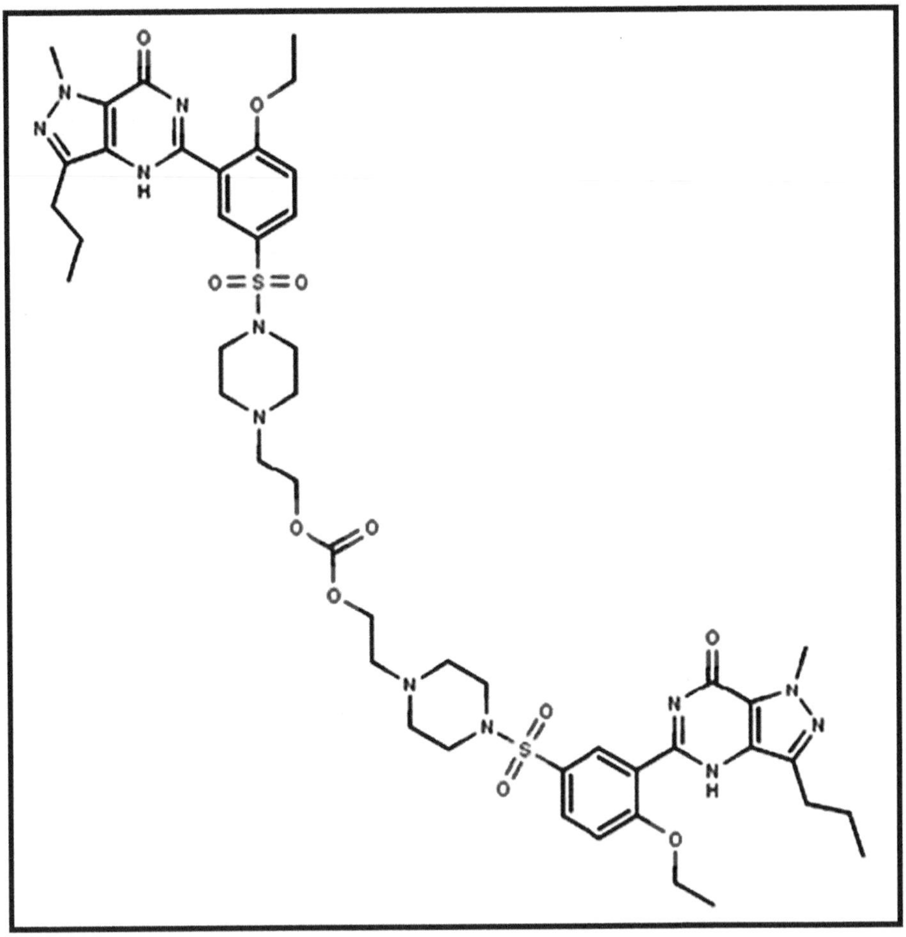

Fig. 4. Lodenafil carbonate chemical structure. (*Data from* Glina S, Fonseca GN, Bertero EB, et al. Efficacy and tolerability of lodenafil carbonate for oral therapy of erectile dysfunction: a phase III clinical trial. J Sex Med 2010;7(5):1928–36.)

SLx-2081. In preclinical studies the drug maintained therapeutic levels greater than 24 hours.[34] Efficacy and safety have been demonstrated in a double-blind, randomized, single-dose study of healthy male volunteers taking 5, 10, 20, 40, and 80 mg. Pharmacokinetic data revealed that the Tmax was 60 minutes for SLx-2101 and 2.8 hours for the metabolite. The half-life was 8 to 13 hours for SLx-2101 and 9 to 14 hours for SLx-2081.[35] This drug may appeal to men who prefer tadalafil because of the frequency of use.

ADVERSE EVENTS

Adverse event profiles for all of the PDE5i are similar and result from incomplete selectivity of the PDE5i, thus because of the homology of receptor structure other isoenzymes can be blocked resulting in unwanted clinical effects. PDE-6 and PDE-11 are the two most common families affected by this cross reactivity. Interference with PDE6 (sildenafil)

at high serum levels contributes to visual disturbances. Partial inhibition of PDE11 has been postulated to be the cause of the back pain that can result with tadalafil ingestion, although this has not been demonstrated to be the mechanism of action responsible for this adverse effect. Relaxation of smooth muscle in the vascular bed may cause headache, flushing, and rhinitis; these side effects are reduced significantly after the first few weeks.[36] Relaxation of the gastroesophageal sphincter may result in dyspepsia. There is less than a 5% dropout rate secondary to side effects.[37,38] The newer PDE5i still need to be evaluated in large studies, but preliminary studies show that side-effect profiles are similar to the approved PDE5i (**Table 1**).

SAFETY

All 3 commercially available PDE5i are contraindicated in patients using nitrates in any form. If patients have ingested sildenafil or vardenafil, the

Table 1
Comparison of approved PDE-5 inhibitors and new PDE-5 inhibitors

Drug	Onset of Action	t 1/2	Dose	Additional Information	Contraindications
Sildenafil	Tmax 30–120 m Onset 20 min High-fat meal decreases absorption Ethanol (ETOH) may affect efficacy	3–5 h	25–100 mg Starting dose 50 mg	Side effects: headache, flushing, rhinitis, dyspepsia, abnormal vision[39]	Nitrates Hypotension CV risk factors Retinitis pigmentosa Change dose with some antiretrovirals Should be on stable dose of α-blockers
Vardenafil	Tmax 45 min Onset 10 min High-fat meal decreases absorption ETOH may affect efficacy	4–5 h	5–10 mg	Side effects: headache, flushing, rhinitis, dyspepsia[39]	Same as sildenafil May have minor prolongation of QT interval Concomitant use of class I antiarrhythmic
Tadalafil	Tmax 30–60 min Onset 20 min Plasma concentration not affected by food or ETOH	17.5 h	10, 20 mg 2.5 or 5.0 mg for daily dose	Side effects: headache, flushing, rhinitis, dyspepsia, myalgias[39]	—
Avanafil[39,40]	Tmax 35 min Onset 20 min	≤1.5 h	50, 100, 200 mg	May be taken within 12 h of nitrate[41]	—
Udenafil [25,41]	Tmax 60 min	11–13 h	—	Several placebo-controlled studies show efficacy May be effective in diabetic ED	—
Lodenafil	Tmax 80 min	2.4 h	—	—	—
Mirodenafil[33]	Tmax 90 min	2.4 h	50, 100 mg	—	—
SLx2101 SLx2081[42]	Tmax 60 min Tmax 2.8 h	8–13 h 9–14 h	5, 10, 20, 40, 80 mg	Metabolite, which remains active for a longer period of time	—

Data from Hatzimouratidis K, Hatzichristou DG. Looking to the future for erectile dysfunction therapies. Drugs 2008; 68(2): 231–50; and Ellsworth P, Kirshenbaum EM. Current concepts in the evaluation and management of erectile dysfunction. Urol Nurs 2008;28(5):357–69.

recommended period before it is safe to administer nitrates is 24 hours and when tadalafil has been used, 48 hours is recommended. The coadministration of PDE5i and nitrates may result in severe systemic hypotension.

Visual changes can be mild and transient; however, a nonrelated condition, nonarteritic anterior ischemic optic neuropathy (NAION), has been observed in users of PDE5i. This link was first made after a few cases were reported in a series of men using sildenafil.[43] NAION is an ischemic event leading to optic nerve injury and occurs in men with the comorbidities often seen in conjunction with ED: diabetes, hypercholesterolemia, hypertension, and cardiovascular disease. It is independent of any effect of PDE5i on retinal PDE-6. A review of all the available clinical trials with more than 13,000 men analyzed has shown no causation. Current recommendations in the product labeling for these products advises no change in prescription; however, patients are advised to seek medical attention and discontinue use of the drugs if they experience visual changes while taking a PDE5i.[44]

Shortly after the introduction of sildenafil concerns were raised about the cardiovascular safety of this drug. It is clear now that the PDE5i do not represent a threat to cardiovascular health; this has been confirmed in multiple controlled trials. There is no increase in incidence of myocardial ischemic events nor overall mortality with PDE5i use compared with the general population.[45–47] Additional concerns arose about possible orthostatic hypotension with concomitant use of α-blockers. The use of PDE5i is not contraindicated in men who are also on α-blockers; however, care must be taken to stabilize on α-blockers before initiation of therapy with PDE5i. Although there has been no increase of cardiovascular events associated with the use of these drugs, it is important to do a thorough cardiovascular history and examination before prescribing PDE5i as the risk factors are shared for ED and cardiovascular disease.

SUMMARY: FUTURE OF ORAL THERAPY

Scientists and physicians continue to move forward in the search for newer and better treatment for erectile dysfunction. The demonstrated efficacy and safety of the 3 PDE5i available since the introduction of oral pharmacotherapy in 1998 sets a high standard, making it difficult to demonstrate that new agents are clearly superior. PDE5i are the initial drugs of choice for men with ED today. Differences in pharmacokinetic and adverse-event profiles may provide an opportunity for one of the newer PDE5i to serve as a superior alternative to current agents. Current and future clinical trials of new agents in this class will establish the evidentiary base that will allow health care providers to better tailor care for these men. Proper evaluation and treatment of erectile dysfunction includes a patient-centered approach that provides all the appropriate options and a physician who is willing to work with patients to meet his goals.

REFERENCES

1. Jardin A. Recommendations of the 1st international consultation on erectile dysfunction. Erectile dysfunction. Plymouth (UK): Health Publications Ltd; 2000.
2. Wessells H, Joyce GF, Wise M, et al. Erectile dysfunction. J Urol 2007;177(5):1675–81.
3. Rosen RC, Hatzichristou D, Broderick G. Clinical evaluation and symptom scales: sexual dysfunction assessment in men. In: Lue T, Basson R, Rosen R, editors. Sexual medicine: sexual dysfunctions in men and women. Paris (France): Health Publications; 2004.
4. Lue TF. Erectile dysfunction. N Engl J Med 2000; 342(24):1802–13.
5. Montague DK, Jarow JP, Broderick GA, et al. Chapter 1: the management of erectile dysfunction: an AUA update. J Urol 2005;174(1):230–9.
6. Wespes E, Amar E, Hatzichristou DG, et al. EAU Guidelines on erectile dysfunction: an update. Eur Urol 2006;49(5):806–15.
7. Feldman HA, Goldstien I, Hatzichristou DG, et al. Impotence and its medical and psychosocial correlates: results of the Massachusetts Male Aging Study. J Urol 1994;151(1):54–61.
8. Burnett AL, Lowenstein CJ, Bredt DS, et al. Nitric oxide: a physiologic mediator of penile erection. Science 1992;257(5068):401–3.
9. Corbin JD, Francis SH. Pharmacology of phosphodiesterase-5 inhibitors. Int J Clin Pract 2002;56(6):453–9.
10. Rajfer J, Aronson WJ, Bush PJ, et al. Nitric oxide as a mediator of relaxation of the corpus cavernosum in response to nonadrenergic, noncholinergic neurotransmission. N Engl J Med 1992;326(2):90–4.
11. Goldstein I, Lue TF, Padma-Nathan H, et al. Oral sildenafil in the treatment of erectile dysfunction. Sildenafil Study Group. N Engl J Med 1998;338(20):1397–404.
12. Padma-Nathan H, Stecher VJ, Sweeny M, et al. Minimal time to successful intercourse after sildenafil citrate: results of a randomized, double-blind, placebo-controlled trial. Urology 2003;62(3):400–3.
13. Gupta M, Kovar A, Meibohm B. The clinical pharmacokinetics of phosphodiesterase-5 inhibitors for erectile dysfunction. J Clin Pharmacol 2005;45(9):987–1003.
14. Nichols DJ, Muirhead GJ, Harness JA. Pharmacokinetics of sildenafil after single oral doses in healthy male subjects: absolute bioavailability, food effects and dose proportionality. Br J Clin Pharmacol 2002;53(Suppl 1):5S–12S.
15. Hellstrom WJ, Gittelman M, Karlin G, et al. Vardenafil for treatment of men with erectile dysfunction: efficacy and safety in a randomized, double-blind, placebo-controlled trial. J Androl 2002;23(6):763–71.
16. Hellstrom WJ, Gittelman M, Karlin G, et al. Sustained efficacy and tolerability of vardenafil, a highly potent selective phosphodiesterase type 5 inhibitor, in men with erectile dysfunction: results of a randomized, double-blind, 26-week placebo-controlled pivotal trial. Urology 2003;61(4 Suppl 1):8–14.
17. Montorsi F, Padma-Nathan H, Buvat J, et al. Earliest time to onset of action leading to successful intercourse with vardenafil determined in an at-home setting: a randomized, double-blind, placebo-controlled trial. J Sex Med 2004;1(2):168–78.
18. Rajagopalan P, Mazzu A, Xia C, et al. Effect of high-fat breakfast and moderate-fat evening meal on the pharmacokinetics of vardenafil, an oral phosphodiesterase-5 inhibitor for the treatment of erectile dysfunction. J Clin Pharmacol 2003;43(3):260–7.

19. Porst H, Padma-Nathan H, Giuliano F, et al. Efficacy of tadalafil for the treatment of erectile dysfunction at 24 and 36 hours after dosing: a randomized controlled trial. Urology 2003;62(1):121–5 [discussion: 125–6].

20. Brock GB, McMahon CG, Chen KK, et al. Efficacy and safety of tadalafil for the treatment of erectile dysfunction: results of integrated analyses. J Urol 2002;168(4 Pt 1):1332–6.

21. Lewis RW, Sadovsky R, Eardley I, et al. The efficacy of tadalafil in clinical populations. J Sex Med 2005; 2(4):517–31.

22. Peterson C. Pharmacokinetics of avanafil, a new PDE5 inhibitor being developed for erectile dysfunction. J Sex Med 2006;3(Suppl 3):253–4.

23. Limin M, Johnsen N, Hellstrom WJ. Avanafil, a new rapid-onset phosphodiesterase 5 inhibitor for the treatment of erectile dysfunction. Expert Opin Investig Drugs 2010;19(11):1427–37.

24. Jung J, Choi C, Cho SH, et al. Tolerability and pharmacokinetics of avanafil, a phosphodiesterase type 5 inhibitor: a single- and multiple-dose, double-blind, randomized, placebo-controlled, dose-escalation study in healthy Korean male volunteers. Clin Ther 2010;32(6):1178–87.

25. Kim BH, Lim HS, Chung JY, et al. Safety, tolerability and pharmacokinetics of udenafil, a novel PDE-5 inhibitor, in healthy young Korean subjects. Br J Clin Pharmacol 2008;65(6):848–54.

26. Ahn GJ, Chung HK, Lee CH, et al. Increased expression of the nitric oxide synthase gene and protein in corpus cavernosum by repeated dosing of udenafil in a rat model of chemical diabetogenesis. Asian J Androl 2009;11(4):435–42.

27. Lee CH, Shin JH, Ahn GJ, et al. Udenafil enhances the recovery of erectile function and ameliorates the pathophysiological consequences of cavernous nerve resection. J Sex Med 2010;7(7):2564–71.

28. Paick JS, Kim SW, Park YK, et al. The efficacy and safety of udenafil [Zydena] for the treatment of erectile dysfunction in hypertensive men taking concomitant antihypertensive agents. J Sex Med 2009; 6(11):3166–76.

29. Glina S, Toscano I, Gomatzky C, et al. Efficacy and tolerability of lodenafil carbonate for oral therapy in erectile dysfunction: a phase II clinical trial. J Sex Med 2009;6(2):553–7.

30. Glina S, Fonseca GN, Bertero EB, et al. Efficacy and tolerability of lodenafil carbonate for oral therapy of erectile dysfunction: a phase III clinical trial. J Sex Med 2010;7(5):1928–36.

31. Lee SK, Kim Y, Kim TK, et al. Determination of mirodenafil and sildenafil in the plasma and corpus cavernous of SD male rats. J Pharm Biomed Anal 2009;49(2):513–8.

32. Choi YH, Lee YS, Bae SH, et al. Dose-dependent pharmacokinetics and first-pass effects of mirodenafil, a new erectogenic, in rats. Biopharm Drug Dispos 2009;30(6):305–17.

33. Paick JS, Ahn TY, Choi HK, et al. Efficacy and safety of mirodenafil, a new oral phosphodiesterase type 5 inhibitor, for treatment of erectile dysfunction. J Sex Med 2008;5(11):2672–80.

34. Hatzimouratidis K, Hatzichristou DG. Looking to the future for erectile dysfunction therapies. Drugs 2008; 68(2):231–50.

35. Prince W. SLx-2101, a new long-acting PDE5 inhibitor: preliminary safety, tolerability, PK and endothelial function effects in healthy subjects. J Sex Med 2006;3(Suppl 1):29–30.

36. Stief C, Porst H, Saenz De Tejada I, et al. Sustained efficacy and tolerability with vardenafil over 2 years of treatment in men with erectile dysfunction. Int J Clin Pract 2004;58(3):230–9.

37. Klotz T, Mathers M, Klotz R, et al. Why do patients with erectile dysfunction abandon effective therapy with sildenafil (Viagra)? Int J Impot Res 2005;17(1):2–4.

38. Carson CC 3rd. Phosphodiesterase type 5 inhibitors: state of the therapeutic class. Urol Clin North Am 2007;34(4):507–15, vi.

39. Kaufman J, Dietrich J. Safety and efficacy of avanafil, a new PDE5 inhibitor for treating erectile dysfunction. J Urol 2006;175(Suppl 4):299.

40. Nehra A. Hemodynamic effects of co-administration of avanafil and glyceryl trinitrate. J Sex Med 2006; 3(Suppl 3):209.

41. Paick JS, Kim SW, Yang DY, et al. The efficacy and safety of udenafil, a new selective phosphodiesterase type 5 inhibitor, in patients with erectile dysfunction. J Sex Med 2008;5(4):946–53.

42. Prince WT, Campbell AS, Tong W. SLx-2101, a new long-acting PDE5 inhibitor: preliminary safety, tolerability, PK and endothelial function effects in healthy subjects. J Sex Med 2006;3(Suppl 1):29–30.

43. Pomeranz HD, Bhavsar AR. Nonarteritic ischemic optic neuropathy developing soon after use of sildenafil (Viagra): a report of seven new cases. J Neuro-ophthalmol 2005;25(1):9–13.

44. Carter JE. Anterior ischemic optic neuropathy and stroke with use of PDE-5 inhibitors for erectile dysfunction: cause or coincidence? J Neurol Sci 2007;262(1–2):89–97.

45. Padma-Nathan H, Eardly I, Kloner RA, et al. A 4-year update on the safety of sildenafil citrate (Viagra). Urology 2002;60(2 Suppl 2):67–90.

46. Kloner RA, Eardley I, Kloner RA, et al. Cardiovascular safety update of tadalafil: retrospective analysis of data from placebo-controlled and open-label clinical trials of tadalafil with as needed, three times-per-week or once-a-day dosing. Am J Cardiol 2006;97(12):1778–84.

47. Reffelmann T, Kieback A, Kloner RA. The cardiovascular safety of tadalafil. Expert Opin Drug Saf 2008; 7(1):43–52.

Central Nervous System Agents and Erectile Dysfunction

Rajeev Kumar, MD, MCh[a], Ajay Nehra, MD[b],*

KEYWORDS

- Apomorphine • Melanocortin • Serotonin
- Erectile dysfunction • Central agents

Cortical regions act as centers for integration of sensory stimuli and hormonal influences to initiate sexual desire and libido. These stimuli and hormones then act through sympathetic and parasympathetic pathways to control the peripheral activities that result in a penile erection. These cortical pathways explain the occurrence of erections without genital stimulation such as those occurring during fantasy, visual stimuli, and sleep. Whereas the role of nitric oxide (NO) as an end effector has been well established, the role of the central nervous system (CNS) in mediating penile erections remains unclear despite several laboratory and animal studies attesting to its importance. Initial studies were based on animal models with retrograde labeling of pathways, but more recent reports have used newer techniques such as the positron emission tomographic scan.[1,2]

Among a large variety of areas that may potentially be involved within the cortex, the medial preoptic area and the paraventricular nucleus (PVN) of the hypothalamus along with the hippocampus seem to be the principal areas of interest.[3] The PVN contains dopaminergic neurons whose stimulation is associated with penile erection. Whereas injection of dopaminergic agents in this region potentiates erections, lesions in this region result in a loss of erectile ability.[4,5] In further attempts to characterize the role of the PVN in erectile functioning, Richards and colleagues[6] recorded potentials from individual neurons in the PVN as well as local field potential activity in anesthetized rats during erectile activity. Apomorphine in erectogenic doses was injected peripherally and resulted in variable firing patterns of the neurons in the preerectile and erectile phases (**Figs. 1** and **2**).

The melanocortinergic system also has multiple sites of action within this complex network. This system consists of neuropeptides such as adrenocorticotropic hormone, β-endorphin, and α, β and γ melanocyte-stimulating hormones (MSHs) apart from their receptors and various antagonists. The melanocortins are posttranslational products of the prohormone pro-opiomelanocortin (POMC), which produces 8 different peptides based on the site of cleavage. POMC messenger RNA exists in several human tissues including the genitourinary tract. Among the various melanocortin receptors (MCRs), MCR3 and MCR4 have been found in the hypothalamus and MCR4 primarily has been seen to be involved in modulating sexual function.[7,8]

The CNS administration of α-MSH induces penile erections and yawning, somewhat similar to that seen with apomorphine. Mizusawa and colleagues[9] implanted catheters in the lateral cerebral ventricle or the subarachnoid space in 78 male Sprague-Dawley rats and injected α-MSH. These injections resulted in penile erections and an increase in intracavernosal pressure, which was abolished by the administration of NO inhibitors. Similar responses were produced by intracerebroventricular oxytocin, but intrathecal α-MSH did not produce any erectile response, suggesting a central role for α-MSH.

The authors have nothing to disclose.

[a] Department of Urology, All India Institute of Medical Sciences, New Delhi, India
[b] Department of Urology, Mayo Clinic College of Medicine, Mayo Clinic, 200 First Street Southwest, Rochester, MN 55905, USA
* Corresponding author.
E-mail address: Nehra.ajay@mayo.edu

Urol Clin N Am 38 (2011) 165–173
doi:10.1016/j.ucl.2011.03.006
0094-0143/11/$ – see front matter © 2011 Published by Elsevier Inc.

Supraspinal
Control and Integration

Spinal Reflexes

Autonomic Nervous

System

Erection

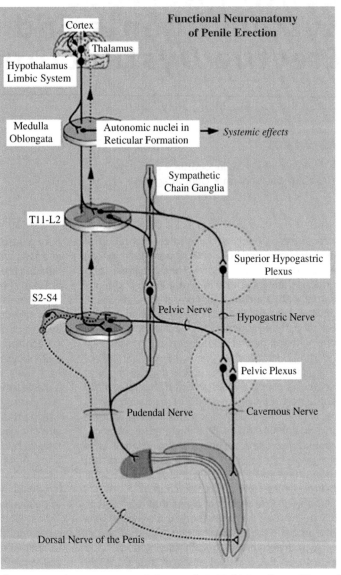

Fig. 1. Functional neuroanatomy of penile erection. (*From* Graugaard C, Hertoft P, Møhl B, editors. Hjerne & Seksualitet: Aspekter af Teori & Klinik. Copenhagen: Munksgaard Denmark 1997; with permission.)

Centrally acting agents are not among the currently recommended treatments for erectile dysfunction (ED) in the guidelines of the American Urological Association and the European Association of Urology.[10,11] These guidelines recommend phosphodiesterase 5 inhibitors (PDE5i) sildenafil, tadalafil, and vardenafil as first-line therapies with options including prostaglandin E_1, intracavernosal vasoactive agents, vacuum constriction devices, and penile prosthesis. The guidelines recommended switching from an oral to an alternate therapy among nonresponders.

PDE5i have a significant failure rate, including both primary and secondary failures among patients who may have initially responded to therapy. Further, some patient groups, such as in those after radical prostatectomy, have poorer outcomes with PDE5i. Adverse effects, time to onset of action, and lack of spontaneity are additional concerns with these agents. The current guidelines leave little oral options for these men, and there is clearly a potential for the development of alternative therapies. The principal reason for the recommendation against centrally acting

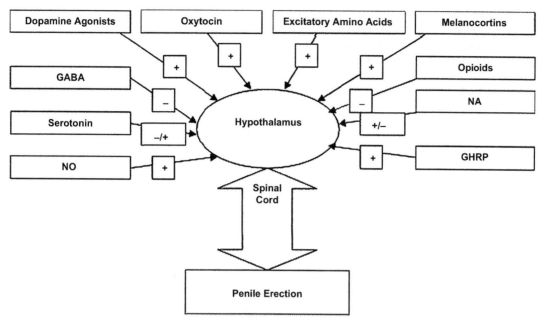

Fig. 2. The various biochemical pathways modulating hypothalamic control of penile erection and sexual behavior. Serotonin facilitates penile responses through 5-hydroxytryptamine receptor (5-HT_{1C}) and inhibits sexual behavior through 5-HT_{1A}. Excitatory amino acids, N-methyl-D-aspartate and L-aspartate; GABA, γ-aminobutyric acid; GHRP, growth hormone–releasing peptide; NA, noradrenaline (α_1-adrenergic receptor produces stimulation and inhibits sexual behavior); NO, nitric oxide. (*From* Kendirci M, Walls MM, Hellstrom WH. Central nervous system agents in the treatment of erectile dysfunction. Urol Clin North Am 2005;32:488; with permission.)

agents is the lack of adequate scientific data on their efficacy and safety.[10] This article reviews the centrally acting agents and the data on their efficacy.

DOPAMINERGIC AGENTS: APOMORPHINE

In one of the earliest clinical reports on the use of apomorphine, Lal and colleagues[12] reported reproducible erections in 7 of 9 men injected subcutaneously with varying doses of the drug. Apart from suggesting the efficacy of apomorphine, this study also showed that these actions were not mediated through cholinergic mechanisms because they were not inhibited by benztropine. Apomorphine has been shown to induce erections even without physical stimulation, solely through visual erotic stimuli. In a randomized blinded study, Danjou and colleagues[13] injected subcutaneous apomorphine in 10 healthy male volunteers at a dose of 9 μg/kg and found that erections were induced starting from the fourth minute after the injection and that this erection was potentiated by visual stimuli in the form of erotic slides.

One of the major hurdles in the use of apomorphine was the lack of an oral formulation. In the pre-PDE5 inhibitor era, this hurdle was a major limitation to the use of drugs in the management of ED. Apomorphine is highly soluble in lipids, has a wide volume of distribution, and undergoes rapid metabolism, thus limiting its actions when administered orally. Although the transmucosal absorption of apomorphine had been documented as early as 1935, the adverse events associated with the large dose limited its clinical usefulness.[14] In 1995, Heaton and colleagues[15] reported a series of experiments using various doses and routes of administration of apomorphine in men without an organic cause of ED. The investigators found excellent outcomes with a sublingual sustained release formulation, which had the least side effects (primarily yawning) when compared with the liquid or oral tablet formulations. After discovery of the sublingual route of administration, several studies evaluated the ideal dose and safety of this preparation. In one of the largest reported studies, 569 men and their partners were enrolled in 1 of 4 arms of a randomized study using dose escalation protocols, fixed doses of apomorphine, or placebo at 51 centers.[4] A total of 444 men completed the 8-week study. A statistically significant higher proportion of men in all the 3 treatment arms attained and maintained an erection compared with the placebo group. The international index of erectile function (IIEF) score in all the treatment groups was higher than the score in the placebo group. Between 30% and 50% patients reported nausea that increased with the dose, but this decreased with increasing period of drug use.

Attempts to formulate an ideal route of administration that minimizes side effects of apomorphine continue. Lu and colleagues[16] showed that intranasal delivery of apomorphine resulted in similar brain and cerebrospinal fluid concentrations of the drug when compared with subcutaneous administration, whereas its plasma concentration was only half. Further, brain concentrations were achieved faster with nasal administration than with subcutaneous injections, leading the investigators to suggest a nose-to-brain pathway for apomorphine. Riley and colleagues[17] recently reported the safety and efficacy of a novel nasal formulation delivered at low doses in men with mild to severe ED. These 2 phase 2b dose-finding studies included a total of 600 patients who were randomized to receive 1 of 3 fixed doses (between 100 and 300 µg) of either apomorphine or placebo on an as-required basis for up to 12 weeks during which they were to attempt intercourse at least 12 times. Changes in the Sexual Encounter Profile (SEP) questions 2 and 3 formed the primary end points. At all tested doses, patients showed an improvement in the ability to achieve vaginal penetration and maintain an erection. The onset of action was within 10 minutes for most responders. The most common adverse effects were headache, nasopharyngitis, and dyspepsia. About 6% of the randomized patients withdrew because of adverse effects. The investigators concluded that nasal apomorphine may become a first-line management for ED because of rapid onset of action and reproducible efficacy.

In direct comparison with existing PDE5i as primary therapy for ED, apomorphine continues to show poorer outcomes.[18–20] Giammusso and colleagues[21] reported a 20-week, open label, randomized crossover study using flexible dosing. The primary outcome was the sexual domain questions (questions 1–5 and 15) of the IIEF, whereas various efficacy and satisfaction questionnaires formed the secondary end points. Treatment preference was determined at the end of the study among subjects who received both treatments. A total of 130 patients were randomized. In the intent-to-treat analysis, there was significantly greater improvement with sildenafil than with apomorphine. A statistical difference in favor of sildenafil was maintained in the per-protocol analysis. Sildenafil was significantly superior to apomorphine in all

secondary parameters evaluated with a much higher events log than apomorphine. It was also superior, significantly, in terms of patient preference. Similar outcomes were reported in a study of 108 patients at 12 centers in Brazil in which sildenafil scored higher in all evaluated parameters.[22] Lack of effectiveness was also reported as the commonest reason for discontinuation of apomorphine in a survey of 11,185 patients in the United Kingdom who had been prescribed this drug as the first-line therapy for ED.[23]

MELANOCORTINS

Several highly potent and selective agonists and antagonists of the melanocortins have been developed to study the effect of this substance on human sexual function. These include melanotan II (MT-II), which is a cyclic peptide analogue of α-MSH and expresses agonistic activity at the MCR4 receptor.[24] PT-141, a metabolite of MT-II, is another synthetic agonist peptide analogue, as is tetrahydroisoquinoline, which has more than 100-fold selectivity for the MCR4 receptor.[25,26]

The development of erections in men given subcutaneous melatonin for pigmentation disorders led to a single-blind placebo-controlled trial with the superpotent MT-II in 3 normal male volunteers.[27,28] All subjects noted intermittent penile erections along with stretching and yawning about 1 to 5 hours after the injections. Spurred by these findings, Wessells and colleagues[29] conducted a randomized, controlled, crossover study in 10 men with psychogenic ED. Subcutaneous injections of MT-II were alternated with saline as placebo. A Rigiscan (Timm Medical Technologies, Inc, Eden Prairie, MN, USA) device was used to monitor erections for 6 hours after the injection, with the patient awake during this entire period. Of the 10 men, 8 reported erections within the 6-hour study period after the MT-II injection compared with none after the placebo. The onset of erection varied from 15 to 270 minutes, with 144 minutes being the mean duration of erections.

The investigators continued their evaluation by extending it to men with organic causes of ED.[30] A total of 10 men with an average of 2.2 organic causes for ED were randomized in a double-blind, crossover placebo-controlled study of MT-II (0.025 mg/kg) or placebo. Of the 10 men, 9 reported improved erections on at least 1 of the 2 injections of the drug, with 12 of 19 injections resulting in an erection compared with 1 of 21 of the placebo. The erections occurred for an average of 64 minutes. The Rigiscan device confirmed the subjective findings. Further, the investigators noted an increased desire after

10 of the drug injections. Nausea was the commonest side effect in the drug group.

Based on these initial reports, PT-141 (bremelanotide), a synthetic peptide analogue of α-MSH was developed as an agonist to melanocortin receptors, including MCR4. Its systemic administration in rats activates neurons in the hypothalamus and in normal men results in a dose-dependent increase in erectile activity.[25]

Rosen and colleagues[31] reported the results of 2 simultaneous studies using subcutaneous PT-141 in healthy men and sildenafil nonresponders. In the first study, a phase 1 evaluation, 48 healthy men received varying doses of PT-141 or placebo, whereas in the second phase 2a study, fixed doses of PT-141 or placebo were administered in a crossover, blinded, randomized manner to men with ED. Healthy men were not provided visual stimulation, whereas men with ED were. Rigiscan-monitored erectile responses were statistically significant in both groups of PT-141–treated men.

Subsequently, an intranasal formulation of PT-141 was developed and tested in healthy male subjects and in patients with sildenafil-responsive ED. Using a Rigiscan, with or without sexual stimulation, Diamond and colleagues[32] reported a statistically significant erectile response in men receiving PT-141 compared with those receiving placebo.

Salvage of PDE5 inhibitor failures is one of the most likely scenarios for the use of melanocortin agents. Safarinejad and Hosseini[33] reported a randomized controlled trial using bremelanotide, 10 mg, as an intranasal spray, 45 minutes to 2 hours before sexual intercourse, versus placebo in 342 men who failed to respond to sildenafil even after a reeducation program. The patients were asked to assess at least 16 attempts with the therapy. Most men had an organic cause for their ED. About 33% men who took bremelanotide responded to treatment compared with 8% taking placebo. Around 86% patients achieved erections within an hour of treatment, with the mean duration of rigidity sufficient for penetration being more than 10 minutes in men with even severe ED. The mean frequency of intercourse increased to 2.2 per week from 1.2 at baseline in the bremelanotide group. Around 16.3% patients on bremelanotide reported adverse effects with nausea, flushing, and sweating being the commonest.

ADRENERGIC AGENTS

The sympathetic nervous system has a key role in maintaining smooth muscle tone. It is thus clearly understandable that it has a role to play in erectile function. Noradrenergic agents modulate sexual activity by their actions on the α_1- and α_2-adrenergic receptors. Whereas the former is generally prosexual in its activity, the latter is associated with the inhibition of sexual behavior. The inhibition of α_2-adrenergic receptors may thus theoretically promote sexual activity.[34–36] The problem with using adrenergic agents is their wide field of action on most organ systems of the body.

Phentolamine, a nonspecific adrenoceptor blocker, has been used both as an intracavernosal agent as well as an oral drug for promoting erections.[37] Goldstein and colleagues[38] reported the outcomes of oral phentolamine in 2 randomized placebo-controlled trials as well as in 2 open label studies. In one study, 311 men received 40 mg of the oral drug in a crossover with placebo, whereas in the other parallel group study, 139 men received 40 mg drug, 146 received 80 mg drug, and another 139 received placebo. In both studies, men who completed the study showed significant improvement in the IIEF scores in the drug arms. Men on the 40-mg drug arm achieved higher vaginal penetration, although this was not statistically significant in the crossover study. Adverse events occurred in 27% of men in the drug groups. Similarly, Padma-Nathan and colleagues[39] reported a multicenter study on the efficacy and safety of oral phentolamine mesylate in 2 doses of 40 mg and 80 mg in men with ED. After an in-office test dose, men were dispensed tablets for home use and efficacy was assessed using the IIEF and the SEP questionnaires. A total of 2003 men received the 40-mg test dose, 1927 went on to receive the 40-mg dose initially, and 691 men further received the 80-mg dose. A total of 404 men completed the study, whereas 51% reported some adverse effect. Among men who completed the study, 87% reported improvements in their erectile function; the mean improvement in IIEF scores with the 40- and 80-mg doses was 6.3 and 5.7 points, respectively.

Yohimbine is a selective antagonist of α_2-adrenoceptors. It is an alkaloid derived from the bark of the yohimbe tree and has been used as an aphrodisiac. Initial reports in the 1960s after uncontrolled studies in men with ED suggested a potential role for this drug in the management of both organic and psychogenic dysfunction.[40] In 2002, Guay and colleagues reported the outcomes of a study with oral yohimbine using the Florida Sexual Health Questionnaire and Rigiscan readings as the primary outcome measure.[41] Men received oral yohimbine hydrochloride, 5.4 mg, thrice a day for 4 weeks followed by a dose escalation to 10.8 mg a day for a similar period. A total of 18 men completed the study.

Nine of them were considered responders because they achieved a successful intercourse in more than 75% of the attempts. There were no significant side effects. In another double-blind, placebo-controlled, 3-way crossover study evaluating yohimbine hydrochloride, 6 mg, with the combination of yohimbine, 6 mg, and L-arginine glutamate, 6 mg, or placebo, Lebret and colleagues[42] included 45 men with ED. The arginine-yohimbine combination was superior to placebo, particularly in men with mild ED.

A fixed dose combination of yohimbine and L-arginine (yohimbine tartrate, 7.7 mg, and L-arginine glutamate, 6 g) was evaluated for its safety, including use with nitrates, in 2 placebo-controlled, randomized, double-blind, 2-way crossover studies. The combination was found to be safe, with no significant decline in blood pressure even with a simultaneous glycerin trinitrite infusion.[43]

Considering a potential role for yohimbine in sildenafil failures, Senbel and colleagues[44] recorded intracavernosal and systemic arterial pressures and changes in sexual arousal and copulatory performance in rats after the intravenous administration of sildenafil, yohimbine, or a combination of both drugs. Although yohimbine alone failed to improve erectile responses, it significantly potentiated the effect of sildenafil such that the effect of the combination was greater than the sum of the effects of the 2 individual drugs with no additive hypotensive effect.

AMINO ACIDS AND NO

Apart from its well-known and well-documented role in the peripheral causation of erections, NO has also been shown to have significant central actions within the CNS.[45] Injection of NO inhibitors within the cerebral ventricles or the PVN inhibits erections induced by dopaminergic agents.[46] Additional support for the central action of NO comes from observations that injection of NO donors within the cerebral ventricles induces erections and yawning.[47]

The amino acid N-methyl-D-aspartic acid (NMDA) acts through its receptors within the PVN to activate neuronal NO synthase (nNOS) resulting in the synthesis and release of NO. This is associated with induction of penile erection and yawning in rats. These responses are blunted by the administration of N-monomethyl-L-arginine, which acts to block NO synthase.[46] These properties of NMDA have been used to study the potential role of central nNOS in penile erections. In a series of experiments on rats with streptozotocin-induced diabetes, Zheng and colleagues[48] reported reduced erections and yawning after NMDA

injections in the PVN of diabetic rats compared with controls. These effects were associated with a reduction in nNOS levels in the brains of these animals. Further, the responses in diabetic rats in which nNOS was restored using adenoviral transfection were normal. This result supports a central role in diabetes-induced ED.

Sanna and colleagues[49] evaluated the central action of PDE5i in another experimental study on rats. The agents were injected within the cerebral ventricles, peritoneum, or ventral tegmental area (VTA) of the brain. The extracellular dopamine level within the brain was simultaneously measured during VTA injections. Noncontact erections were counted after each injection. The PDE5i caused a significant increase in noncontact erections along with a concomitant increase in extracellular dopamine levels, suggesting a central action of these agents. Similarly, oxytocin injected into the VTA induces cyclic GMP–mediated penile erection, probably by activating NO synthase in the cell bodies of mesolimbic dopaminergic neurons.[50]

SEROTONIN

Serotonin seems to have an inhibitory effect on sexual function both at the periphery and within the CNS.[36,51] There is conflicting evidence about the action of selective serotonin reuptake inhibitors (SSRIs) such as trazodone in sexual function. Centrally, these agents may affect the transport of dopamine, its transmission, or its availability, thus resulting in decreased erections. SSRIs may also retard ejaculation, a property that has been exploited in the management of premature ejaculation.[52] On the other hand, Azadzoi and colleagues[53] reported improved erectile function in humans and rats after the peripheral administration of trazodone. However, these agents have not been significantly evaluated or used in the management of ED.[54]

Bupropion is a non-SSRI antidepressant that has been used to salvage SSRI-induced ED with mixed outcomes. Masand and colleagues[55] randomized 31 men with ED and on SSRI therapy for at least 6 weeks and to receive sustained-release low-dose (150 mg/d) of bupropion or placebo for 3 weeks. They found an improvement in the erectile function in both groups but no difference between the groups. On the other hand, Safarinejad,[56] using a similar dose and formulation in a 12-week, double-blind, randomized study of 234 men found significantly better outcomes in erectile function in the bupropion group compared with the placebo group. The improvement in the IIEF score was 54% in the drug arm compared with 1% in the placebo arm and the Erectile Dysfunction Inventory Treatment Satisfaction scores were significantly higher.

SUMMARY

Several centrally acting agents have shown potential to improve erectile function in men with ED. They still lack adequate data in efficacy and tolerability. Nasal formulations of apomorphine and bremelanotide seem to be the most likely candidates for future approval. They may play a role, specifically in men who fail PDE5 therapy, are unable to take PDE5i because of side effects, or are on nitrate therapy.

REFERENCES

1. Chuang AT, Steers WS. Neurophysiology of penile erection. In: Carson C, Kirby R, Goldstein I, editors. Textbook of erectile dysfunction. Oxford (United Kingdom): Isis Medical Media; 1999. p. 59–72.
2. Stoléru S, Grégoire MC, Gérard D, et al. Neuroanatomical correlates of visually evoked sexual arousal inhuman males. Arch Sex Behav 1999;28(1):1–21.
3. Giuliano F. Control of penile erection by the melanocortinergic system: experimental evidences and therapeutic perspectives. J Androl 2004;25(5):683–91.
4. Dula E, Keating W, Siami PF, et al. Efficacy and safety of fixed-dose and dose-optimization regimens of sublingual apomorphine versus placebo in men with erectile dysfunction. The Apomorphine Study Group. Urology 2000;56(1):130–5.
5. Argiolas A, Melis MR, Mauri A, et al. Paraventricular nucleus lesion prevents yawning and penile erection induced by apomorphine and oxytocin but not by ACTH in rats. Brain Res 1987;421:349–52.
6. Richards N, Wayman C, Allers KA. Electrophysiological actions of the dopamine agonist apomorphine in the paraventricular nucleus during penile erection. Neurosci Lett 2009;465(3):242–7.
7. Mountjoy KG, Mortrud MT, Low MJ, et al. Localization of the melanocortin-4 receptor (MC4-R) in neuroendocrine and autonomic control circuits in the brain. Mol Endocrinol 1994;8(10):1298–308.
8. Van der Ploeg LH, Martin WJ, Howard AD, et al. A role for the melanocortin 4 receptor in sexual function. Proc Natl Acad Sci U S A 2002;99(17):11381–6.
9. Mizusawa H, Hedlund P, Andersson KE. Alpha-melanocyte stimulating hormone and oxytocin induced penile erections, and intracavernous pressure increases in the rat. J Urol 2002;167(2 Pt 1):757–60.
10. Montague DK, Jarow JP, Broderick GA, et al. The management of erectile dysfunction: an AUA update. J Urol 2005;174:230–9.
11. Hatzimouratidis K, Amar E, Eardley I, et al. Guidelines on male sexual dysfunction: erectile dysfunction and premature ejaculation. Eur Urol 2010;57(5):804–14.
12. Lal S, Ackman D, Thavundayil JX, et al. Effect of apomorphine, a dopamine receptor agonist, on penile tumescence in normal subjects. Prog Neuropsychopharmacol Biol Psychiatry 1984;8(4–6):695–9.
13. Danjou P, Alexandre L, Warot D, et al. Assessment of erectogenic properties of apomorphine and yohimbine in man. Br J Clin Pharmacol 1988;26(6):733–9.
14. Walton RP, Lacey C. Absorption of drugs through the oral mucosa. J Pharmacol Exp Ther 1935;54:61–76.
15. Heaton JP, Morales A, Adams MA, et al. Recovery of erectile function by the oral administration of apomorphine. Urology 1995;45:200–6.
16. Lu W, Jiang W, Chen J, et al. Modulation of brain delivery and copulation by intranasal apomorphine hydrochloride. Int J Pharm 2008;349(1–2):196–205.
17. Riley A, Main M, Morgan F. Inhalation device allows novel administration of apomorphine in men with erectile dysfunction—efficacy and safety findings. J Sex Med 2010;7:1508–17.
18. Porst H, Behre HM, Jungwirth A, et al. Comparative trial of treatment satisfaction, efficacy and tolerability of sildenafil versus apomorphine in erectile dysfunction–an open, randomized cross-over study with flexible dosing. Eur J Med Res 2007;12(2):61–7.
19. Pavone C, Curto F, Anello G, et al. Prospective, randomized, crossover comparison of sublingual apomorphine (3 mg) with oral sildenafil (50 mg) for male erectile dysfunction. J Urol 2004;172(6 Pt 1):2347–9.
20. Eardley I, Wright P, MacDonagh R, et al. An open-label, randomized, flexible-dose, crossover study to assess the comparative efficacy and safety of sildenafil citrate and apomorphine hydrochloride in men with erectile dysfunction. BJU Int 2004;93:1271–5.
21. Giammusso B, Colpi GM, Cormio L, et al. An open-label, randomized, flexible-dose, crossover study to assess the comparative efficacy and safety of sildenafil citrate and apomorphine hydrochloride in men with erectile dysfunction. Urol Int 2008;81(4):409–15.
22. Afif-Abdo J, Teloken C, Damião R, et al. Comparative cross-over study of sildenafil and apomorphine for treating erectile dysfunction. BJU Int 2008;102(7):829–34.
23. Maclennan KM, Boshier A, Wilton LV, et al. Examination of the safety and use of apomorphine prescribed in general practice in England as a treatment for erectile dysfunction. BJU Int 2006;98(1):125–31.
24. Wikberg JE, Muceniece R, Mandrika I, et al. New aspects on the melanocortins and their receptors. Pharm Res 2000;42:393–420.

25. Molinoff PB, Shadiack AM, Earle D, et al. PT-141: a melanocortin agonist for the treatment of sexual dysfunction. Ann N Y Acad Sci 2003;994:96–102.

26. Sebhat IK, Martin WJ, Ye Z, et al. Design and pharmacology of N-[(3R)-1,2,3,4-tetrahydroiso-quinolinium-3-ylcarbonyl]-(1R)-1-(4-chlorobenzyl)-2-[4-cyclohexyl-4-(1H-1,2,4-triazol-1-ylmethyl) piperidin-1-yl]-2-oxoethylamine (1), a potent, selective, melanocortin subtype-4 receptor agonist. J Med Chem 2002;45:4589–93.

27. Hadley ME. Discovery that a melanocortin regulates sexual functions in male and female humans. Peptides 2005;26(10):1687–9.

28. Dorr RT, Lines R, Levine N, et al. Evaluation of Melanotan-II, a superpotent cyclic melanotropic peptide in a pilot phase-I clinical study. Life Sci 1996;58:1777.

29. Wessells H, Fuciarelli K, Hansen J, et al. Synthetic melanotropic peptide initiates erections in men with psychogenic erectile dysfunction (double blind placebo controlled crossover study). J Urol 1998; 160:389–93.

30. Wessells H, Gralnek D, Dorr R, et al. Effect of an alpha-melanocyte stimulating hormone analog on penile erection and sexual desire in men with organic erectile dysfunction. Urology 2000;56:641–6.

31. Rosen RC, Diamond LE, Earle DC, et al. Evaluation of the safety, pharmacokinetics and pharmacodynamic effects of subcutaneously administered PT-141, a melanocortin receptor agonist, in healthy male subjects and in patients with an inadequate response to Viagra. Int J Impot Res 2004;16(2):135–42.

32. Diamond LE, Earle DC, Rosen RC, et al. Double-blind, placebo-controlled evaluation of the safety, pharmacokinetic properties and pharmacodynamic effects of intranasal PT-141, a melanocortin receptor agonist, in healthy males and patients with mild-to-moderate erectile dysfunction. Int J Impot Res 2004;16:51–9.

33. Safarinejad MR, Hosseini SY. Salvage of sildenafil failures with bremelanotide: a randomized, double-blind, placebo controlled study. J Urol 2008;179(3): 1066–71.

34. Bitran D, Hull EM. Pharmacological analysis of male rat sexual behavior. Neurosci Biobehav Rev 1987; 11(4):365–89.

35. Miner MM, Seftel AD. Centrally acting mechanisms for the treatment of male sexual dysfunction. Urol Clin North Am 2007;34(4):483–96.

36. Andersson KE. Pharmacology of erectile function and dysfunction. Urol Clin North Am 2001;28(2):233–47.

37. Andersson KE, Stief C. Oral alpha adrenoceptor blockade as a treatment of erectile dysfunction. World J Urol 2001;19(1):9–13.

38. Goldstein I, Carson C, Rosen R, et al. Vasomax for the treatment of male erectile dysfunction. World J Urol 2001;19(1):51–6.

39. Padma-Nathan H, Goldstein I, Klimberg I, et al. Long-term safety and efficacy of oral phentolamine mesylate (Vasomax) in men with mild to moderate erectile dysfunction. Int J Impot Res 2002;14(4): 266–70.

40. Morales A. Yohimbine in erectile dysfunction: would an orphan drug ever be properly assessed? World J Urol 2001;19(4):251–5.

41. Guay AT, Spark RF, Jacobson J, et al. Yohimbine treatment of organic erectile dysfunction in a dose-escalation trial. Int J Impot Res 2002;14:25–31.

42. Lebret T, Hervé JM, Gorny P, et al. Efficacy and safety of a novel combination of L-arginine glutamate and yohimbine hydrochloride: a new oral therapy for erectile dysfunction. Eur Urol 2002; 41(6):608–13 [discussion: 613].

43. Kernohan AF, McIntyre M, Hughes DM, et al. An oral yohimbine/L-arginine combination (NMI 861) for the treatment of male erectile dysfunction: a pharmaco-kinetic, pharmacodynamic and interaction study with intravenous nitroglycerine in healthy male subjects. Br J Clin Pharmacol 2005;59(1):85–93.

44. Senbel AM, Mostafa T. Yohimbine enhances the effect of sildenafil on erectile process in rats. Int J Impot Res 2008;20(4):409–17.

45. Melis MR, Argiolas A. Role of central nitric oxide in the control of penile erection and yawning. Prog Neuropsychopharmacol Biol Psychiatry 1997;21(6): 899–922.

46. Melis MR, Stancampiano R, Argiolas A. Nitric oxide synthase inhibitors prevent N-methyl-D-aspartic acid-induced penile erection and yawning in male rats. Neurosci Lett 1994;179(1–2):9–12.

47. Melis MR, Argiolas A. Nitric oxide donors induce penile erection and yawning when injected in the central nervous system of male rats. Eur J Pharmacol 1995;294(1):1–9.

48. Zheng H, Bidasee KR, Mayhan WG, et al. Lack of central nitric oxide triggers erectile dysfunction in diabetes. Am J Physiol Regul Integr Comp Physiol 2007;292(3):R1158–64.

49. Sanna F, Succu S, Boi A, et al. Phosphodies-terase type 5 inhibitors facilitate noncontact erections in male rats: site of action in the brain and mechanism of action. J Sex Med 2009;6(10): 2680–9.

50. Succu S, Sanna F, Cocco C, et al. Oxytocin induces penile erection when injected into the ventral tegmental area of male rats: role of nitric oxide and cyclic GMP. Eur J Neurosci 2008;28(4):813–21.

51. Tang Y, Rampin O, Calas A, et al. Oxytocinergic and serotonergic innervation of identified lumbosacral nuclei controlling penile erection in the male rat. Neuroscience 1998;82(1):241–54.

52. Hellstrom WJ. Clinical applications of centrally acting agents in male sexual dysfunction. Int J Impot Res 2008;20(Suppl 1):S17–23.

53. Azadzoi KM, Payton T, Krane RJ, et al. Effects of intracavernosal trazodone hydrochloride: animal and human studies. J Urol 1990;144(5):1277–82.

54. Kendirci M, Walls MM, Hellstrom WH. Central nervous system agents in the treatment of erectile dysfunction. Urol Clin North Am 2005;32:487–501.

55. Masand PS, Ashton AK, Gupta S, et al. Sustained-release bupropion for selective serotonin reuptake inhibitor-induced sexual dysfunction: a randomized, double-blind, placebo-controlled, parallel-group study. Am J Psychiatry 2001;158(5):805–7.

56. Safarinejad MR. The effects of the adjunctive bupropion on male sexual dysfunction induced by a selective serotonin reuptake inhibitor: a double-blind placebo-controlled and randomized study. BJU Int 2010;106(6):840–7.

Testosterone Deficiency and Risk Factors in the Metabolic Syndrome: Implications for Erectile Dysfunction

Andre T. Guay, MD[a,b,*], Abdulmaged Traish, PhD[c,d]

KEYWORDS
- Hypogonadism • Metabolic syndrome
- Endothelial dysfunction • Erectile dysfunction
- Testosterone

Although multiple factors converge and contribute to development of metabolic syndrome (MetS), reduced testosterone (T) and sex hormone-binding globulin (SHBG) levels are considered significant risk factors in men.[1–4]

RELATIONSHIP BETWEEN TESTOSTERONE DEFICIENCY AND METS

Testosterone deficiency (TD) is strongly associated with MetS, and may be a risk factor for type 2 diabetes mellitus (T2DM) and cardiovascular (CV) disease.[5] The fact that androgens decline with age in men is a well established observation. However, whether the decline in androgens per se or the aging process itself accounts for the increased risk of MetS is a subject of continuous debate.[6,7] The effects of declining dehydroepiandrosterone sulfate on the metabolic profile are age dependent, but those of T are not according to Blouin and colleagues.[6,7] The investigators observed that patients with higher T values were more likely to have less than three components of MetS as opposed to those having lower T values. Laaksonen and colleagues[8] further supported a role for declining T levels in MetS, suggesting an inverse relationship between total T levels and odds ratios for having MetS. This correlates with the observations made by Kaplan and colleagues,[9] in which they noted that an inverse relationship exists between mean baseline total T levels and number of National Cholesterol Education Program-Adult Treatment Panel III (NCEP-ATP III) components, expressed in over 864 men with a mean age of 52 years. The Baltimore Longitudinal Study of Aging followed men for a mean of

Funding: This manuscript was not supported by any organization or pharmaceutical company.
Financial Disclosure: Andre Guay MD: Consultant and Advisory Board member: Auxilium, Bayer/Schering AG, Endo Pharmaceuticals, Repros Therapeutics.
Abdulmaged Traish PhD: nothing to disclose.
[a] Center for Sexual Function/Department of Endocrinology, Lahey Clinic, Northshore One Essex Center Drive, Peabody, MA 01960, USA
[b] Tufts University School of Medicine, Boston, MA, USA
[c] Department of Biochemistry, Boston University School of Medicine, 715 Albany Street, A502, Boston, MA 02118, USA
[d] Department of Urology, Boston University School of Medicine, 715 Albany Street, A502, Boston, MA 02118, USA
* Corresponding author. Center for Sexual Function/Department of Endocrinology, Lahey Clinic, Northshore One Essex Center Drive, Peabody, MA 02118.
E-mail address: Andre.T.Guay@Lahey.org

Urol Clin N Am 38 (2011) 175–183
doi:10.1016/j.ucl.2011.02.004

5.8 years[10] and confirmed that the prevalence of MetS increased with age and was associated with lower androgen levels. Lower total T and SHBG levels predicted higher incidence of MetS, according to the aforementioned study.

Clearly, low circulating androgen levels are a risk factor for MetS, and Laaksonen and colleagues[11] showed the reverse relationship to be true as well—namely, that patients with MetS at baseline, by various definitions of MetS, exhibited increased odds of developing TD during an 11-year follow-up period. In contrast, Chen and colleagues[12] confirmed that total T levels were inversely related to the likelihood of having MetS, but questioned the role in the development of T2DM. However, insulin resistance (IR) is part of the definition of T2DM as well as being the central component of MetS; thus it is significant that increasing insulin levels are associated with a statistically significant increase in the prevalence of MetS components.[13] The investigators, in the Diabetes Epidemiology: Collaborative Analysis of Diagnostic Criteria in Europe (DECODE) study (6156 men from 11 European cohort studies, mean follow-up 8.8 years), showed that the prevalence of individual components of MetS increased significantly with an increase in insulin levels.

ASSOCIATION BETWEEN TD AND INDIVIDUAL COMPONENTS OF METS
Relationship Between TD and T2DM

As discussed previously, T2DM and IR are two important components of MetS. The prevalence of T2DM has increased dramatically, probably related, in part, to the increased prevalence of obesity, and it is estimated that the number of individuals diagnosed with T2DM in the United States exceeded 15 million in 2004.[14] This trend has been emerging during the past 5 decades.[15] The prevalence of MetS, and its core component of IR, a key component of MetS, is approximately 4.5% in adolescents,[16] and represents a serious public health concern.

Men with low T are at a greater risk of developing T2DM.[17–19] A meta-analysis by Ding and colleagues[20] of 43 studies including 6427 men confirmed this, and four studies were even powered high enough to show that TD might predict the onset of diabetes. A relationship between low SHBG and T exists such that low T predicts higher glucose and insulin levels as well as increased obesity.[21,22] Low levels of T and SHBG were thought to play a role in the development of IR and subsequently T2DM, based on the findings of the longitudinal Massachusetts Male Aging Study.[18] Fukui and colleagues[23]

demonstrated similar findings in Japanese patients with T2DM when compared with healthy men and suggested that T supplementation in hypogonadal men could decrease IR and atherosclerosis.

A significant inverse relationship between total T and IR in men was noted in a number of studies.[24–26] Simon and colleagues[24] reported that total T concentrations were significantly associated with fasting plasma insulin, as well as 2-hour plasma insulin levels. Taken together, these findings raise the possibility that T may have a protective function against development or progression of T2DM in men.

Relationship Between TD and Hypertension

Hypertension, dyslipidemia, obesity, and IR comprise the major components of MetS with serious implications on CV disease risk. The relationship among these various components is complex and understanding their underlying pathophysiology requires a comprehensive framework of investigation. Lower total T values were found in men less than 25-years-old presenting with hypertension; and this is independent of age.[27,28] Conversely, Phillips and colleagues[29] reported that T levels correlated inversely with blood pressure in hypogonadal obese men. Smith and colleagues[30] found that, after 3 months of treatment of prostate cancer patients with GnRH antagonists, T levels predictably decreased into the hypogonadal range, with the consequence that diastolic pressure was elevated, along with mean pulse pressure.

On the other hand, hypogonadal men treated with T replacement therapy experienced amelioration of their high blood pressure. T treatment of abdominally obese men for 9 months reduced diastolic blood pressure significantly.[31] Similar findings were reported in which both resting systolic and diastolic blood pressure were significantly lowered during treatment with intramuscular T undecanoate in 66 hypogonadal men for up to 9.5 years.[32] The investigators noted that the most significant reductions occurred between 6 to 9 months. In addition, Anderson and colleagues[33] reported a significant favorable change in diastolic blood pressure in men treated for 6 months with T-replacement therapy. Given the fact that the relationship between hypertension and TD is complex and poorly investigated, the limited data available still suggest that T-replacement therapy tends to normalize blood pressure; however, this remains to be investigated.

Relationship Between TD and Dyslipidemia

Emerging evidence on the role of T in vascular function is challenging the traditional notion that androgens are atherogenic.[34,35] This notion stemmed from the fact that women seem to be protected from CV disease in their premenopausal years because of the estrogens they produce. It was then deduced that the higher risk of CV disease in men attributed to T, a postulate that was never proven scientifically. The current thinking is just the reverse; that is, that CV risk is related to low-T levels in men. Further, androgen deficiency has been considered a primary risk factor for dyslipidemia.[36–40] Reduced-T concentrations are thought to be associated with an atherogenic lipoprotein profile, with increased low-density lipoprotein (LDL) and triglyceride levels.[41] Increased total cholesterol (TC) and LDL cholesterol (LDL-C) have also been associated with lower T levels, in epidemiologic studies.[24,42,43] Interestingly, T therapy reduced TC and LDL-C levels, and positive association between high-density lipoprotein (HDL)-C levels and testosterone was noted in several studies.[44–46]

Increased HDL-C levels were associated with normalizing testosterone levels in patients with TD.[32,47] However, other studies showed either no changes in HDL-C levels[48,49] or reduced HDL-C levels.[50,51] The discrepancies among the various reported studies may be explained by the nature of the study design, doses, and formulations of androgens used for replacement; route and frequency of administration; patient age and hypogonadal states; body fat distribution; or methods of analysis of the lipoproteins and lipids. The observed decline in HDL level in some studies with androgen treatment may have been due to supraphysiological levels of T often seen with intramuscular depot long-acting T esters as suggested in a recent meta-analysis.[52]

T stimulates the activities of several lipoprotein-modifying enzymes involved in HDL metabolism, thus leading to efficient catabolism of plasma HDL and hence efficient reverse cholesterol transport.[53] Estradiol and testosterone have been suggested to exert opposite effects on lipid profiles, in particular HDL-C,[54] and estrogens are associated with unfavorable lipid profiles in men. This observation supports the conclusion of Tivesten and colleagues[55] who suggested that low T levels in conjunction with elevated estradiol levels in men are likely to be associated with lower extremity peripheral vascular disease (PAD).

TD and Obesity

Obesity is an independent risk of CV disease and a cornerstone of other CV risks, especially MetS and IR. Men with MetS had significantly higher prevalence of TD, with waist circumference (WC)

and hyperglycemia most strongly predicting such condition.[56,57] The investigators noted that lower total T levels contributed to elevated insulin levels and hypothesized that body fat distribution influences this relationship. Wannamethee and colleagues[58] studied 2924 men with no history of T2DM or CV disease, and found that both body mass index (BMI) and WC had the strongest association with MetS; whereas percentage body fat had the weakest association. WC, BMI, insulin, and homeostatic model assessment (HOMA) of IR were significantly and negatively correlated to T levels.[59]

Reduced total T levels have been related to central or abdominal obesity, and increased WC in a number of studies.[8,39,59,60] These findings were confirmed and amplified in a study by Svartberg and colleagues[27,28] who demonstrated that free-T and SHBG levels were inversely related to WC in 1548 community-dwelling men (age 25–84 years).

Elevated leptin levels may interfere with LH-hCG–stimulated androgen production, thus suppressing androgenic hormone formation in obese individuals.[61] Similarly, elevated cortisol levels may cause central suppression of central gonadotropins.[62] In addition, increased aromatase activity, in visceral adipose tissue, results in elevated circulating levels of estradiol, which suppresses T production via negative feedback mechanism. Decreased SHBG or cytokine-mediated inhibition of testicular steroid production is among the other possible mechanisms by which obesity contributes to reduced T levels.[39]

Relationship Between TD, MetS, and Erectile Dysfunction

Men with MetS have increased risk of erectile dysfunction (ED).[63] Because MetS increases CV risk, it is not surprising that ED may also be a predictor of subsequent CV disease. This is not surprising since medical conditions that comprise the components of MetS are also thought to be the major causes of ED. The prevalence of ED among men with MetS increases with the number of MetS components.[63] Patients with three to five components of MetS exhibited 20%, 30%, and 35% incidence of ED, respectively. This finding is consistent with the suggestion that MetS is an independent risk factor for ED,[64] and the more specific risk factor of WC[65] has also been found to be an independent predictor. A recent study by Zhody and colleagues[66] investigated androgen deficiency in relation to ED and MetS by analyzing BMI measurements in 158 obese men. The investigators found a significant statistical association between increasing BMI and the following parameters: increased systolic blood pressure, reduced serum T, reduced penile duplex parameters, increased triglycerides, decreased HDL, and increased LDL. With increasing BMI, the frequency of TD and ED increased, whereas total serum T showed a strong negative correlation. To assess the effect of BMI on vasculogenic ED, the investigators examined this relationship in the absence of other risk factors and found that for a BMI less than 25, 3 out of 13 men (23.1%) had vasculogenic ED, as compared with 32 out of 54 men (59.3%) with a BMI greater than 25, suggesting that TD is related to both ED and MetS.

Based on basic research and clinical studies, androgens regulate multiple signaling pathways and the structural integrity of penile cavernosal tissue and cellular components. These include: (1) regulation of nitric oxide synthase expression and activity, (2) regulation of phosphodiesterase type 5 expression and activity, (3) regulation of the alpha adrenoceptor expression and function, (4) regulation of smooth muscle cell metabolism and responses, (5) regulation of connective tissue synthesis and deposition, (6) regulation of differentiation of progenitor vascular-stroma cells into myogenic and adipogenic lineages, and (7) maintaining nerve fiber network function. Alterations in these functions are manifested as changes in tissue response to endogenous vasodilators causing diminished blood inflow (failure to fill); alterations in the fibroelastic properties and expandability with inadequate compliance of the corpus cavernosum, concomitant with increased blood outflow (failure to accumulate blood under pressure); and dysfunctional venoocclusive mechanism, contributing to ED (failure to contain blood).[67]

RELATIONSHIP BETWEEN TD, METS, AND ENDOTHELIAL DYSFUNCTION

Endothelial dysfunction is the fundamental pathologic process common to CV disease and ED (**Fig. 1**). The link between TD and endothelial dysfunction has been investigated.[68,69] However, more studies are needed to delineate the mechanisms underlying these pathways. Endothelial dysfunction in men with TD has been shown to be independent of other risk factors, suggesting a protective effect of T on the endothelium.[70]

Endothelial dysfunction is an early step in the progression of atherosclerotic vascular disease. Low serum free T is inversely related to intima media thickness.[71,72] Castration in animals produced significant endothelium damage represented by structural alterations, including

a crumpled cell surface, which was, rough, adhesive, and ruptured.[73] T or dihydrotestosterone treatment of castrated animals partially restored the endothelium ultrastructure, suggesting a direct role of androgens in endothelial function. Mäkinen and colleagues[74] hypothesized that normal T offers protection against the development or progression of atherosclerosis in middle-aged men with TD.

Significant reduction in total cholesterol was demonstrated with T therapy and a shift in the cytokine balance to a state of reduced inflammation was also reported by Malkin and colleagues[75,76] suggesting that T modulated the immune-response and that T is important in inhibiting atheroma formation and progression to acute coronary syndrome. Measurement of flow-mediated vasodilation (FMD) of the brachial artery using ultrasonography in 187 consecutive male outpatients, total and free T significantly correlated with percent of FMD. The percent of FMD was 1.7-fold higher in patients with the highest quartile of free testosterone than in patients in the lowest quartile. The findings indicate that low T levels were associated with endothelial dysfunction in men independent of other risk factors, and further suggest a protective effect of endogenous T on the endothelium.[70] It has been further shown that low T levels are independent determinants of endothelial dysfunction in men.

POTENTIAL IMPLICATIONS FOR T THERAPY IN PATIENTS WITH TD, METS, AND ED

Makhsida and colleagues[77] argued that TD is a central feature of MetS and that T treatment may have a beneficial impact on MetS itself, slowing the progression to diabetes and CVD, in addition to restoring eugonadal hormone concentrations. Early studies indicate that T treatment in TD may decrease the risk of CV disease by ameliorating components of the MetS. In a small study of men who had both T2DM and TD who were treated with intermediate-acting T esters by injection every 2 weeks for 3 months, T replacement showed significant decrease in fasting glucose and hemoglobin A1c (HbA1$_C$) levels, fasting insulin, HOMA index for insulin resistance, as well as a decrease in WC and visceral adiposity, even though the treatment was for a short time.[78] Heufelder and colleagues[79] studied the effects of diet and exercise with or without T treatment in 32 men who had new onset T2DM, TD, and IR. No specific medications were used for the T2DM. Both groups were treated with diet and exercise, while one group received T replacement with a gel formulation. Fasting glucose, HbA1$_C$ levels, HDL cholesterol,

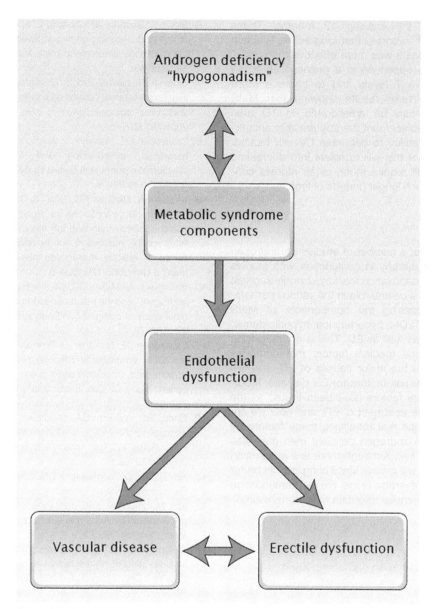

Fig. 1. The relationship between androgen deficiency (hypogonadism) and components of the metabolic syndrome is depicted as bidirectional. The metabolic syndrome components impact adversely endothelial function and in turn contribute to pathologies underlying cardiovascular disease and erectile dysfunction, as they share a common risk factor of endothelial dysfunction with concomitant diminished blood flow.

triglycerides, and WC improved significantly in both groups, but the addition of T replacement to the diet and exercise further improved such parameters positively, over diet and exercise alone. Further, in the T-treated group, the percentage of men who no longer met the diagnosis of MetS decreased by 81.3% versus the 31.3% of the diet and exercise alone group. Aversa and colleagues[80] investigated the effects of T replacement in men with MetS and TD, the majority of whom did not exhibit T2DM, for 2 years, in a placebo-controlled format. The

treatment with a long-acting T-ester injection every 12 weeks demonstrated significant changes within 12 months with marked and significant improvement in HOMA index for IR, C-reactive protein, as well as fasting glucose and HbA1$_C$ levels. More importantly, a significant decrease in carotid intima media thickness was recorded, a finding that had been suggested by data in a previous report.[81] The results prompted the investigators to transfer all patients to the T-treatment group after 12 months, with the same positive findings observed in the ensuing 12 months. These investigators[82] reported that long-acting injection of T undecanoate was more effective than oral T undecanoate, based on in a previous study, to reach effective T levels and to improve MetS parameters. These results showing that MetS components can be ameliorated in TD men receiving T-replacement therapy are very encouraging in the ability to decrease CV risk factors. Whether or not this will translate into decreased CV events will require much larger studies conducted for much longer periods of time.

SUMMARY

The findings of a number of studies on androgen replacement therapy in conjunction with studies on androgen deprivation therapy strongly suggest that TD plays a central role in the various pathologies encompassing the components of MetS including IR, T2DM, hypertension, hyperlipidemia, and obesity, as well as ED. This is not surprising since the same medical factors that comprise MetS also are the major causes of ED, and are also the major risk factors for CV disease. Modifying these risk factors have been touted as the first line of the treatment of ED, and now we are seeing evidence that modifying these factors by replacing T in androgen deficient men may also decrease CV risk. Although there is a suggestion that adding T will modify MetS components better than diet and exercise alone, the recommendation is to use all avenues to obtain maximum results.

REFERENCES

1. Muller M, Grobbee DE, den Tonkelar I, et al. Endogenous sex hormones and metabolic syndrome in aging men. J Clin Endocrinol Metab 2005;90:2618–23.
2. Kupelian V, Page ST, Araujo AB, et al. Low sex hormone-binding globulin, total testosterone, and symptomatic androgen deficiency are associated with development of the metabolic syndrome in nonobese men. J Clin Endocrinol Metab 2006;91: 843–50.
3. Kupelian V, Shabsigh R, Araujo AB, et al. Erectile dysfunction as a predictor of the metabolic syndrome in aging men: results from the Massachusetts Male Aging Study. J Urol 2006;176:222–6.
4. Miner MM, Sadovsky R. Evolving issues in male hypogonadism: evaluation, management, and related comorbidities. Cleve Clin J Med 2007;74:S38–46.
5. Miner MM, Seftel AD. Testosterone and aging: what we have learned since the Institute of Medicine and what lies ahead. Int J Clin Pract 2007;61:622–32.
6. Blouin K, Despres JP, Couillard C, et al. Contribution of age and declining androgen levels to features of the metabolic syndrome in men. Metabolism 2005; 54:1034–40.
7. Blouin K, Richard C, Brochu G, et al. Androgen inactivation and steroid converting enzyme expression in abdominal adipose tissue in men. J Endocrinol 2006;191:637–49.
8. Laaksonen DE, Niskanen L, Punnonen K, et al. Sex hormones, inflammation and the metabolic syndrome: a population-based study. Eur J Endocrinol 2003;149:601–8.
9. Kaplan SA, Meehan AG, Shah A. The age related decrease in testosterone is significantly exacerbated in obese men with the metabolic syndrome. What are the implications for the relatively high incidence of erectile dysfunction observed in these men? J Urol 2006;176:1524–8.
10. Rodriguez A, Muller DC, Metter EJ, et al. Aging, androgens, and the metabolic syndrome in a longitudinal study of aging. J Clin Endocrinol Metab 2007; 92:3568–72.
11. Laaksonen DE, Niskanen L, Punnonen K, et al. The metabolic syndrome and smoking in relation to hypogonadism in middle-aged men: a prospective cohort study. J Clin Endocrinol Metab 2005;90: 712–9.
12. Chen RY, Wittert GA, Andrews GR. Relative androgen deficiency in relation to obesity and metabolic status in older men. Diabetes Obes Metab 2006;8:429–35.
13. Hu G, Qiao Q, Tuomilehto J. DECODE Study Group. Prevalence of the metabolic syndrome and its relation to all-cause and cardiovascular mortality in nondiabetic European men and women. Arch Intern Med 2004;164:1066–76.
14. Steinbrook R. Facing the diabetes epidemic—mandatory reporting of glycosylated hemoglobin values in New York City. N Engl J Med 2006;354:545–8.
15. Parikh NI, Pencine MJ, Wang TJ, et al. Increasing trends in incidence of overweight and obesity over 5 decades. Am J Med 2007;120:242–50.
16. Ford ES, Li C, Zhao G, et al. Prevalence of the metabolic syndrome among US adolescents using the definition from the International Diabetes Federation. Diabetes Care 2008;31:587–9.
17. Haffner SM, Miettinen H, Karhapää P, et al. Leptin concentrations, sex hormones, and cortisol in nondiabetic men. J Clin Endocrinol Metab 1997;82:1807–9.
18. Stellato RK, Feldman HA, Hamdy O, et al. Testosterone, sex hormone-binding globulin, and the development of type 2 diabetes in middle-aged men: prospective results from the Massachusetts male aging study. Diabetes Care 2000;23:490–4.
19. Selvin E, Feinleib M, Zhang L, et al. Androgens and diabetes in men. Diabetes Care 2007;30: 234–8.

20. Ding EL, Song Y, Malik VS, et al. Sex differences of endogenous sex hormones and risk of type 2 diabetes: a systematic review and meta-analysis. JAMA 2006;295:1288–99.

21. Haffner SM, Shaten J, Stern MP, et al. Low levels of sex hormone-binding globulin and testosterone predict the development of non-insulin-dependent diabetes mellitus in men. MRFIT Research Group. Multiple Risk Factor Intervention Trial. Am J Epidemiol 1996;143:889–97.

22. Grossman M, Thomas MC, Panagiotopoulos S, et al. Low testosterone levels are common and associated with insulin resistance in men with diabetes. J Clin Endocrinol Metab 2008;93(5):1834–40.

23. Fukui M, Soh J, Tanaka M, et al. Low serum testosterone concentration in middle-aged men with type 2 diabetes. Endocr J 2007;54:871–7.

24. Simon D, Charles MA, Nahoul K, et al. Association between plasma total testosterone and cardiovascular risk factors in healthy adult men: the Telecom Study. J Clin Endocrinol Metab 1997;82:682–5.

25. Pitteloud N, Hardin M, Dwyer AA, et al. Increasing insulin resistance is associated with a decrease in Leydig cell testosterone secretion in men. J Clin Endocrinol Metab 2005;90:2636–41.

26. Basaria S, Muller DC, Carducci MA, et al. Hyperglycemia and insulin resistance in men with prostate carcinoma who receive androgen-deprivation therapy. Cancer 2006;106:581–8.

27. Svartberg J, von Muhlen D, Schirmer H, et al. Association of endogenous testosterone with blood pressure and left ventricular mass in men. The Tromsø Study. Eur J Endocrinol 2004;150:65–71.

28. Svartberg J, von Muhlen D, Sundsfjord J, et al. Waist circumference and testosterone levels in community dwelling men. The Tromsø Study. Eur J Epidemiol 2004;19:657–63.

29. Phillips GB, Jing TY, Resnick LM, et al. Sex hormones and hemostatic risk factors for coronary heart disease in men with hypertension. J Hypertens 1993;11:699–702.

30. Smith MR, Bennett S, Evans L, et al. The effects of induced hypogonadism on arterial stiffness, body composition, and metabolic parameters in males with prostate cancer. J Clin Endocrinol Metab 2001;86:4261–7.

31. Marin P, Holmang S, Gustafsson C, et al. Androgen treatment of abdominally obese men. Obes Res 1993;1:245–51.

32. Zitzmann M, Nieschlag E. Androgen receptor gene CAG repeat length and body mass index modulate the safety of long term intramuscular testosterone undecanoate therapy in hypogonadal men. J Clin Endocrinol Metab 2007;92:3844–53.

33. Anderson FH, Francis RM, Faulkner K. Androgen supplementation in eugonadal men with osteoporosis-effects of 6 months of treatment on bone mineral density and cardiovascular risk factors. Bone 1996;18:171–7.

34. Kaufman JM, Vermeulen A. The decline of androgen levels in elderly men and its clinical and therapeutic implications. Endocr Rev 2005;26:833–76.

35. Ng MK. New perspectives on Mars and Venus: unraveling the role of androgens in gender differences in cardiovascular biology and disease. Heart Lung Circ 2007;16:185–92.

36. Traish AM, Guay A, Feely R, et al. The dark side of testosterone deficiency: I. metabolic syndrome and erectile dysfunction. J Androl 2009;30:10–22.

37. Traish AM, Saad F, Guay A. The dark side of testosterone deficiency: II. type 2 diabetes and insulin resistance. J Androl 2009;30:23–32.

38. Traish AM, Guay A, Feely R, et al. The dark side of testosterone deficiency: III. vascular disease. J Androl 2009;30:477–94.

39. Kalyani RR, Dobs AS. Androgen deficiency, diabetes, and the metabolic syndrome in men. Curr Opin Endocrinol Diabetes Obes 2007;14:226–34.

40. Kapoor D, Jones TH. Androgen deficiency as a predictor of metabolic syndrome in aging men: an opportunity for investigation? Drugs Aging 2008;5:357–69.

41. Wu FC, von Eckardstein A. Androgens and coronary artery disease. Endocr Rev 2003;24:183–217.

42. Barrett-Connor E. Lower endogenous androgen levels and dyslipidemia in men with non-insulin-dependent diabetes mellitus. Ann Intern Med 1992;117:807–11.

43. Haffner SM, Mykkänen L, Valdez RA, et al. Relationship of sex hormones to lipids and lipoproteins in nondiabetic men. J Clin Endocrinol Metab 1993;77:1610–5.

44. Saad F, Gooren LJ, Haider A, et al. A dose-response study of testosterone on sexual dysfunction and features of the metabolic syndrome using testosterone gel and parenteral testosterone undecanoate. J Androl 2008;29:102–5.

45. Tenover JS. Effects of testosterone supplementation in the aging male. J Clin Endocrinol Metab 1992; 75(4):1092–8.

46. Ly LP, Jimenez M, Zhuang TN, et al. A double-blind, placebo-controlled, randomized clinical trial of transdermal dihydrotestosterone gel on muscular strength, mobility, and quality of life in older men with partial androgen deficiency. J Clin Endocrinol Metab 2001;86:4078–88.

47. Saad F, Gooren L, Haider A, et al. An exploratory study of the effects of 12-month administration of the novel long-acting testosterone undecanoate on measures of sexual function and the metabolic syndrome. Arch Androl 2007;53:353–7.

48. Zgliczynski S, Ossowski M, Slowinska-Srzednicka J, et al. Effect of testosterone replacement therapy on lipids and lipoproteins in hypogonadal and elderly men. Atherosclerosis 1996;121:35–43.

49. Uyanik BS, Ari Z, Gumus B, et al. Beneficial effects of testosterone undecanoate on the lipoprotein profiles in healthy elderly men. Jpn Heart J 1997; 38:73–82.

50. Thompson PD, Cullinane EM, Sady SP, et al. Contrasting effects of testosterone and stanozolol on serum lipoprotein levels. JAMA 1989;261:1165–8.

51. Bagatell CJ, Heiman JR, Matsumoto AM, et al. Metabolic and behavioral effects of high dose exogenous testosterone in healthy men. J Clin Endocrinol Metab 1994;79:561–7.

52. Isidori AM, Giannetta E, Greco EA, et al. Effects of testosterone on body composition, bone metabolism and serum lipid profile in middle-aged men: a meta-analysis. Clin Endocrinol 2005;63:280–93.

53. Traish AM, Abdou R, Kypreos KE. Androgen deficiency and atherosclerosis: the lipid link. Vascul Pharmacol 2009;51:303–13.

54. Tomaszewski M, Charchar FJ, Maric C, et al. Association between lipid profile and circulating concentrations of estrogens in young men. Atherosclerosis 2009;203:257–62.

55. Tivesten A, Mellström D, Jutberger H, et al. Low serum testosterone and high serum estradiol associate with lower extremity peripheral arterial disease in elderly men. The MrOS Study in Sweden. J Am Coll Cardiol 2007;50:1070–6.

56. Corona G, Mannucci E, Petrone L, et al. A comparison of NCEP ATPIII and IDF metabolic syndrome definitions with relation to metabolic syndrome-associated sexual dysfunction. J Sex Med 2007;4:789–96.

57. Corona G, Mannucci E, Schulman C, et al. Psychobiologic correlates of the metabolic syndrome and associated sexual dysfunction. Eur Urol 2006;50: 595–604.

58. Wannamethee SG, Shaper AG, Morris RW, et al. Measures of adiposity in the identification of metabolic abnormalities in elderly men. Am J Clin Nutr 2005;81:1313–21.

59. Osuna JA, Gomez-Perez R, Arata-Bellabarba G, et al. Relationship between BMI, total testosterone, sex hormonebinding-globulin, leptin, insulin and insulin resistance in obese men. Arch Androl 2006; 52:355–61.

60. Pasquali R, Macor C, Vicennati V, et al. Effects of acute hyperinsulinemia on testosterone serum concentrations in adult obese and normal weight men. Metabolism 1997;46:526–9.

61. Isidori AM, Caprio M, Strollo F, et al. Leptin and androgens in male obesity: evidence for leptin contribution to reduced androgen levels. J Clin Endocrinol Metab 1999;84:3673–80.

62. Rosmond R, Wallerius S, Wanger P, et al. A 5 year follow-up study of disease incidence in men with an abnormal hormone pattern. J Intern Med 2003; 254:386–90.

63. Esposito K, Giugliano F, Martedi E, et al. High proportions of erectile dysfunction in men with the metabolic syndrome. Diabetes Care 2004;28:1201–3.

64. Heidler S, Temml C, Broessner C, et al. Is the metabolic syndrome an independent risk factor for erectile dysfunction? J Urol 2007;177:651–4.

65. Demir T, Demir O, Kefi A, et al. Prevalence of erectile dysfunction in patients with metabolic syndrome. Int J Urol 2006;13:385–8.

66. Zhody W, Kamal EE, Ibrahim Y. Androgen deficiency and abnormal penile duplex parameters in obese men with erectile dysfunction. J Sex Med 2007;4: 797–808.

67. Traish AM, Guay AT. Are androgens critical for penile erections in humans? Examining the clinical and preclinical evidence. J Sex Med 2006; 3:382–407.

68. Miller VM, Mulvagh SL. Sex steroids and endothelial function: translating basic science to clinical practice. Trends Pharmacol Sci 2007;28:263–70.

69. Sader MA, Griffiths KA, Skilton MR, et al. Physiological testosterone replacement and arterial endothelial function in men. Clin Endocrinol (Oxf) 2003; 59:62–7.

70. Akishita M, Hashimoto M, Ohike Y, et al. Low testosterone level is an independent determinant of endothelial dysfunction in men. Hypertens Res 2007;30: 1029–34.

71. Van den Beld AW, Bots ML, Janssen JA, et al. Endogenous hormones and carotid atherosclerosis in elderly men. Am J Epidemiol 2003;157:25–31.

72. Demirbag R, Yilmaz R, Ulucay A, et al. The inverse relationship between thoracic aortic intima media thickness and testosterone level. Endocr Res 2005; 31:335–44.

73. Lu YL, Zhu H, Wu H, et al. Changes in aortic endothelium ultrastructure in male rats following castration, replacement with testosterone and administration of 5-alpha-reductase inhibitor. Asian J Androl 2007;9: 843–7.

74. Mäkinen J, Järvisalo MJ, Pöllänen P, et al. Increased carotid atherosclerosis in andropausal middle-aged men. J Am Coll Cardiol 2005;45:1603–8.

75. Malkin CJ, Pugh PJ, Jones RD, et al. Testosterone as a protective factor against atherosclerosis–immunomodulation and influence upon plaque development and stability. J Endocrinol 2003;178:373–80.

76. Malkin CJ, Pugh PJ, Jones RD, et al. The effect of testosterone replacement on endogenous inflammatory cytokines and lipid profiles in hypogonadal men. J Clin Endocrinol Metab 2004;89:3313–8.

77. Makhsida N, Shah J, Yan G, et al. Hypogonadism and metabolic syndrome: implications for testosterone therapy. J Urol 2005;174:827–34.

78. Kapoor D, Goodwin E, Channer KS, et al. Testosterone replacement therapy improves insulin resistance, glycaemic control, visceral adiposity and

hypercholesterolemia in hypogonadal men with type 2 diabetes. Eur J Endocrinol 2006;154:899–906.

79. Heufelder AE, Saad F, Bunck MC, et al. Fifty-two-week treatment with diet and exercise plus transdermal testosterone reverses the metabolic syndrome and improves glycemic control in men with newly diagnosed type 2 diabetes and subnormal plasma testosterone. J Androl 2009;30:726–33.

80. Aversa A, Bruzziches R, Francomano D, et al. Effects of testosterone undecanoate on cardiovascular risk factors and atherosclerosis in Middle-aged men with late-onset hypogonadism and metabolic syndrome: results from a 24-month, randomized, double-blind, placebo-controlled study. J Sex Med 2010;7:3495–503.

81. Mathur A, Malkin C, Saeed B, et al. Long-term benefits of testosterone replacement therapy on angina threshold and atheroma in men. Eur J Endocrinol 2009;161:443–9.

82. Aversa A, Bruzziches R, Francomano D, et al. Efficacy and safety of two different testosterone undecanoate formulations in hypogonadal men with metabolic syndrome. J Endocrinol Invest 2010; 33(11):776–83.

Priapism: New Concepts in Medical and Surgical Management

Arthur L. Burnett, MD, MBA[a],*,
Trinity J. Bivalacqua, MD, PhD[b]

KEYWORDS

- Ischemic priapism • Erectile dysfunction • Penis • Erection

References to priapism as a trivial erection problem misrepresent its importance as a true clinical disorder of male sexual function. The presumably limited frequency and population extent of this disorder largely influences this misconception, although its pathophysiologic obscurity, the dearth of remedies for it, and its self-remitting tendency also are contributing factors in this regard. Unlike the widespread emphasis placed on male erectile dysfunction (ED), less attention has historically been given to priapism despite this erectile disorder also carrying adverse health risks. It is therefore heartening to observe that, at this time when recent advances have been made in the scientific understanding and clinical practice of male ED, a similar aim toward establishing effective, evidence-based therapeutics for priapism is gaining momentum. This article reviews recent clinical developments in the medical and surgical management of priapism and surveys scientific research activity in this rapidly evolving field of study that conceivably will pave the way for further innovations in its treatment. In addition, the relevance of health care administration and policy to this field is evaluated, particularly as this area relates to the sickle cell disease population, and some health care programmatic areas are proposed for improving health outcomes of individuals with priapism.

DISEASE PROFILE

In a clinical context, priapism connotes abnormally persistent penile erection unrelated to sexual provocation or purpose.[1–3] An occurrence of 4 hours is often applied as a diagnostic criterion, although the existence of the disorder is accepted for episodes of shorter durations. The penis is readily recognized as the diseased bodily organ, although priapism of the clitoris has also been reported.[4] The abnormality typically involves the main erectile bodies, the corpora cavernosa, although involvement of the corpus spongiosum has also been observed.[5,6] The disorder represents a dysfunctional process of prolonged genital organ erection.

Many different clinical conditions have been associated with priapism. A basic categorization of these associations is clinically practical and also lends insight into the causal origins of the disorder (**Box 1**).[1–3] Categories include hematologic dyscrasias, ED pharmacotherapeutic complications, pharmacologic exposures, nonhematologic malignancies, pelvic or genital trauma, and neurologic conditions. An idiopathic category presently exists,

This work was supported by grant nos. DK067223 and HL068160 from the National Institutes of Health.
Disclosures: Pfizer Inc (ALB).

[a] Division of Sexual Medicine, Department of Urology, The James Buchanan Brady Urological Institute, Johns Hopkins Medical Institutions, Johns Hopkins Hospital, Marburg 407, 600 North Wolfe Street, Baltimore, MD 21287, USA
[b] Department of Urology, The James Buchanan Brady Urological Institute, Johns Hopkins Medical Institutions, Johns Hopkins Hospital, Marburg 409, 600 North Wolfe Street, Baltimore, MD 21287, USA
* Corresponding author.
E-mail address: aburnett@jhmi.edu

Urol Clin N Am 38 (2011) 185–194
doi:10.1016/j.ucl.2011.02.005

Box 1
Causes of priapism

Ischemic priapism

Hematologic dyscrasias

Sickle cell disease, thalassemia, leukemia, multiple myeloma, hemoglobin Olmsted variant, fat emboli associated with hyperalimentation, hemodialysis, glucose-6-phosphate dehydrogenase deficiency

Vasoactive erectile agents

Papaverine, phentolamine, prostaglandin E1, combination therapy

Medications

α-Adrenergic receptor antagonists

Prazosin, terazosin, doxazosin, tamsulosin

Antianxiety agents

Hydroxyzine

Anticoagulants

Heparin, warfarin

Antidepressants and antipsychotics

Trazodone, bupropion, fluoxetine, sertraline, lithium, clozapine, risperidone, olanzapine, chlorpromazine, thioridazine, phenothiazines

Antihypertensives

Hydralazine, guanethidine, propranolol

Drugs (recreational)

Alcohol, cocaine (intranasal and topical), crack cocaine, marijuana

Hormones

Gonadotropin-releasing hormone (in hypogonadal men), testosterone

Infectious (toxin mediated)

Scorpion sting, spider bite, rabies, malaria

Metabolic

Amyloidosis, Fabry disease, gout

Neoplastic (metastatic or regional infiltration)

Prostate, urethra, testis, bladder, colorectal, lung, kidney, penis

Neurogenic

Syphilis, spinal cord injury, cauda equina compression, autonomic neuropathy, lumbar disc herniation, spinal stenosis, cerebral vascular accident, brain tumor, spinal anesthesia, cauda equina syndrome

Anxiety disorders

Anesthesia (general, regional)

Nonischemic priapism

Trauma

Straddle injury, coital injury, pelvic trauma, kick to penis/perineum

Intracavernous injection needle laceration

Penile revascularization surgery

Vasoactive erectile agents/drugs

Neurologic conditions

Treatment-refractory ischemic priapism

NB: Categories are assigned according to the clinicopathologic division of priapism forms.

although it is suspected that future scientific investigations of idiopathic presentations will eventually reveal their etiopathogenic sources. Disease associations are additionally relevant for discerning the epidemiology of priapism. A major at-risk population for the disorder consists of individuals with sickle cell disease or other hematologic and coagulative dyscrasias, including thrombophilia and thalassemia. Cohort studies of these populations assign the lifetime probability of developing priapism to be between 29% and 42%.[7–10] Men with ED receiving vasoactive pharmacotherapies also comprise a major at-risk population, and high rates of priapism occurrences have historically coincided with the clinical introduction of these therapies.

PATHOLOGIC BASIS OF DISEASE

Advances in the clinical management of priapism, as for any medical disorder, derive practically from a solid core of knowledge of its pathogenesis. Study of the dynamics and mechanisms of disease involved in priapism conceivably assures the identification of biologic targets toward which therapeutic objectives for the disorder are aimed. Approaches to this investigation include clinical and basic scientific research work.

Clinicopathologic Observations

The natural course of priapism varies, although characteristic clinical patterns and outcomes of the disorder are commonly recognized. The disorder may occur briefly and abate in some individuals with little apparent adverse health consequence, although in others it persists for long durations with major clinicopathologic significance. Two standard forms of priapism are recognized, and this division offers a useful classification system for the disorder. Ischemic priapism, also termed venoocclusive or low-flow priapism, characteristically features absent intracorporal blood flow. This form of priapism represents an actual compartment syndrome localized to the corpora cavernosa and is associated with penile rigidity and pain. Nonischemic priapism, also termed arterial or high-flow priapism, features increased vascular flow within the corpora cavernosa without rendering a compartment syndrome effect. This classification system is also relevant to clinical management. Accordingly, ischemic priapism, which occurs more commonly, represents a medically emergent condition and prompts immediate clinical action, whereas nonischemic priapism, occurring less commonly, can be managed nonemergently.

A major episode of ischemic priapism is generally defined if it has been present for more than a few hours; if it is not treated promptly, pathologic changes of the erectile tissue can be expected, resulting from the prolonged ischemic conditions. Priapism recurrences, in which repeated prolonged erectile events occur but characteristically last less than 3 hours and spontaneously remit, are also observed.[7,8,10,11] These recurrent episodes, often termed stuttering attacks, also are ischemic in quality. A frequent clinical pattern of priapism is the display of recurrences as short-lived episodes that, in time, progress in duration before a major episode occurs. Whether major or recurrent, ischemic priapism implies a risk for development of metabolic derangements in the penis caused by lack of intracorporal circulation. At 4 hours of ischemia, significant acidosis and glucopenia develop in the penis, and thereafter erectile tissue reactivity begins to become irreversibly impaired.[12–16] Nonischemic priapism follows a distinct natural course that either resolves spontaneously or persists without resolution for extended durations. It also differs pathologically from its ischemic counterpart by maintaining normoxic, metabolically intact intracorporal circulation.

Genital complications of ischemic priapism occur both structurally and functionally. Tissue edema with cellular loss is observed within the penis after several hours of unrelieved ischemia.[17] Penile tissue necrosis and progressive fibrosis represent end-stage pathologic changes.[18] The gross pathologic feature of this course is penile disfigurement, with morphologic defects that range from megalophallic deformity to major penile tissue destruction and sloughing.[19,20] These changes are responsible for loss of erectile function, directly because of the inability of the penis to achieve physiologic blood engorgement. Complete ED rates of 30% to 90% are documented in men who have experienced major ischemic priapism episodes.[2,10,21] As much as a 25% ED rate has been reported in men sustaining recurrent ischemic priapism.[10] Although it is generally believed that individuals with nonischemic priapism escape pathologic effects of the penis that reduce erectile ability, descriptions of ED have been documented for this group.[22] Penile tissue damage associated with the traumatic development of this form of priapism may explain this phenomenon.

Besides its physical complications, the adverse effects of priapism extend to psychosocial and relational realms. Psychological study of the effect of priapism on patients with sickle cell disease has shown its association with despair, embarrassment, and isolation (lack of relationships) as significant health burdens.[23]

Pathophysiology

The pathophysiologic description of priapism has undergone considerable evolution in recent years. Early study of priapism established the features of vascular stasis within the penis and decreased venous outflow from the organ, which correlated with the finding of dark and viscous blood that is surgically drained from the priapic penis.[18] These observations contributed to notions of the ischemic nature of priapism and supported the early hypothesis that penile congestion explained the disorder. This early way of thinking specified the pathophysiology to be that of obstructive processes interfering with penile rheology, a concept modeled by priapism associated with sickle cell disease, in which misshapen erythrocytes were conceived to impede intracorporal blood flow.[18,24] The causative basis of sickle cell disease–associated priapism, as well as that likely involved in other hematologic dyscrasias, is now suggested to be more scientifically complex than solely a matter of obstructive intravascular phenomena (as described later). The phenomena of venous congestion and heightened blood viscosity within the penis may well be contributive or otherwise simply an effect of the pathophysiologic condition, rather than representing its true cause. However, it remains plausible that mechanical obstruction of blood flow in the penis leading to priapism is causative in some instances of the disorder, such as local primary or metastatic neoplasms involving the penis.

The pathophysiology of nonischemic priapism is characterized as having a traumatic basis. The mechanism fundamentally involves excessive arterial inflow to the penis, resulting from structural damage of its arterial circulation.[22,25,26] Physical trauma to the penis classically involves a straddle injury to the perineum, although other forms of genital trauma, including needle lacerations associated with intracavernosal pharmacotherapy for ED, have also been described.[27] The pathognomonic feature of this form of priapism is the formation of a fistula between the cavernosal artery and lacunar spaces of the cavernous tissue. This defect then allows blood to bypass the helicine arteriolar bed, which regularly serves as a vascular resistance mechanism in the penis. A nonischemic priapism variant is recognized in which a high-flow hemodynamic state of the cavernosal arteries exists in the absence of fistula formation.[28,29] This variant commonly is observed as a refractory presentation of priapism after medical or surgical treatment of ischemic priapism, and in similar fashion to the fistula type of nonischemic priapism ostensibly results from cavernosal arterial dysregulated inflow.

Recent discoveries in priapism research suggest that the pathogenesis of ischemic priapism is explained by molecular science and involves altered vascular homeostatic actions in the penis coupled with deficient erection control mechanisms.[30,31] A dysregulatory erection physiology hypothesis equates with the evolution of understanding in this field.[32] The range of dysregulatory erection physiologic mechanisms likely exists at multiple control levels of penile erection, including central and peripheral neurotransmission, paracrine agency within the corporal tissue, as well as the hormonal axis. Major molecular determinants of erection physiology are currently proposed to be principally involved, and recent descriptions have centered on aberrant nitric oxide (NO), RhoA/Rho-kinase and adenosine signaling pathways as primary mechanisms acting at a local penile level.[3] Consistent with other factors contributing to the pathophysiology of the condition, ongoing investigative work has centered on mechanisms of ischemia-reperfusion injury, inflammation and oxidative stress, and tissue fibrosis. Scientific progress in this field exemplifies the rapidly changing molecular science of erection physiology, and, as much as this evolution has led to the introduction of new therapies for ED, similar innovations in molecularly based clinical therapeutics for priapism are anticipated.

CLINICAL MANAGEMENT: CURRENT PRACTICE GUIDELINES
Principles

In the modern era of sexual medicine, the purpose of advancing a standardized approach for the management of priapism has been affirmed.[3,21] Several consensus body efforts have generated practical guidelines for the contemporary evaluation and treatment of the disorder. At present, expert opinion has mainly supported these guidelines, although their direction is also derived from the best available scientific evidence. A fundamental objective of managing priapism is to reduce the extent of physical damage of the penis and erectile loss as well as associated psychosocial complications as much as possible. To this end, appropriate management at a minimum involves the prompt recognition of the disorder and timely initiation of clinical interventions that alleviate recognized dangers such as penile ischemia and anoxia. As scientific progress in the field is further achieved, management objectives should turn to applying preventive or corrective approaches for the disorder that are consistent with maximal preservation of sexual health.[33]

Diagnosis

The physical conspicuousness of the unintentionally erect penis of excessive duration is immediate grounds for making the diagnosis. The evaluation proceeds with the execution of clinical history, physical examination, and other diagnostic procedures to define the clinical presentation and construct a treatment plan. Most importantly, the diagnostic evaluation keys on distinguishing between ischemic and nonischemic priapism because the former represents a urological emergency. Treatment of ischemic priapism may be initiated early based on differentiating clinical features even when confirmatory laboratory and radiologic study results are awaited (**Box 2**).

The clinical history and physical examination are useful to delineate the features of the presentation. The clinical practitioner should query the presence or absence of pain, duration of priapism, role of antecedent factors, prior priapism episodes, use and success of relieving maneuvers or prior clinical treatments, existence of causal conditions including use of any erectogenic therapies by prescription or nonprescription sources, and erectile function status before the priapism episode. The presence of pain generally suggests the likelihood of ischemic priapism. Physical examination should involve both inspection and palpation of the penis, which may be informative with respect to the extent of tumescence or rigidity, corporal body involvement (ie, whether rigidity involves only the corpora cavernosa with a soft glans penis and corpus spongiosum or all 3 corporal bodies), and the presence and extent of tenderness. The corpora cavernosa usually are rigid and tender to palpation as suspected conditions of ischemic priapism. In contrast, the presentation of only tumescent or partially erect, nontender corpora cavernosa is suggestive of nonischemic priapism. Abdominal, perineal, and rectal examinations may reveal signs of trauma or malignancy.

Laboratory testing is incorporated in the diagnostic evaluation and commonly involves several test procedures. Complete blood count, white blood cell differential, and platelet count may reveal the presence of acute infections or hematologic abnormalities. Reticulocyte count and hemoglobin electrophoresis may signify the presence of sickle cell disease or trait or other hemoglobinopathies. These tests are recommended in all men unless another cause of priapism is obvious, acknowledging that hemoglobinopathies are not restricted to men of African American descent and may be found in nonsuspected ethnic groups, including men of Mediterranean ancestry. Other hematologic tests, such as serum lactic dehydrogenase level, a marker of intravascular hemolysis, and glucose-6-phosphate dehydrogenase testing, may also be informative. Urine and plasma toxicology may be performed to screen for the potential pharmacologic influences of psychoactive medications and recreational drugs, particularly if the involvement of these agents is suspected based on clinical history.

Penile diagnostics also serve an important role in the diagnostic evaluation. Initially aspirated blood from the affected corpora yields information both by visual inspection and blood gas testing. The appearance of blood that is darkly colored and evidently hypoxic suggests ischemic priapism; in contrast, its appearance as oxygenated (bright red in color) suggests nonischemic priapism. Blood gas testing offers a direct, quantitative assessment of the extent of cavernous blood oxygenation that would be helpful in assigning the form of priapism. Measurements of hypoxia, hypercarbia, and acidosis suggest the clinical presentation of ischemic priapism, in contrast with those of normal arterial blood observed at room air conditions that suggest the clinical presentation of nonischemic priapism (**Table 1**).

Penile imaging also is applied diagnostically, although it should not delay timely clinical management. Color duplex ultrasonography (CDU) of the penis and perineum is useful to evaluate intracorporal blood flow, and it complements cavernous blood gas testing as a tool to differentiate ischemic from nonischemic priapism. The finding of absent blood flow in the cavernosal arteries of the corpora cavernosa characterizes ischemic priapism. The finding of normal to high

Table 1
Blood gas values

Source	Po$_2$ (mm Hg)	Pco$_2$ (mm Hg)	pH
Normal arterial blood (room air)	>90	<40	7.4
Normal mixed venous blood (room air)	40	50	7.35
Ischemic priapism (first corporal aspirate)	<30	>60	<7.25

Data from Montague DK, Jarow J, Broderick GA, et al. American Urological Association guideline on the management of priapism. J Urol 2003;170:1320.

blood flow velocities in the cavernosal arteries of the corpora cavernosa characterizes nonischemic priapism. CDU may also reveal anatomic abnormalities such as an arteriolar-sinusoidal fistula or pseudoaneurysm, which is diagnostic of nonischemic priapism. CDU may also be advantageously performed to evaluate the effect of treatments for ischemic priapism in the incompletely detumescent penis. In this case, the evaluation may guide further intervention if necessary because of the finding of persistent ischemia, or determine other diagnostic possibilities such as resolved ischemia with penile edema or conversion to high-flow priapism. The study should be done with the patient placed in lithotomy or frog leg position, to scan the perineum first and then the entire penile shaft. This technical aspect acknowledges the possibility that an abnormality could exist in the perineal portion of the corpora cavernosa in conditions of a straddle injury or direct scrotal trauma.

Penile arteriography may be used adjunctively to identify the presence and location of an arteriolar-sinusoidal fistula in the patient suspected to have nonischemic priapism based on initial tests. It has a secondary role in the diagnosis of priapism and is applied commonly only as a part of an embolization procedure. Other radiographic studies, such as penile scintigraphy, cavernosography, and magnetic resonance imaging, also serve secondary roles.

Treatment

Treatment approaches for priapism are practically applied according to diagnostic category, differing in whether the form of priapism is ischemic or nonischemic. Ischemic priapism is straightforwardly managed with the objective of eliminating the ischemic effects of the compartment syndrome involving the penis. For a major episode (ischemic priapism lasting more than 4 hours), initial intervention consists of penile aspiration, and the drainage of blood serves to relieve pain and counteract local acidotic and anoxic metabolic derangements (in addition to providing a sample for cavernous blood gas testing). The technique of penile blood aspiration is variably done and alternatively involves transglanular intracorporal angiocatheter (16 gauge) insertion in the manner of a percutaneous corporoglanular shunt (see later discussion) or proximal penile shaft needle access.[34] This procedure can be extended to include vigorous blood evacuation from the corpora cavernosa with irrigation, possibly in combination with intracavernous injection of an α-adrenergic sympathomimetic agent

(ie, phenylephrine, etilefrine, ephedrine, norepinephrine, metaraminol). A dorsal nerve block or local penile shaft block may precede this more invasive aspect of the procedure as a penile anesthetic maneuver. The pharmacologic component is intended to exploit the potential smooth muscle contractile responsiveness of the cavernosal tissue and facilitate the recovery of basal penile flaccidity. These first-line treatments may be repeated as necessary in accordance with clinician judgment. Priapism resolution following aspiration with or without irrigation is approximately 30%, and after the concomitant use of sympathomimetic agents with or without irrigation it may range up to 80%.[2] In the absence of literature support for applying oral sympathomimetic agents (eg, terbutaline, pseudoephedrine) for major ischemic priapism, these treatments are eschewed in the current guidelines for management of this disorder.[2] The concomitant management of an identified underlying causal condition (eg, analgesia, hydration, oxygenation, alkalinization, and even exchange transfusion for sickle cell disease in association with priapism) has generally been offered, although such medical management should not supplant first-line intracavernous procedures for the treatment of major ischemic priapism.[2,3]

If first-line management for major ischemic priapism fails or is contraindicated (eg, cardiovascular side effects secondary to the use of sympathomimetic medications), definitive surgical management may be appropriately pursued. Second-line intervention generally refers to penile shunt surgery, which describes the surgical creation of a vent for blood egress from the corpora cavernosa. The efficacy of this intervention for recovering erectile function is controversial, and its role for major ischemic priapism of sufficiently long duration (eg, ≥36 hours) may only be to mitigate local pathologic effects. Four subdivisions of shunt procedures are described by various contributors: (1) percutaneous distal (corporoglanular) shunts (ie, Winter[35]; Ebbehoj[36]; Lue[37]); (2) open distal (corporoglanular) shunts (ie, Al-Ghorab[38]; Burnett[39]); (3) open proximal (corporospongiosal) shunts (ie, Quackles[40]; Sacher[41]); and vein anastomoses/shunts (ie, saphenous; [Grayhack[42]]; superficial or deep dorsal vein [Barry[43]]). Surgeon preference and familiarity may dictate the selection of shunt procedure, although conventional practice has shown that distal shunts are typically done first, whereas proximal shunts are performed in situations of distal shunt failures as determined by clinical indicators (ie, clinical assessment, cavernous blood gas testing, penile CDU, or intracavernosal pressure monitoring).[3]

Recent modifications of distal shunt techniques that use intracorporal instrumentation have been shown to be highly effective and safe monotherapies, possibly obviating the need for multimodal intervention.[37,39] Their proposed advantages include a more complete evacuation of stagnant blood from the corporal bodies and thereby better preservation of shunt patency than standard shunting (distally or proximally), application of the anatomically favorable venous drainage system of the glans penis and corpus spongiosum, feasible combination of local penile block anesthesia, and limited complication risks.

Penile prosthesis surgery is also advocated in the management of major ischemic priapism with purposes in various settings. It has been done in the acute setting for priapism relief when the duration of the priapism episode is prolonged (ie, ≥ 72 hours) and it is predictable that complete erection loss will occur irrespective of penile shunting success.[44,45] It may also be done nonacutely to facilitate the resumption of sexual intercourse for the individual whose priapism has resulted in erection loss or significant penile deformity.[46,47] Penile reconstructive approaches, applied many times in the course of penile prosthesis surgery, may also be required to address a complicated deformity or possibly penile tissue loss resulting from major ischemic priapism.[48,49]

Although considered to be distinct from major ischemic priapism, recurrent or stuttering priapism warrants management that also acknowledges the ischemic feature of this clinical presentation. Preventative strategies have been considered for the purpose of limiting priapism recurrences and possibly risks of its evolution into a major episode. Several strategies have been advanced to include systemic therapies (eg, hormonal agents, baclofen, digoxin, terbutaline, phosphodiesterase type 5 [PDE5] inhibitors), intracavernous self-injection of sympathomimetic agents, and penile prosthesis surgery.[3] Most widely used are hormonal treatments (eg, gonadotropin-releasing hormone agonists, androgen receptor antagonists, 5-α-reductase inhibitors), although they carry the potential drawbacks as antiandrogenic agents of negatively affecting sexual function and physical composition.[50] Intracavernously administered sympathomimetic agents also are not ideal, and they require proper instruction and safety precautions.[51] Long-term, low-dose PDE5 inhibitor therapy has shown some success, in accordance with recent scientific evidence showing that ischemic priapism involves aberrant NO signaling in the penis, although practical use of this treatment for this indication is hindered by the requirement for patient adherence to a specific therapeutic regimen.[52] These obstacles suggest that ongoing work is necessary to develop and implement therapy that effectively and uncomplicatedly controls the disorder.

Nonischemic priapism invokes a wholly different approach to management. The generally held primary intervention for this form of priapism is clinical surveillance, in accordance with reports that spontaneous resolution occurs in nearly two-thirds of cases.[2] Alternative interventions, including embolization, in combination with penile arteriography, and surgery (ie, arterial ligation), in combination with intraoperative CDU, offer a more immediate resolution (at a rate that approximates 75%).[2] However, these clearly more invasive options are usually deferred because of their potential complication risks. Most notable among the reported risks is ED, occurring in as much as 50% of procedures, although others include penile gangrene, gluteal ischemia, purulent cavernositis, and perineal abscess.[2,3]

Risk Management

A review of current management in this field should include a discussion of its potential medicolegal challenges, because of the possible adverse sequelae (eg, decreased natural sexual function, psychological distress, loss of sexual relationships) that may arise in the course of this activity. Delayed diagnosis and management, improper diagnosis, and complications from treatment are all possibly hazardous scenarios for clinical practitioners, and the worst outcomes are feared irrespective of clinical intervention because of the disorder's inherent pathologic risks. Several recommendations for clinical practice are offered. Practitioners should be advised to promptly recognize priapism and initiate standard clinical management on its clinical presentation. When instituting procedures to treat the disorder, they should counsel patients that the damage sustained in the course of their management may be a consequence of the priapism and not the intervention, particularly when the presentation to the clinical practitioner is delayed. When instituting procedures to treat ED caused by prior priapism episodes, practitioners should inform patients of the standard risks of ED therapeutic interventions and also the chance that these interventions may provoke a priapism occurrence.

CLINICAL THERAPEUTICS: NEW PROSPECTS

Scientific progress in priapism has moved forward greatly in recent years. At this time, a molecular pathophysiologic basis for many of the clinical presentations of priapism is increasingly appreciated, consistent with the notion that the disorder is explained by derangements in molecular factors that are involved in the regulatory biology or biologic function of the erectile response. Ischemic priapism is the main form of priapism featured in this investigation; the pathogenesis of ischemic priapism is generally well understood and largely relates to mechanical mechanisms affecting intracorporal hemodynamics. The exciting trajectory of this area of investigative work fosters translational opportunities for molecular target–based therapies for the management of priapism that may meet such ideal objectives as prevention or correction. Recurrent ischemic priapism takes central importance for prevention prospects because these presentations often herald subsequent major episodes and their repetitive nature presents opportunities to intervene preventatively. However, with consideration of ischemic priapism in general with a view toward patients with sickle cell disease who are most affected by this disorder, corrective prospects remain purposeful given the high incidence of priapism in this population. It is reasonable to propose the usefulness of a therapy in the future that is administered to all at-risk individuals for priapism to reduce their overall risk of developing priapism.

Current preclinical investigations have suggested the roles of the NO, RhoA/Rho-kinase, and adenosine signaling pathways as primary intracorporal mechanisms for priapism. At the clinical level, PDE5 inhibitor therapy, which is based on aberrant NO function in the penis, has been studied in noncontrolled trials and shown to have preliminary success in the treatment of recurrent ischemic priapism.[52] Further investigation of this therapeutic option in the form of a randomized, placebo-controlled, clinical trial is currently underway in hopes of establishing its true efficacy. Therapeutic proposals stemming from newly described molecular signaling pathways and also past scientific research (eg, oral sympathomimetic agents) warrant similar levels of investigation to support their clinical roles. Other investigative studies (eg, comparator trials for distal shunting techniques, delayed management vs immediate interventions for nonischemic priapism) are also needed to establish an evidence basis for priapism treatments.[3]

HEALTH POLICY

Issues of health administration and policy are considerations in the management of priapism, particularly its ischemic form, which disproportionately affects individuals with sickle cell disease and related hemoglobinopathies. This concern is legitimate given various socioeconomic, behavioral, and cultural factors, all of which negatively affect the acquisition of medical services and therefore the best possible health outcomes for this population. In addition, deficiencies persist in several aspects of medical and research services, ranging from access to resource allocation to quality of care for patients with sickle cell disease, relative to other genetic diseases, and this concern extends to sexual health matters in this population.[33] Priapism may receive less emphasis among health complications of sickle cell disease by health care providers, possibly owing to its taboo subject area and perceptions of its unimpressive health adversity risk. Further efforts initiated at a health care programmatic level will serve a critical purpose to improve the sexual wellness outcomes of individuals affected by priapism, particularly those having sickle cell disease. Such efforts encompass improvement of educational and clinical training programs, support of interdisciplinary health care delivery services, diffusion of clinical advances, promotion of best practice guidelines, and expansion of governmental and private foundation funding for facilitating scientific advancements.

SUMMARY

Priapism holds a rightful place in the modern province of sexual medicine, and all clinical practitioners should recognize its importance and be prepared to provide appropriate clinical management for patients afflicted by it. Advances have recently been made in both medical and surgical management, and these offer improvements in the level of care historically afforded such patients. Further developments can be expected in the future based on ongoing progress, particularly in the area of molecular science, which is inarguably the primary source for driving novel therapeutic approaches. Along with focus brought to the scientific and clinical activities of the field, continued action to address the health care administrative concerns of those most commonly affected by priapism, specifically individuals with sickle cell disease, is also appropriate. All successes in these arenas ensure that afflicted individuals avoid the health burdens of priapism and preserve sexual function.

REFERENCES

1. Berger R, Billups K, Brock G, et al. Report of the American Foundation for Urologic Disease (AFUD) Thought Leader Panel for evaluation and treatment

of priapism. Int J Impot Res 2001;13(Suppl 5): S39–43.

2. Montague DK, Jarow J, Broderick GA, et al. American Urological Association guideline on the management of priapism. J Urol 2003;170:1318–24.

3. Broderick GA, Kadioglu A, Bivalacqua TJ, et al. Priapism: pathogenesis, epidemiology, and management. J Sex Med 2010;7:476–500.

4. Monllor J, Taño F, Arteaga PR, et al. Priapism of the clitoris. Eur Urol 1996;30:521–2.

5. Hashmat AI, Raju S, Singh I, et al. 99mTc penile scan: an investigative modality in priapism. Urol Radiol 1989;11:58–60.

6. Sharpsteen JR Jr, Powars D, Johnson C, et al. Multisystem damage associated with tricorporal priapism in sickle cell disease. Am J Med 1993;94:289–95.

7. Emond AM, Holman R, Hayes RJ, et al. Priapism and impotence in homozygous sickle cell disease. Arch Intern Med 1980;140:1434–7.

8. Fowler JE Jr, Koshy M, Strub M, et al. Priapism associated with the sickle cell hemoglobinopathies: prevalence, natural history and sequelae. J Urol 1991;145:65–8.

9. Mantadakis E, Cavender JD, Rogers ZR, et al. Prevalence of priapism in children and adolescents with sickle cell anemia. J Pediatr Hematol Oncol 1999;21:518–22.

10. Adeyoju AB, Olujohungbe AB, Morris J, et al. Priapism in sickle-cell disease; incidence, risk factors and complications-an international multicentre study. BJU Int 2002;90:898–902.

11. Sergeant GR, de Ceulaer K, Maude GH. Stilboestrol and stuttering priapism in homozygous sickle-cell disease. Lancet 1985;2:1274–6.

12. Kim NN, Kim JJ, Hypolite J, et al. Altered contractility of rabbit penile corpus cavernosum smooth muscle by hypoxia. J Urol 1996;155:772–8.

13. Broderick GA, Harkaway R. Pharmacologic erection: time-dependent changes in the corporal environment. Int J Impot Res 1994;6:9–16.

14. Saenz de Tejada I, Kim NN, Daley JT, et al. Acidosis impairs rabbit trabecular smooth muscle contractility. J Urol 1997;157:722–6.

15. Moon DG, Lee DS, Kim JJ. Altered contractile response of penis under hypoxia with metabolic acidosis. Int J Impot Res 1999;11:265–71.

16. Liu SP, Mogavero LJ, Levin RM. Correlation of calcium-activated ATPase activity, lipid peroxidation, and the contractile response of rabbit corporal smooth muscle treated with in vitro ischemia. Gen Pharmacol 1999;32:345–9.

17. Spycher MA, Hauri D. The ultrastructure of the erectile tissue in priapism. J Urol 1986;135:142–7.

18. Hinman F Jr. Priapism; reasons for failure of therapy. J Urol 1960;83:420–8.

19. Datta NS. Megalophallus in sickle cell disease. J Urol 1977;117:672–3.

20. Burnett AL, Allen RP, Tempany CM, et al. Evaluation of erectile function in men with sickle cell disease. Urology 1995;45:657–63.

21. Pryor J, Akkus E, Alter G, et al. Priapism. J Sex Med 2004;1:116–20.

22. Brock G, Breza J, Lue TF, et al. High flow priapism: a spectrum of disease. J Urol 1993;150:968–71.

23. Addis G, Spector R, Shaw E, et al. The physical, social and psychological impact of priapism on adult males with sickle cell disorder. Chronic Illn 2007;3:145–54.

24. Winter CC, McDowell G. Experience with 105 patients with priapism: update review of all aspects. J Urol 1988;140:980–3.

25. Hauri D, Spycher M, Brühlmann W. Erection and priapism: a new physiopathological concept. Urol Int 1983;38:138–45.

26. Hakim LS, Kulaksizoglu H, Mulligan R, et al. Evolving concepts in the diagnosis and treatment of arterial high flow priapism. J Urol 1996;155:541–8.

27. Witt MA, Goldstein I, Saenz de Tejada I, et al. Traumatic laceration of intracavernosal arteries: the pathophysiology of nonischemic, high flow, arterial priapism. J Urol 1990;143:129–32.

28. Seftel AD, Haas CA, Brown SL, et al. High flow priapism complicating veno-occlusive priapism: pathophysiology of recurrent idiopathic priapism? J Urol 1998;159:1300–1.

29. Rodriguez J, Cuadrado JM, Frances A, et al. High-flow priapism as a complication of a veno-occlusive priapism: two case reports. Int J Impot Res 2006;18:215–7.

30. Bivalacqua TJ, Burnett AL. Priapism: new concepts in the pathophysiology and new treatment strategies. Curr Urol Rep 2006;7:497–502.

31. Burnett AL, Musicki B, Bivalacqua TJ. Molecular science of priapism. Curr Sex Health Rep 2007;4:9–14.

32. Burnett AL. Pathophysiology of priapism: dysregulatory erection physiology thesis. J Urol 2003;170:26–34.

33. Burnett AL. Sexual health outcomes improvement in sickle cell disease: a matter of health policy? J Sex Med, in press.

34. Chung SY, Stein RJ, Cannon TW, et al. Novel technique in the management of low flow priapism. J Urol 2003;170:1952.

35. Winter CC. Cure of idiopathic priapism: new procedure for creating fistula between glans penis corpora cavernosa. Urology 1976;8:389–91.

36. Ebbehoj J. A new operation for priapism. Scand J Plast Reconstr Surg 1974;8:241–2.

37. Brant WO, Garcia MM, Bella AJ, et al. T-shaped shunt and intracavernous tunneling for prolonged ischemic priapism. J Urol 2009;181:1699–705.

38. Hanafy HM, Saad SM, El-Rifaie M, et al. Early Arabian medicine: contribution to urology. Urology 1976;8:63–7.

39. Burnett AL, Pierorazio PM. Corporal "snake" maneuver: corporoglanular shunt surgical modification for ischemic priapism. J Sex Med 2009;6: 1171–6.

40. Quackels R. Treatment of a case of priapism by cavernospongious anastomosis. Acta Urol Belg 1964; 32:5–13.

41. Sacher EC, Sayegh E, Frensilli F, et al. Cavernospongiosum shunt in the treatment of priapism. J Urol 1972;108:97–100.

42. Grayhack JT, McCullough W, O'Conor VJ Jr, et al. Venous bypass to control priapism. Invest Urol 1964;1:509–13.

43. Barry JM. Priapism: treatment with corpus cavernosum to dorsal vein of penis shunts. J Urol 1976;116: 754–6.

44. Upadhyay J, Shekarriz B, Dhabuwala CB. Penile implant for intractable priapism associated with sickle cell disease. Urology 1998;51:638–9.

45. Ralph DJ, Garaffa G, Muneer A, et al. The immediate insertion of a penile prosthesis for acute ischemic priapism. Eur Urol 2009;56:1033–8.

46. Bertram RA, Carson CC 3rd, Webster GD. Implantation of penile prostheses in patients impotent after priapism. Urology 1985;26:325–7.

47. Douglas L, Fletcher H, Serjeant GR. Penile prostheses in the management of impotence in sickle cell disease. Br J Urol 1990;65:533–5.

48. Monga M, Broderick GA, Hellstrom WJ. Priapism in sickle cell disease: the case for early implantation of the penile prosthesis. Eur Urol 1996;30:54–9.

49. Montague DK, Angermeier KW. Corporeal excavation: new technique for penile prosthesis implantation in men with severe corporeal fibrosis. Urology 2006;67:1072–5.

50. Dahm P, Rao DS, Donatucci CF. Antiandrogens in the treatment of priapism. Urology 2002;59:138.

51. van Driel MF, Joosten EA, Mensink HJ. Intracorporeal self-injection with epinephrine as treatment for idiopathic recurrent priapism. Eur Urol 1990;17:95–6.

52. Burnett AL, Bivalacqua TJ, Champion HC, et al. Feasibility of the use of phosphodiesterase type 5 inhibitors in a pharmacologic prevention program for recurrent priapism. J Sex Med 2006;3:1077–84.

Peyronie's Disease: Review of Nonsurgical Treatment Options

Stephen M. Larsen, MD, Laurence A. Levine, MD*

KEYWORDS

- Peyronie's disease • Traction • Intralesional injection
- Oral therapy • Nonsurgical

In 1743 Francois de la Peyronie described and was the first to offer treatment for *induration penis plastica,* which subsequently became known as Peyronie's disease (PD).[1] PD is most simply referred to as a fibrotic wound-healing disorder of the tunica albuginea. It is both a physically and psychologically devastating disorder that causes penile deformity, curvature, hinging, narrowing, shortening, and painful erections. Despite a myriad of treatment options, PD remains a considerable therapeutic dilemma because of the paucity of randomized, placebo-controlled trials. The number of medical treatments and arguably their efficacy likely relates to the fact that the true etiopathophysiology of PD and the mechanism of plaque formation are largely unknown. One paradigm is that PD is a disorder in which genetically susceptible individuals experience a localized response to endogenous factors, such as transforming growth factor (TGF)-beta, which are released in response to repeated microtrauma. This response can lead to biologic transformation of cells within the tunica albuginea; cell-cycle dysregulation; genotypic changes; and increased expression of cytokines and free radicals that can lead to unregulated extracellular matrix deposition, including fibronectin and collagen, and ultimately plaque formation, which does not appear to undergo proper scar remodeling, leaving an inelastic segment in the involved tunica albuginea.[2–8] Del Carlo and colleagues[9] investigated the role of matrix metalloproteinases (MMP), the major identified antifibrotic enzymes, and tissue inhibitors of matrix metalloproteinases (TIMP) in the pathogenesis of PD using harvested plaque from human subjects with PD. PD tissue samples were found to have reduced or absent levels of MMP 1, 8, and 13 when compared with subject-matched perilesional tunica. PD fibroblasts were then cultured with soluble MMP and TIMP after treatment with either TGF-1 or interleukin (IL)-1. They found that IL-1 stimulation increased the production of MMP 1, 2, 8, 9, 10, and 13 in PD fibroblasts; whereas, TGF-1 increased the production of only MMP 10 and decreased the production of MMP-13, but markedly increased the production of all TIMPs. These findings suggest that PD fibroblasts may be manipulated to encourage scar remodeling in the final phase of wound healing.

NONSURGICAL THERAPY FOR PD

Several nonsurgical options are currently being employed in the treatment of PD that may reduce or stabilize objective measures, such as penile curvature, and also improve subjective measures, such sexual function, pain, and partner satisfaction. PD data outcomes are difficult to interpret without a validated questionnaire and this is further complicated by a reported spontaneous improvement rate of 13% to 39%.[10–13] A review of the

Larsen has nothing to disclose.

Disclosures: Auxilium consultant, investigator, speaker; AMS consultant, speaker; Coloplast consultant, speaker; US Physiomed consultant; Pfizer consultant; Slate pharmaceutical consultant (L.A.L).

Department of Urology, Rush University Medical Center, 1725 West Harrison Street, Suite 352, Chicago, IL 60612, USA

* Corresponding author.

E-mail address: drlevine@hotmail.com

Urol Clin N Am 38 (2011) 195–205

doi:10.1016/j.ucl.2011.02.006

latest literature on nonsurgical options, including oral, topical, intralesional, and external energy, is presented. For further review of PD, the reader is directed to such articles by Akin-olgubade, Trost, and Taylor.[14–16] The purpose of this article is to review the contemporary literature on nonsurgical therapies for PD, and where possible, focus on randomized, placebo-controlled trials. The recently published guidelines on PD treatment by the International Consultation on Sexual Medicine (ICSM) are noted[17] along with the authors' expert opinion.

ORAL THERAPIES
Vitamin E

Vitamin E is one of the oldest described oral treatments for the treatment of PD and there does appear to be a biochemical mechanism to support its use.[18] Vitamin E, a fat-soluble vitamin metabolized in the liver, excreted in bile is an antioxidant that is thought to limit oxidative stress of reactive oxygen species (ROS) known to be increased during the acute and proliferative phases of wound healing.[19] Increased free-radical expression and a prolonged inflammatory phase of wound healing has been demonstrated in PD.[4,19] In 1983, Pryor and colleagues[20] conducted a double-blind, placebo-controlled crossover study evaluating vitamin E for the treatment of PD in 40 subjects. No significant improvements were noted in plaque size or penile curvature. Gelbard and colleagues[12] compared vitamin E therapy to the natural history of PD in 97 subjects with disease duration ranging from 3 months to 8 years; no significant differences were found between the 2 groups in terms of curvature, pain, or the ability to have intercourse. In 2007, Safarinejad and colleagues[21] compared the effects of vitamin E to L-carnitine, separately or in combination to placebo, and found no significant difference in the improvement in pain, curvature, or plaque size. The study involved 236 subjects with early chronic PD, which was defined as pain during erection, penile curvature not interfering with vaginal penetration, palpable scar that is not painful, hyperechoic lesions, plaque total area less than 2 cm^2 and without calcification. Subjects had received 2 or more previous treatments for PD, including potassium aminobenzoate, tamoxifen, colchicine, systemic steroids, and intralesional verapamil. To date no placebo-controlled trials using vitamin E have demonstrated any clinical benefit in the treatment of PD. Because there is evidence that vitamin E may also increase the risk of cerebrovascular events[22] and no evidence of clinical improvement,

the authors do not recommend the use of vitamin E for PD.

Colchicine

Colchicine inhibits fibrosis and collagen deposition primarily by inhibiting neutrophil microtubules.[23] Colchicine has been used both as a primary oral therapy for PD as well as in combination with other modalities. Akkus and colleagues[24] administered an escalating dose of colchicine in a nonrandomized, nonplacebo-controlled fashion to 19 subjects with PD over a 3- to 5-month period. Of these subjects, 36% noted a reduction in curvature and 63% reported an improvement in the palpable plaque. Of the subjects that were experiencing painful erections at the time of treatment initiation, 78% had resolution of this symptom. Kadioglu and colleagues[25] treated 60 subjects in the acute phase of PD (mean duration 5.7 months $\pm$ 4.3 months) using 1 mg of colchicine twice daily, with a mean follow-up of 11 months. They found significant improvement of pain in 95% of men. However, 30% of subjects reported improved curvature; whereas, 22% of subjects reported worsened curvature. Safarinejad performed a randomized, placebo-controlled trial of colchicine in 2004 with 84 men with PD.[26] Mean disease duration was 15 months (range 6–42 months) and 73.8% had previously received 1 or more treatments for PD, including potassium aminobenzoate, vitamin E, and tamoxifen, which had no effect. It was demonstrated that colchicine was no better than placebo in improving pain, curvature, or plaque size as measured by ultrasound. This trial is the only randomized trial looking at the effects of colchicine as a monotherapy. Because of the lack of demonstrable efficacy and a significant side-effect profile (gastrointestinal distress, diarrhea, aplastic anemia) colchicine is currently not recommended by the authors as therapy for PD.

Potassium Aminobenzoate (Potaba)

Zarafonetis and Horrax[27] were the first to describe the use of potassium aminobenzoate (Potaba) for the treatment of PD. It appears to have both an anti-inflammatory and an antifibrotic effect caused by stabilization of the tissue serotonin-monoamine oxidase activity and a direct inhibitory effect on fibroblast glycosaminoglycan secretion.[27,28] In 1999, Weidner and colleagues[29] published a randomized, placebo-controlled trial of potassium aminobenzoate. Subjects were given 3 g orally 4 times per day for 1 year. A significant reduction in plaque size was demonstrated in the treatment group. This finding, however, was not correlated with a decrease in penile curvature. A 2005 follow-up study also by Weidner and colleagues[30] included 103 subjects with disease duration of no greater than 12 months. Subjects were therapy naïve and could not have calcified plaques. This trial was randomized, double-blind, and placebo-controlled, and showed that the use of potassium aminobenzoate may protect against the progression of penile curvature. The study also suggested that penile deviation may be prevented with the use of potassium aminobenzoate in patients with Peyronie's plaque without penile deviation. In the 13 subjects with an initial straight penis, no subjects developed a deviation while taking potassium para-aminobenzoate. However, 6 of 8 subjects (75%) receiving placebo developed a new penile curvature. There were no relevant differences between potassium aminobenzoate and placebo with regard to improvement of preexisting penile deviation. The authors do not support the use of potassium aminobenzoate as a result of its limited evidence of benefit, side-effect profile, and inconvenient administration (24 tabs/d).

Tamoxifen Citrate

Tamoxifen is a selective estrogen receptor modulator that has both agonist and antagonist effects on target tissues depending on tissue-specific estrogen receptor expression. In addition, tamoxifen is reported to affect the release of TGF from fibroblasts, and blocks TGF-receptors, thus potentially reducing fibrogenesis.[31,32] A study in 1999 by Teloken and colleagues[33] failed to show any statistically significant difference between tamoxifen and placebo. This study included 25 subjects who were given tamoxifen 20 mg twice daily for 3 months. There was no demonstrable improvement in pain, curvature, or plaque size. Thus, again, the authors do not recommend the use of tamoxifen for the treatment of PD.

Carnitine

Carnitine is a naturally occurring metabolic intermediate. Carnitine facilitates the entry of long-chain fatty acids into muscle mitochondria, which are then used as an energy substrate. Carnitine is hypothesized to inhibit acetyl coenzyme-A, which may help in the repair of damaged cells.[34] Safarinejad and colleagues,[21] in a double-blind, placebo-controlled trial compared L-carnitine, L-carnitine plus vitamin E, and vitamin E alone with placebo. A total of 236 men with PD were randomized amongst the 4 groups for a total of 6 months. The study failed to demonstrate improvement in pain, curvature, or plaque size.

Pentoxifylline

Pentoxifylline (PTX) has been shown in vitro to attenuate both collagen fiber deposition and elastogenesis through an alpha 1 antitrypsin-related mechanism in normal tunica albuginea-derived fibroblasts exposed to TGF-β1 suggesting a possible role for pentoxifylline in the management of PD.[35,36] PTX is a nonspecific phosphodiesterase inhibitor, with combined anti-inflammatory and antifibrogenic properties by downregulating TGF-β and increasing fibrinolytic activity. In the only double-blind placebo-controlled study of the efficacy and safety of pentoxifylline, 228 subjects with early chronic PD, Safarinejad and colleagues[37] demonstrated improvement in penile curvature and plaque volume when compared with placebo. The study population was comprised mostly of subjects who had failed previous oral therapies, including potassium aminobenzoate, carnitine, colchicine, tamoxifen, and vitamin E, or combination thereof. When treated with pentoxifylline, ventral, dorsal, and lateral curvature decreased by 40.0%, 22.2%, and 20.0%, respectively. Curvature was measured using dynamic penile duplex ultrasound (DUS) before and after an intracavernous injection with 20 μg of prostaglandin E1. A second injection was administered as necessary to achieve a maximum erectile response. Within the placebo group, ventral, dorsal, and lateral curvature was shown to increase by 26.9%, 31.4%, and 22.2%, respectively. Treatment satisfaction was assessed using the Erectile Dysfunction Inventory of Treatment Satisfaction (EDITS) questionnaire developed by Althof and colleagues.[38] Mean EDITS scores after 6 months of treatment were significantly higher when compared with placebo, 64.2 versus 38.3, respectively. Subjects in the treatment group experienced significantly more nausea, vomiting, dyspepsia, and diarrhea.[37] Because this is a single-center study, further randomized, placebo-controlled trials are necessary to optimize treatment regimens and confirm these results. In the authors' own extensive yet nonrandomized evaluation of pentoxifylline, subjective and objective improvement is limited.

Overall, there appears to be no oral therapy that has been shown to reliably reduce penile deformity in a clinically meaningful way. The authors agree with the recently published guidelines on PD by Ralph and colleagues,[17] which states that, "There is evidence that there is no benefit with respect to deformity reduction with any oral therapy, including vitamin E, potassium aminobenzoate, colchicine, tamoxifen, and carnitine." Refer to **Table 1** for a summary of oral treatments for PD.

Table 1
Oral therapies

Treatment	Mechanism of Action	Clinical Benefit	Side Effects	ICSM Guidelines[17]
Vitamin E	Antioxidant limits oxidative stress of ROS shown to be increased in PD	No benefit	Possible cerebrovascular events, nausea, vomiting, diarrhea, headache, dizziness	No benefit with respect to deformity
Colchicine	Inhibits fibrosis and collagen deposition primarily by inhibiting neutrophil microtubules	No benefit	Myelosuppression, diarrhea, nausea, vomiting	No benefit with respect to deformity
Potassium aminobenzoate	Stabilizes tissue serotonin monoamine oxidase activity; antifibrotic effect caused by a direct inhibitory effect on fibroblast glycosaminoglycan secretion	Possible scar stabilization	Anorexia, nausea, fever, skin rash, hypoglycemia	No benefit with respect to deformity
Tamoxifen	Affects the release of TGF from fibroblasts and blocks TGF receptors, reducing fibrogenesis	No benefit	Alopecia, retinopathy, thromboembolism, pancytopenia	No benefit with respect to deformity
Carnitine	Attenuate both collagen fiber deposition and elastogenesis	No benefit	Seizure, diarrhea, nausea, stomach cramps, vomiting	No benefit with respect to deformity
Pentoxifylline	Nonspecific phosphodiesterase inhibitor, attenuate both collagen fiber deposition and elastogenesis	One trial demonstrating decrease in curvature	Indigestion, nausea, vomiting, dizziness, headache, angina, aplastic anemia, leucopenia, thrombocytopenia	Further studies required to confirm findings

INTRALESIONAL THERAPIES
Collagenase

Collagenase is an enzyme that catalyzes the breakdown of collagen, the primary component of the dense, fibrotic PD plaque and, therefore, appears to be a sensible injectable agent to lyse the collagen types I and III found in PD plaques. Gelbard and colleagues[39,40] were the first to study clostridial collagenase in vitro for the treatment of PD in 1982. A double-blind, placebo-controlled trial by Gelbard and colleagues[41] in 1993 composed of 49 men showed a statistically significant improvement in vacuum-induced curvature in the treatment group when compared with placebo; however, maximal improvement ranged from 15° to 20° and was only seen in the subjects with curvature of less than 30° and plaques of less than 2 cm in length. Jordan assessed the efficacy and safety of intralesional clostridial collagenase injection therapy in a noncontrolled trial with 25 men with PD.[42] Mean duration of PD was 39.2 months, average penile deviation was 53°, and no alternative treatment could be used within 1 month before study entry. Subjects were treated with 3 injections of clostridial collagenase 10,000 untis/0.25 mL per injection administered over 7 to 10 days. A repeat treatment (ie, 3 injections of collagenase 10,000 untis/0.25 mL per injection) was administered over 7 to 10 days at 3 months. Angle of deformity was measured under vacuum-induced erection at baseline, 3, 6, and 9 months and demonstrated a positive treatment response as defined by a decrease in curvature of 25% from baseline in 57%. Positive treatment results peaked at 3 months and declined progressively at 9 months. The study investigator attributed this to a loss of successful subjects to follow up, with nonresponders remaining in the study pool. Collagenase therapy was generally safe and well tolerated. Adverse events occurred in 20 (80%) subjects, with edema, penile pain, and ecchymosis as the most common. Currently this agent is in a large scale, multicenter, multination, randomized, placebo-controlled trial,[43] which may become the first US Food and Drug Administration (FDA)-approved treatment for PD.

Calcium Channel Blockers

Verapamil is a calcium channel blocker that in vitro has been shown to inhibit local extracellular matrix production by fibroblasts, reduce fibroblast proliferation, increase local collagenase activity, and alter the cytokine milieu of fibroblasts.[4,44] Levine and colleagues[45] were the first to introduce intralesional verapamil in 1994. This study was the first of 3 published, nonrandomized trials by this group.

The first study evaluated the response to dose escalation for efficacy and toxicity in 14 men. No adverse effects were noted and, subjectively, there was significant improvement in plaque-associated penile narrowing (100%) and curvature (42%). Objectively, a decreased plaque volume of greater than 50% was noted in 30% of the subjects. Plaque softening was noted in all subjects, and 83% noticed that plaque-related changes in erectile function had arrested or improved.[45] The second trial of 38 men demonstrated in subjects with early stage disease defined as PD for less than 1 year, a rapid reduction of pain after a mean of 2.5 injections in 97% of men, improvement in sexual function, reduction in deformity, and a mean reduction of 21° in 65%. In late stage disease, defined as PD for greater than 1 year, intralesional verapamil decreased curvature in 8 men (44%), with a mean reduction in curvature of 23°.[46] The third trial was the largest published single-center study of intralesional verapamil.[47] This was a prospective nonrandomized study of 140 subjects with mean duration of disease of 17.7 months and 77.5% of subjects had received previous therapy, including vitamin E, potassium aminobenzoate, or colchicine. All subjects received a standardized dose of 10 mg verapamil (5 mg/2 mL) diluted to 10 mL total volume with injectable saline. The solution was distributed throughout the plaque. Each set of injections was administered at a prescribed interval of 2 weeks for a total of 12 treatment sessions. Of the subjects who completed therapy, 121 were evaluated with a second duplex ultrasound, which revealed that curvature decreased in 73 (60%, mean decrease in curvature from baseline of 30°, range 5°–90°), increased in 10 (8%, mean increase of 26°, range 5°–45°), and remained unchanged in 38 (31%).[47] In these 3 studies, subjects received 12 biweekly injections over 6 months. The rationale is that scar remodeling occurs at glacial speed. Therefore, repeated treatment over time would encourage better results. This approach is in contradistinction to the study by Bennett and colleagues[48] where 94 subjects received 10 mg of intralesional verapamil biweekly but for only 6 injections over 3 months. The investigators concluded that intralesional verapamil in this regimen resulted in curve improvement in 22%, but 60% showed no disease progression, suggesting a stabilizing effect. This finding is important because those investigators previously reported that 48% of subjects had curvature progression in a natural history observation study.[49] The first randomized, single-blind trial of intralesional verapamil was published in 1998 by Rehman and colleagues.[50] Significant improvements were noted in terms of erection quality and plaque volume. A trend toward improvement in curvature was also noted. Recently nicardipine, a calcium channel blocker, was compared with saline injection as a potential treatment for PD.[51] Soh and colleagues[51] assigned 74 subjects randomly to nicardipine or saline injection. Subjects were administered a total of 6 biweekly injections. Objective outcomes included change in International Index of Erectile Function (IIEF-5) score, an international pain scale, plaque size, and penile curvature as measured by photographs of a pharmacologically induced erection. The study demonstrated significant reduction in IIEF-5 score and in plaque size only in the nicardipine group. Significant improvement in penile curvature was seen in both the nicardipine and saline groups. The article, however, does not provide specific values for degrees or percentage of curve reduction. No severe side effects were observed in the treatment group. In 2009, Shirazi and colleagues[52] performed a randomized, single-blind, placebo-controlled trial comparing intralesional verapamil to saline. The study included 80 subjects who received 10 mg of intralesional verapamil for only 6 biweekly injections. The study failed to demonstrate any significant differences/improvements in penile deformity, pain, plaque softening, or sexual function between the 2 groups.

Although there is limited controlled trial data showing evidence of benefit with intralesional verapamil, the larger scale quasi-experimental design trials show a consistent curvature improvement rate in 50% to 60% of men completing 12 injections, which is supported by the drug's mechanism of action noted in PD derived fibroblasts.

Interferons

Duncan and colleagues[53] reported in 1991 that interferon (IFN) α, β, and γ decrease the rate of proliferation of fibroblasts in Peyronie's plaques in vitro, reduce the production of extracellular collagen, and increase the activity of collagenase. Initial studies performed by Wegner and colleagues[54,55] demonstrated low rates of improvement using IFN-α2b, but a high incidence of side effects, including myalgia and fever. In 2006, Hellstrom and colleagues[56] reported in a multicenter, placebo-controlled trial of 117 men with PD for more than 12 months, who underwent 6 biweekly injections of either IFN-α2b or saline for a total of 12 weeks. Average curvature in the treatment group improved 13° versus 4° in the placebo arm. Pain resolution was noted in 67% of the treatment subjects versus 28% for the placebo. This

trial was the first placebo-controlled trial of intralesional injection therapy for PD, which offered evidence of treatment benefit. Later in 2006, Inal and colleagues[57] compared intralesional IFN-α 2b injections with and without vitamin E versus vitamin E alone in 30 men. Mean duration of disease was 10.8 months (range 6–18), and all subjects were treatment naive before entry into the study. Curvature was measured during duplex ultrasound of a pharmacologically induced erection. The study showed no statistically significant difference in penile curvature when compared with the initial measurements of the individual groups or among the 3 groups.

As with all PD treatment, IFN therapy requires further investigation to define efficacy, dosing regimens, and side-effect profiles. Intralesional therapy with verapamil or interferon appears to make scientific sense but trial outcomes do not suggest a robust, reliable, or consistently effective therapy. However, reduction or stabilization of deformity and improved sexual function can be expected in 50% of men undergoing this option. The ICSM guidelines regarding intralesional therapy states there are, "No objective measures of therapeutic benefit" for intralesional steroids. On collagenase the ICSM guidelines states, "Several small noncontrolled trials showed limited benefit. It is currently being studied in a phase 3 trial." "Verapamil appears to make scientific sense but there are no large scale placebo controlled trials." On IFN, the ICSM guidelines states, "One placebo-controlled trial showed an outcome benefit with interferon over saline."[38] Refer to **Table 2** for a summary on intralesional therapy.

EXTERNAL ENERGY THERAPIES
Penile Electroshock Wave Therapy

Local penile electroshock wave therapy (ESWT) has been suggested to be of benefit for the treatment of PD. Various hypotheses about its mechanism of action exist, including direct damage to the plaque resulting in an inflammatory reaction with increased macrophage activity leading to plaque lysis, improved vascularity resulting in plaque resorption, and the creation of contralateral scarring of the penis resulting in false straightening.[58] Palmieri and colleagues[59] randomized 100 subjects to ESWT or placebo shocks that were delivered via a nonfunctioning transducer. This trial is the only published placebo-controlled trial of ESWT. Four weekly treatments of 2000 shocks were administered to the treatment group. They reported a disappearance of pain in 53% in the treatment group versus 7% in the placebo group. At 24 weeks follow-up there was no significant

Table 2
Intralesional therapies

Treatment	Mechanism	Clinical Benefit	Side Effects	ICSM Guidelines[17]
Collagenase	Lyses collagen, the primary component of PD plaques	25% reduced curvature in 57%, currently large-scale trial ongoing	Penile pain, swelling, contusions, ecchymoses	Several small, noncontrolled trials showed limited benefit
Verapamil	Inhibits local extracellular matrix production, reduces fibroblast proliferation, increases local collagenase activity	Improvement in curvature in 50%–60%, improvement in pain, prevent disease progression	Nausea, lightheadedness, penile pain, ecchymoses, no cardiovascular events	Appears to make scientific sense but no large-scale, placebo-controlled trials
Nicardipine	Ca^{2+} channel blocker, mechanism likely similar to verapamil	Improvement in IIEF scores, reduction in curvature, although no specific values	Headache, no hypotension or cardiovascular events	No guidelines
Interferons	Decrease fibroblast proliferation in vitro, reduce extracellular matrix production, and increase collagenase	Some improvement in pain and curvature when compared with saline	Myalgia, flulike symptoms, fever	One placebo-controlled trial showed an outcome benefit with interferon over saline

difference in plaque size or curvature in the ESWT group, but the placebo group showed a statistically significant increase in both plaque size and curvature. The study authors concluded that ESWT appears to stabilize deformity progression. However, the differences between the 2 treatment arms of 2° to 4° do not appear clinically significant. Hauck and colleagues[60] randomized 43 men to ESWT or oral placebo for 6 months. No significant effect was noted in terms of curvature, plaque size, or subjective improvement in sexual function or rigidity. The authors do not support ESWT for PD as studies have not shown reliable clinical benefit. Furthermore, the ICSM guidelines state, "There is evidence that ESWT does not improve PD-related deformity."[38]

Iontophoresis

Iontophoresis involves the transport of ions through tissue by means of an electric current. Stancik and colleagues[61] recently demonstrated the decreased expression of bFGF mRNA and bFGF protein expression in excised Peyronie's plaques after having undergone electromotive drug therapy with dexamethasone, verapamil,

and lidocaine when compared with therapy naïve plaques. This study also showed an overexpression of TGF-β protein and the TGF-β receptor in those treated using electromotive drug therapy. In 2007, Greenfield and colleagues[62] reported in a randomized, double-blind, placebo-controlled trial of 42 men with PD, which compared verapamil to saline, and showed similar measured curve reduction in both groups. The total number of subjects experiencing significant improvement (20° or greater) was 7 subjects (30%) in the treatment group and 4 (21%) in the saline group. Although a greater percent of subjects treated with verapamil had improved curvature, the results were not statistically significant. The investigators concluded that the positive response may be caused by the electric current, which has been noted in other fields, such as dermatology, to induce wound healing.[63] In 2005, Di Stasi and colleagues[64] compared subjects receiving verapamil and dexamethasone using iontophoresis versus 2% lidocaine iontophoresis in a prospective, randomized, placebo-controlled study of 96 subjects. In the treatment group, plaque volume decreased and mean measured erect penile curvature was reduced from 43° to 21° as measured by photographs and duplex ultrasound during full pharmacologically induced erection. No changes were noted in the lidocaine group. The ICSM guidelines state, "Several controlled trials had evidence of reduced deformity following iontophoresis treatment using verapamil and dexamethasone."[38] The authors think that iontophoresis is nontoxic and noninvasive and it may be most beneficial in those with mild to moderate curvature or those with plaque-related pain.

Penile Traction Devices

Placing tissues under tension has been used in several fields, including orthopedics and maxillofacial and plastic surgery. Much work has gone into elucidating the mechanisms through which mechanical strain can yield a biologic response in several nonpenile models, including bone, muscle, and Dupuytren scar. Mechanical stress modulates cell function through a process called mechanotransduction by activating multiple signal transduction pathways via the internal cytoskeleton and extracellular matrix.[65] Several signaling cascades activated by cellular tension activate downstream signaling pathways, such as cyclin D1-mediated cell cycle proliferation,[65] paracrine signaling via FGF and PDGF,[66] and activation of mechanosensitive calcium channels and the IP3/DAG pathway.[67] On a histologic level, tension has been demonstrated to reorient collagen fibrils parallel to the axis of stress.[68,69] On a genetic level, mechanical shear stress has been shown to cause an upregulation of antifibrotic genes.[70] In the first published pilot study on traction therapy for PD, Levine and colleagues[71] evaluated 11 men with PD, 8 had failed nonsurgical treatments. Mean duration of disease was 29 months (range 8–72 months). Penile traction therapy was then initiated with the FastSize Penile Extender (Aliso Viejo,

Table 3
External energy therapies

Treatment	Mechanism	Clinical Benefits	Side Effects	ICSM Guidelines[17]
Penile ESWT	Local inflammatory reaction leading to plaque lysis, improved vascularity, plaque resorption, and contralateral scarring	No reliable benefit	Bruising, skin hemorrhage, hematoma, urethral bleeding	Evidence that ESWT does not improve PD-related deformity
Electromotive drug administration –iontophoresis	Decreased expression of bFGF mRNA and bFGF protein expression in excised Peyronie's plaques, verapamil same mechanism as intralesional	Decreased curvature in mild/moderate curvature, reduction of pain	Mild erythema	Several controlled trials had evidence of reduced deformity following iontophoresis treatment using verapamil and dexamethasone
Penile traction	Tension-induced cellular proliferation, reorientation collagen fibrils, upregulation of antifibrotic genes	Decreased curvature, increased length	Local irritation	Early evidence from 2 small, noncontrolled prospective trials have reported a reduction of deformity and increased penile length

California) for 2 to 8 hours per day for 6 months. Curvature was reduced in all men with a mean reduction of 22° (range 10°–45°). There was an overall mean reduction of curvature of 33% from an average pretreatment and post-treatment curvature from 51° to 34°. The mean IIEF was found to increase from 44.6 to 55.0 and specifically the IIEF-erectile function domain increased from 18.3 to 23.6 for the treatment group. There was no change in penile sensation or new erectile dysfunction in this group. Also, stretched penile length improved in all subjects with an increase in length up to 2.5 cm. Gontero and colleagues[72] also evaluated the efficacy of traction therapy in PD. Fifteen subjects were evaluated for change in curvature as a primary endpoint. Subject population was composed of those with PD for greater than 12 months, curvature less than 50°, and fibrous plaque diagnosed on physical examination or ultrasound. Traction was performed using the Andropenis (Andromedical, Madrid, Spain) penile extender for 5 to 9 h/d for a total of 6 months. Penile curvature decreased in 6 subjects from a mean baseline value of 31° (standard deviation [SD] 1.55) to 27° (SD 2.79) after 6 months of treatment ($P = .059$). Curvature worsened in 1 subject and remained unchanged in 8 subjects. Both studies reported length gain, which is significant in that shortening is a common occurrence in the natural history of PD. In a critical review of these 2 studies, Greenfield[73] described factors that may account for the different results in these 2 studies, including duration of disease, plaque calcification, and methodology of measuring curvature. The ICSM guidelines states, "Early evidence from two small non-controlled prospective trials have reported a reduction of deformity and increased penile length with traction therapy."[38] The primary limitation of traction is that prolonged daily use is necessary to obtain clinical benefit, which may be beyond what some men can or are willing to do. Refer to **Table 3** for a summary of external energy therapies for PD.

SUMMARY

Nonsurgical treatment of PD has come a long way since the time of de la Peyronie. Yet, a reliable and effective treatment still eludes the practicing urologist. At this time, it appears that a combination of oral agents or intralesional injection with traction therapy may provide a synergy between the chemical effects of the drugs and the mechanical effects of traction. Until a reliable treatment emerges, it does appear that some of the nonsurgical treatments discussed can be used to stabilize the scarring process and may result in some reduction of

deformity with improved sexual function. This treatment seems appropriate given the low adverse event profiles and the risk of more advanced deformity when no treatment is offered.

REFERENCES

1. de la Peyronie F. Sur quelques obstacles qui s'opposent a l'ejaculation naturelle de la semence. Mem Acad Royale Chir 1743;1:337–42.
2. El-Sakka AI, Hassoba HM, Chui RM, et al. An animal model of Peyronie's like condition associated with an increase of transforming growth factor beta mRNA and protein expression. J Urol 1997;158:2284–90.
3. El-Sakka AI, Hassoba HM, Pillarisetty RJ, et al. Peyronie's disease is associated with an increase in transforming growth factor-beta protein expression. J Urol 1997;158:1391–4.
4. Mulhall JP, Anderson MS, Lubrano T, et al. Peyronie's disease cell culture models: phenotypic, genotypic and functional analyses. Int J Impot Res 2002;14: 397–405.
5. Nachtsheim DA, Rearden A. Peyronie's disease is associated with an HLA class II antigen, HLA-DQ5, implying an autoimmune etiology. J Urol 1996;156: 1330–4.
6. Schiavino D, Sasso F, Nucera E, et al. Immunologic findings in Peyronie's disease: a controlled study. Urology 1997;50:764–8.
7. Cantini LP, Ferrini MG, Vernet D, et al. Profibrotic role of myostatin in Peyronie's disease. J Sex Med 2008; 5:1607–22.
8. Ryu JK, Piao S, Shin HY, et al. IN-1130, a novel transforming growth factor-beta type I receptor kinase (activin receptor-like kinase 5) inhibitor, promotes regression of fibrotic plaque and corrects penile curvature in a rat model of Peyronie's disease. J Sex Med 2009;6:1284–96.
9. Del Carlo M, Cole AA, Levine LA. Differential calcium independent regulation of matrix metalloproteinases and tissue inhibitors of matrix metalloproteinases by interleukin-1beta and transforming growth factor-beta in Peyronie's plaque fibroblasts. J Urol 2008; 179:2447–55.
10. Deveci S, Hopps CV, O'Brien K, et al. Defining the clinical characteristics of Peyronie's disease in young men. J Sex Med 2007;4:485–90.
11. Furlow WL, Swenson HE Jr, Lee RE. Peyronie's disease: a study of its natural history and treatment with orthovoltage radiotherapy. J Urol 1975;114(1): 69–71.
12. Gelbard MK, Dorey F, James K. The natural history of Peyronie's disease. J Urol 1990;144:1376–9.
13. Deveci S, Hopps CV, O'Brien K, et al. A retrospective review of 307 men with Peyronie's disease. J Urol 2002;168:1075–9.

14. Akin-Olugbade Y, Mulhall JP. The medical management of Peyronie's disease. Nat Clin Pract Urol 2007;4(2):95–103.

15. Trost LW, Gur S, Hellstrom WJ. Pharmacological management of Peyronie's disease. Drugs 2007; 67(4):527–45.

16. Taylor FL, Levine LA. Non-surgical therapy of Peyronie's disease. Asian J Androl 2008;10(1):79–87.

17. Ralph D, Gonzalez-Cadavid N, Mirone V, et al. The management of Peyronie's disease: evidence-based 2010 guidelines. J Sex Med 2010;7(7): 2359–74.

18. Scott WW, Scardino PL. A new concept in the treatment of Peyronie's disease. South Med J 1948;41: 173–7.

19. Sikka SC, Hellstrom WJ. Role of oxidative stress and antioxidants in Peyronie's disease. Int J Impot Res 2002;14:353–60.

20. Pryor JP, Farell CF. Controlled clinical trial of Vitamin E in Peyronie's disease. Prog Reprod Biol 1983;9:41–5.

21. Safarinejad MR, Hosseini SY, Kolahi AA. Comparison of vitamin E and propionyl-L-carnitine, separately or in combination, in patients with early chronic Peyronie's disease: a double-blind, placebo controlled, randomized study. J Urol 2007; 178(4 Pt 1):1398–403.

22. Brown BG, Zhao XQ, Chait A, et al. Simvastatin and niacin, antioxidant vitamins, or the combination for the prevention of coronary disease. N Engl J Med 2001;345(22):1583–92.

23. Furst DE, Munster T. Nonsteroidal anti-inflammatory drugs, disease-modifying antirheumatic drugs, nonopioid analgesics & drugs used in gout. In: Bertram G, editor. Basic and clinical pharmacology. New York: Katzung Lange; 2001.

24. Akkus E, Carrier S, Rehman J, et al. Is colchicine effective in Peyronie's disease? A pilot study. Urology 1994;44:291–5.

25. Kadioglu A, Tefekli A, Koksal T, et al. Treatment of Peyronie's disease with oral colchicine: long term results and predictive parameters of successful outcome. Int J Impot Res 2000;12:169–75.

26. Safarinejad MR. Therapeutic effects of colchicine in the management of Peyronie's disease: a randomized double-blind, placebo-controlled study. Int J Impot Res 2004;16:238–43.

27. Zarafonetis CJ, Horrax TM. Treatment of Peyronie's disease with potassium para-aminobenzoate (Potaba). J Urol 1959;81:770–2.

28. Griffiths MR, Priestley GC. A comparison of morphoea and lichen sclerosus et atrophicus in vitro: the effects of para-aminobenzoate on skin fibroblasts. Acta Derm Venereol 1992;72(1):15–8.

29. Weidner W, Schroeder-Printzen I, Rudnick J. Randomized prospective placebo controlled therapy of Peyronie's disease (IPP) with Potaba (aminobenzoate potassium). J Urol 1999;6:205.

30. Weidner W, Hauck EW, Schnitker J, et al. Potassium paraaminobenzoate (Potaba) in the treatment of Peyronie's disease: a prospective, placebo-controlled, randomized study. Eur Urol 2005;47: 530–6.

31. Ralph DJ, Brooks MD, Bottazzo GF, et al. The treatment of Peyronie's disease with tamoxifen. Br J Urol 1992;70:648–51.

32. Colletta AA, Wakefield LM, Howell FV, et al. Anti-oestrogens induce the secretion of active transforming growth factor beta from human fetal fibroblasts. Br J Cancer 1990;62:405–9.

33. Teloken C, Rhoden EL, Grazziotin TM, et al. Tamoxifen versus placebo in the treatment of Peyronie's disease. J Urol 1999;162:2003–5.

34. Biagiotti G, Cavallini G. Acetyl-L-carnitine vs tamoxifen in the oral therapy of Peyronie's disease: a preliminary report. BJU Int 2001;88:63–7.

35. Shindel AW, Lin G, Ning H, et al. Pentoxifylline attenuates transforming growth factor-β1-stimulated collagen deposition and elastogenesis in human tunica albuginea-derived fibroblasts part 1: impact on extracellular matrix. J Sex Med 2010;7(6): 2077–85.

36. Lin G, Shindel AW, Banie L, et al. Pentoxifylline attenuates transforming growth factor-beta1-stimulated elastogenesis in human tunica albuginea-derived fibroblasts part 2: interference in a TGF-beta1/Smad-dependent mechanism and downregulation of AAT1. J Sex Med 2010;7(5):1787–97.

37. Safarinejad MR, Asgari MA, Hosseini SY, et al. A double-blind placebo-controlled study of the efficacy and safety of pentoxifylline in early chronic Peyronie's disease. BJU Int 2010;106(2):240–8.

38. Althof SE, Corty EW, Levine SB. EDITS: development of questionnaires for evaluating satisfaction with treatments for erectile dysfunction. Urology 1999; 53:793–9.

39. Gelbard MK, Walsh R, Kaufman JJ. Collagenase for Peyronie's disease experimental studies. Urol Res 1982;10:135–40.

40. Gelbard MK, Linkner A, Kaufman JJ. The use of collagenase in the treatment of Peyronie's disease. J Urol 1985;134:280–3.

41. Gelbard MK, James K, Riach P, et al. Collagenase vs. placebo in the treatment of Peyronie's disease: a double blind study. J Urol 1993;149:56–8.

42. Jordan GH. The use of intralesional clostridial collagenase injection therapy for Peyronie's disease: a prospective, single-center, non-placebo-controlled study. J Sex Med 2008;5(1):180–7.

43. Glina S, Gelbard MK, Akkus E, et al. The use of collagenase in the treatment of Peyronie's disease M.K. Gelbard, A. Lindner, and J.J. Kaufman. J Sex Med 2007;4(5):1209–13.

44. Roth M, Eickelberg O, Kohler E, et al. Ca2+ channel blockers modulate metabolism of collagens within

the extra-cellular matrix. Proc Natl Acad Sci U S A 1996;93:5478–82.

45. Levine LA, Merrick PF, Lee RC. Intralesional verapamil injection for the treatment of Peyronie's disease. J Urol 1994;151(6):1522–4.

46. Levine LA. Treatment of Peyronie's disease with intralesional verapamil injection. J Urol 1997;158(4): 1395–9.

47. Levine LA, Goldman KE, Greenfield JM. Experience with intraplaque injection of verapamil for Peyronie's disease. J Urol 2002;168(2):621–5.

48. Bennett NE, Guhring P, Mulhall JP. Intralesional verapamil prevents the progression of Peyronie's disease. Urology 2007;69(6):1181–4.

49. Mulhall JP, Schiff J, Guhring P. An analysis of the natural history of Peyronie's disease. J Urol 2006; 175(6):2115–8.

50. Rehman J, Benet A, Melman A. Use of intralesional verapamil to dissolve Peyronie's disease plaque: a long-term single-blind study. Urology 1998;51: 620–6, 69:1181–4.

51. Soh J, Kawauchi A, Kanemitsu N, et al. Nicardipine vs. saline injection as treatment for Peyronie's disease: a prospective, randomized, single-blind trial. J Sex Med 2010;7(11):3743–9.

52. Shirazi M, Haghpanah AR, Badiee M, et al. Effect of intralesional verapamil for treatment of Peyronie's disease: a randomized single-blind, placebo-controlled study. Int Urol Nephrol 2009;41(3):467–71.

53. Duncan MR, Berman B, Nseyo UO. Regulation of the proliferation and biosynthetic activities of cultured human Peyronie's disease fibroblasts by interferons-alpha, -beta and -gamma. Scand J Urol Nephrol 1991;25:89–94.

54. Wegner HE, Andreson R, Knipsel HH, et al. Treatment of Peyronie's disease with local interferon-alpha-2b. Eur Urol 1995;28:236–40.

55. Wegner HE, Andresen R, Knipsel HH, et al. Local inter-feron-alpha 2b is not an effective treatment in early-stage Peyronie's disease. Eur Urol 1997;32: 190–3.

56. Hellstrom WJ, Kendirci M, Matern R, et al. Single-blind, multicenter placebo-controlled parallel study to asses the safety and efficacy of intralesional interferon alpha-2B for minimally invasive treatment for Peyronie's disease. J Urol 2006;176:394–8.

57. Inal T, Tokatli Z, Akand M, et al. Effect of intralesional interferon-alpha 2b combined with oral vitamin E for treatment of early stage Peyronie's disease: a randomized and prospective study. Urology 2006;67:1038.

58. Levine LA. Review of current nonsurgical management of Peyronie's disease. Int J Impot Res 2003; 15:S113–20.

59. Palmieri A, Imbimbo C, Longo N, et al. A first prospective, randomized, double-blind, placebo-controlled clinical trial evaluating extracorporeal shock wave therapy for the treatment of Peyronie's disease. Eur Urol 2009;56(2):363–9.

60. Hauck EW, Altinkilic BM, Ludwig M, et al. Extracorporeal shock wave therapy in the treatment of Peyronie's disease. First results of a case-controlled approach. Eur Urol 2000;38:663–70.

61. Stancik I, Schäfer R, Andrukhova O, et al. Effect of transdermal electromotive drug therapy on fibrogenic cytokine expression in Peyronie's disease. Urology 2009;74(3):566–70.

62. Greenfield JM, Shah SJ, Levine LA. Verapamil versus saline in electromotive drug administration (EDMA) for Peyronie's disease: a double blind, placebo controlled trial. J Urol 2007;177:972–5.

63. Weiss DS, Kirsner R, Eaglestein WH. Electrical stimulation and wound healing. Arch Dermatol 1990; 126(2):222–5.

64. Di Stasi SM, Giannantoni A, Capelli G, et al. Transdermal electromotive administration of verapamil and dexamethasone for Peyronie's disease. BJU Int 2003;91(9):825–9.

65. Alenghat FJ, Ingber DE. Mechanotransduction: all signals point to cytoskeleton, matrix, and integrins. Sci STKE 2002;2002(119):PE6.

66. Alman BA, Naber SP, Terek RM, et al. Platelet-derived growth factor in fibrous musculoskeletal disorders: a study of pathologic tissue sections and in vitro primary cell cultures. J Orthop Res 1995;13(1):67–77.

67. Brighton CT, Fisher JR Jr, Levine SE, et al. The biochemical pathway mediating the proliferative response of bone cells to a mechanical stimulus. J Bone Joint Surg Am 1996;78(9):1337–47.

68. Molea G, Schonauer F, Blasi F. Progressive skin extension: clinical and histological evaluation of a modified procedure using Kirschner wires. Br J Plast Surg 1999;52(3):205–8.

69. Shapiro F. Bone development and its relation to fracture repair. The role of mesenchymal osteoblasts and surface osteoblasts. Eur Cell Mater 2008;15: 53–76.

70. Fong KD, Trindade MC, Wang Z, et al. Microarray analysis of mechanical shear effects on flexor tendon cells. Plast Reconstr Surg 2005;116(5): 1393–404.

71. Levine LA, Newell MM. FastSize Medical Extender for the treatment of Peyronie's disease. Expert Rev Med Devices 2008;5(3):305–10.

72. Gontero P, Di Marco M, Giubilei G, et al. Use of penile extender device in the treatment of penile curvature as a result of Peyronie's disease. Results of a phase II prospective study. J Sex Med 2009; 6(2):558–66.

73. Greenfield JM. Penile traction therapy in Peyronie's disease. F1000 Med Rep 2009;1(pii):37.

Peyronie Disease: Plication or Grafting

Joshua P. Langston, MD*, Culley C. Carson III, MD

KEYWORDS

- Peyronie disease • Plication • Grafting • Penile prosthesis

Peyronie disease (PD) is an incurable, fibrotic disease of the tunica albuginea, which causes penile curvature with a loss of coital function in many patients. Scar-like plaques form between layers of the thick fibroelastic tunica, and currently experts hypothesize that the plaques occur as a result of abnormal wound healing in response to repeated microtrauma and/or more obvious traumatic buckling of the rigid phallus.[1] The reported prevalence of PD ranges from 3.2% to 8.9%, with a mean age of 57.4 years and an incidence that clearly increases with aging.[2,3] Clinically the plaques present with penile curvature, hour-glass deformity, and/or erectile dysfunction (ED) often caused by venoocclusive incompetence, or they may be asymptomatic. Presentation can also include penile pain with erection, inability to have intercourse secondary to penile deformity, and a palpable plaque.

The natural history of PD includes both an active and quiescent phase of the disease. The active, or inflammatory, portion of the disease state is characterized by painful erections, an evolving plaque, and progressive development of penile curvature, and usually lasts 12 to 24 months from the time of onset. Studies have shown that almost all men (94%) will experience resolution of coital pain within 18 months.[3] The quiescent phase is characterized by stability of the penile deformity, resolution of penile pain, and in some, the onset of ED. Both early[4] and more current[5] reports have confirmed that without treatment only 12% to 13% of men will improve, roughly 40% to 48% will worsen, and 40% to 47% will maintain a stable deformity. Given these findings, along with the well-documented psychosocial implications of

the disease, men for hundreds of years have sought treatment for this debilitating condition.

Ultimately, treatment is designed to improve coital function and result in a satisfactory, comfortable erection for both patient and partner. Most patients prefer nonsurgical intervention before proceeding with a surgical procedure. Nonsurgical therapies have included: expectorant, oral medications, intralesional injections, extracorporeal shock-wave therapy, and ultrasound. Treatment efforts began with de la Peyronie's original recommendation to bathe in the warm waters of Barèges in southern France.[6,7] Unfortunately, despite the multitude of modalities that have been tried, current medical therapies have offered limited success in producing tangible results for patients.

SURGERY FOR PEYRONIE DISEASE

Surgery is recommended for patients with stable PD and poor coital function. This poor function may result from the penile curvature, from hourglass deformity resulting in distal flaccidity, or from ED caused by the PD plaque or venoocclusive dysfunction. Surgery is usually avoided during the active phase of the disease, and this provides an opportunity for patients to pursue medical therapies. Montorsi and colleagues[8] recommend waiting at least 12 months from the end of the active phase of PD before considering surgery, suggesting in fact that if surgery is undertaken in men with stable disease of less than 6 months' duration, many will suffer from postoperative recurrence.

The choice of a surgical procedure depends on each patient's needs and preferences. Counseling

Division of Urologic Surgery, Department of Surgery, University of North Carolina, 2113 Physicians Office Building, CB 7235, 170 Manning Drive, Chapel Hill, NC 27599-7235, USA
* Corresponding author.
E-mail address: joshua.langston@unc.edu

Urol Clin N Am 38 (2011) 207–216
doi:10.1016/j.ucl.2011.03.001

and decision making should be based on the patient's current coital function as reported in their history, their deformity on physical examination, and their erectile rigidity. Three surgical categories are used for PD patients (**Fig. 1**),[9] and the evaluation process must identify which surgery will best serve each unique patient. Corporoplasty or plication techniques generally have the best outcomes regarding postoperative sexual satisfaction and erectile function,[10] and are the least invasive approach, but are reserved for patients with adequate erections, simple curvature of 60° or less, and adequate penile length to undergo the additional shortening that may occur with the procedure. Plaque incision/excision and grafting procedures are used for more severe or complex curves, hourglass deformities, and in men who have already suffered significant penile shortening secondary to PD, as these procedures will lengthen the tunica. Inflatable penile prosthesis (IPP) implantation is reserved for men with PD and refractory ED, or men who prefer this method of treatment. Men with satisfactory erectile function with or without supportive medications are candidates for straightening procedures using either tunical lengthening or shortening operations.

EVALUATION OF PATIENTS FOR SURGERY

Key factors in evaluating patients for proper placement in the surgical treatment algorithm are degree and complexity of curve, baseline penile length and percent of estimated loss of length with correction, and baseline erectile function. All

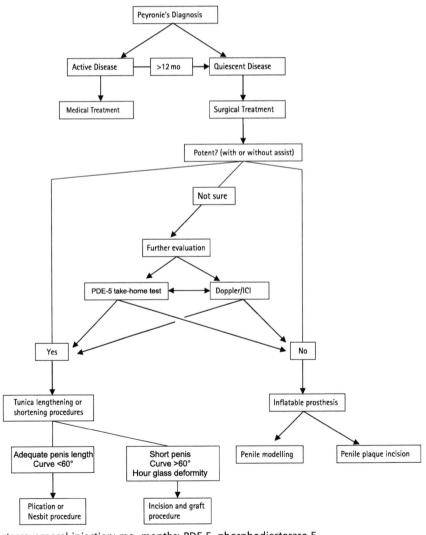

Fig. 1. ICI, intercavernosal injection; mo, months; PDE-5, phosphodiesterase-5.

of these factors are easily evaluated, mostly through physical examination, with the exception of baseline erectile function.

Determining a patient's baseline erectile status is of prime importance in selecting the surgical treatment that will lead to a satisfactory outcome. Potency may be evaluated by sexual history, a phosphodiesterase-5 (PDE-5) inhibitor take-home test, or intercavernosal injection (ICI) ± Doppler ultrasonography (DUS) examination. Because many men with PD have avoided coitus for months to years, they are often uncertain of their potency. Severe curvature may preclude intromission, and patients may not appreciate the quality of their erections or the presence of venoocclusive dysfunction. In these men, a home trial of PDE-5 inhibitors with sexual stimulation and subsequent follow-up history regarding the quality of the erections is helpful in choosing the best surgical procedure. In a report by Mulhall and colleagues,[11] 81% of men who complained of some degree of ED on initial assessment responded to medical therapy with PDE-5 inhibitors or home ICI and were able to avoid implantation of an IPP. When erection quality remains unclear, or ED of some degree is likely, ICI with DUS is helpful in identifying abnormalities in penile hemodynamics, plaque location and size, presence of calcification, and degree of curvature.[12] Others have suggested that subclinical penile abnormalities and aberrant communicating vessels that could contribute to postoperative ED if damaged during surgery are able to be noted on ICI/DUS as well.[8] While dynamic infusion cavernosometry and cavernosography (DICC) has evolved as the gold standard for evaluating penile blood flow, peak-systolic and end-diastolic velocities (PSV and EDV) as well as their resultant resistive index (RI) obtained by DUS have been validated as adjuncts to this time-consuming and cumbersome undertaking.[13,14] A recent article has preliminarily suggested that a RI of less than 0.8 on DUS is predictive of postoperative ED in patients undergoing PD surgery, and thus should be used as the cutoff for recommending IPP rather than corporoplasty or grafting.[15] In any case, severe reduction in blood flow or severe venoocclusive ED should suggest that that prosthesis implantation would be the most successful choice. Digital photography at the time of ICI/DUS can be valuable in determining the severity of PD, planning surgical intervention, and counseling patient and partners as to realistic surgical outcomes.

The importance of proper preoperative assessment of erectile function cannot be overstated. In a recent series, Levine and colleagues[16] reported that among 37 men undergoing grafting

procedures for correction of PD, the only preoperative determinant of postoperative development of frank ED was patient-reported preoperative diminished rigidity. Furthermore, Mulhall and colleagues[11] showed that when grafting was used in patients with preoperative diminished rigidity that was responsive to medical therapy (PDE-5 or ICI with Trimix), overall sexual satisfaction decreased significantly postoperatively, whereas this was not the case with patients who underwent corporoplasty. Thus, baseline erectile function is important not only in the decision to proceed with IPP placement but also in deciding between corporoplasty and grafting.

Tunica-shortening or plication procedures are the least invasive surgically and seem to offer the best results with regard to postoperative ED, but are not advisable for all candidates. Shortening procedures reduce penile length in accordance with the degree of curve being corrected. Therefore, they are only advisable for patients with adequate penile length to undergo additional shortening, and should not be used when the potential loss of length is 20% or more of total penile length.[17] Estimation of the loss of penile length can be made at the time of ICI/DUS by measuring the difference between the concave and convex length of the penis.

Preoperative counseling should include discussions of the patient's and partner's expectations, alternative treatments, and the risks, complications, and potential outcomes of surgery. As discussed by Nelson and colleagues,[18] the significant psychosocial impact of PD leads many men to a depressed state with poor self-image, and thus many will have overly optimistic expectations as to what is attainable with surgical reconstruction. Because of this, the preoperative discussion needs to be frank and include details as to realistic expectations and surgical limitations. Complications, though generally uncommon, should be discussed, and include penile shortening, glans hypoesthesia, ED, recurrence of curvature, hematoma, and graft contraction. Most patients will require the use of PDE-5 inhibitors postoperatively for penile rehabilitation, and this should also be discussed preoperatively.

TUNICA-SHORTENING PROCEDURES (CORPOROPLASTY)
Nesbit and Modified Nesbit

The Nesbit procedure was first described in 1965 for correcting congenital penile curvature caused by corporeal disproportion.[19] Pryor and Fitzpatrick[20] first described the use of the procedure for PD. Plication procedures require that the tunica opposite the Peyronie plaque and penile curvature be excised or plicated, or both, to correct the curvature. After an artificial erection is obtained using injectable saline and the Gittes technique, or with injection of a vasoactive substance into the corpora, an initial circumcising incision is made followed by degloving the penis to the location of the maximal curvature. A ventral penile incision may be used for ventral exposure in very proximal dorsal curvature. Longitudinal penile incisions should be avoided because postoperative scarring can be painful or unsightly, or may even produce further curvature. Buck's fascia is dissected from the tunica albuginea in patients with dorsal curvature, or it is dissected off the dorsal neurovascular bundles for ventral curvature. After induction of an artificial erection, the point of maximal curve is marked on the convex side of the penis. A 5- to 10-mm transverse ellipse of the tunica albuginea may be excised in the classic Nesbit procedure, or approximately 1 mm for each 10° of curvature.

Rehman and colleagues[21] modified this technique by using a partial-thickness shaving of the tunica to avoid possible bleeding and cavernosal injury. Alternatively, a longitudinal incision can be made at the location of the curvature and closed horizontally in the Heinike-Mikulicz fashion.

Next the tunica is closed in a hemostatic horizontal fashion using either running or interrupted locking, nonabsorbable, braided sutures with buried knots. Nonabsorbable sutures are preferred for maintaining correction during healing, as absorbable sutures are more likely to break, causing recurrence of the curvature. Braided sutures result in fewer knot problems beneath penile skin. A circumcision is recommended in men with redundant foreskin, owing to the increased risk for preputial edema, postoperative phimosis, or preputial necrosis. An artificial erection should again be induced after the tunical closure and, if satisfactory straightening has occurred, Buck's fascia and the skin can be closed. If extensive dissection has been required it is the authors' practice to leave a small subcutaneous drain such as the TLS drain (Porex Surgical, Newnan, GA, USA) for 12 to 24 hours to diminish edema. If not adequately straight, subsequent plications or tunical incisions/excisions may be necessary.

A penile block should be administered using long-lasting bupivacaine and a nonpressure dressing and ice pack applied postoperatively. Patients may be discharged home on the same day after this operation. Patients should avoid sexual activity for 6 weeks. The authors' patients are discharged home on 2 weeks of nightly benzodiazepines for suppression of nocturnal erections,

and given amyl nitrate ampoules to be used as needed to suppress additional erections.

Yachia[22] modified the Nesbit procedure by making single or multiple 1- to 1.5-cm incisions longitudinally along the convex side of the tunica, which are subsequently closed horizontally, applying the Heinike-Micwlicz principle. Yachia felt that his modification would reduce injury to the neurovascular bundle and thus reduce glans hypoesthesia, though this known complication is still possible. The authors prefer this approach because tunical deformities and palpable suture lines appear to be fewer. Planning for the tunical incision can be facilitated by placing an Alliss clamp on the tunica to simulate the suture positioning needed to achieve straightening of the penis.

Plication Procedures

Plication of the tunica albuginea is the least invasive technique for correction of PD, and is often performed using only local anesthetic. The predominant techniques used for this include the Lue 16-dot technique, and the tunica albuginea plication (TAP) procedure used by Levine and others. Lue and colleagues[23,24] describe a 16-dot plication method using multiple plication sutures, with a high patient satisfaction rate. Following induction of an artificial erection, a ventral longitudinal or circumcising incision is performed. Longitudinal incisions are reserved for uncircumcised men desiring to keep their foreskin, and are best performed on the ventral aspect of the penis. Buck's fascia is incised medial to the neurovascular bundle, and an intravascular space is developed bluntly between the dorsal vein and arteries with subsequent placement of plication sutures in the developed space in a specific 16-point pattern. For men with a dorsal curvature, a ventral longitudinal incision is made down to Buck's fascia overlying the corpus cavernosum.

After the center-point of the curvature and entry and exit sites for the sutures have been marked, sutures are placed 2 mm lateral to the corpus spongiosum. Two or 3 pairs of 2-0 braided, permanent polyester sutures are placed through the tunica albuginea with 4 entry and exit points per suture. Van der Horst and colleagues[25] found that use of polytetrafluoroethylene sutures resulted in significantly fewer complaints of discomfort by patients than with polypropylene sutures (13% vs 52%) when a similar plication technique was used, whereas Dean and Lue[24] recommend 2-0 braided polyester. The sutures are gradually tied with one surgical knot placed and subsequent clamping. Once all plications are partially tied and clamped, the penis is examined using an artificial erection. If the desired straightening has been achieved the knots are tied and buried, ideally under minimal tension. Buck's fascia is then reapproximated with absorbable suture and the skin is closed. A penile block is administered with bupivacaine, noncompressive dressing and ice pack are applied, and in most cases patients are discharged on the same day.

Gholami and Lue[23] report that 85% of patients maintained a straight erection while 15% suffered slight or severe curve recurrence in a review of 132 patients at a mean follow-up of 2.6 years. Forty-one percent of the patients in their series reported shortening between 0.5 and 1.5 cm, but this caused functional problems in 7% of patients. Twelve percent reported bothersome knots, 11% erectile pain, 9% penile induration, 6% glans hypoesthesia, and 6% worsened ED.

A modification of the original description of plication by Baskin and Duckett[26] was developed and is used by Levine and others. In this technique, parallel incisions each 1.0 to 1.5 cm in length are made in the tunica and then plicated using 2-0 braided polyester suture in a vertical mattress fashion to bury the knot. If the space between the two incisions is too large dog-ear irregularity of the tunica may occur, and it is recommended that the distance be 0.7 to 1.5 cm between the incisions. If the tunica is significantly thick between the incisions, Levine[27] has had success with shaving down the thickness to reduce the bulk of the plicated tissue.

Licht and Lewis[28] compared the Nesbit, modified Nesbit, and tunical incision and grafting procedures, and found the greatest satisfaction (83%) and lowest ED rates (0%) with the modified Nesbit procedure, but this did not include comparison with plication procedures. More recent studies have echoed these findings, showing satisfaction rates of 67% to 100% with rates of complete straightening of 79% to 100%.[20,28–31] Similar rates of satisfaction (78%–83%) and straightening (93%) have been found with the Yachia modification to the Nesbit procedure.[22,32,33]

Despite these high satisfaction and successful straightening rates, penile shortening remains an unwelcome outcome of the Nesbit, modified Nesbit, and other plication procedures. In a study involving 359 men, Pryor and Fitzpatrick[20] reported shortening of less than 1 cm in 86.6% of men, between 1 and 2 cm in 8.6%, and greater than 2 cm in 4.7% of men. Similarly, in another large study of 157 men with PD, Savoca and colleagues[30] reported shortening of less than 1.5 cm in 86% of men and between 1.5 and 3 cm in 14% of men. Pryor and Fitzpatrick[20]

suggest that the degree of penile shortening rarely precludes sexual activity, noting this outcome in only 1.7% of the men in their study. Analysis of other studies shows that the range for reported sexual dysfunction secondary to shortening is 1.3% to 11.9% for the Nesbit and modified Nesbit procedures.[20,28,30,31,33] Greenfield and colleagues[34] analyzed the factors affecting the loss of length in their cohort of 102 patients and found preoperative stretched length and degree of curvature to be predictive of the severity of length lost, with an average length lost of 2.4%.

Results vary for plication procedures, with straightening rates ranging from 58% to 100%.[23,35–39] Chahal and colleagues[36] reported significantly worse outcomes than Gholami and Lue,[23] with 57% of patients reporting deterioration of their quality of life, 55% severe penile shortening, 48% glans hypoesthesia, and 34% bothersome suture knot nodules.

Known complications with these procedures include curve recurrence (7.7%–10.6%), ED (0%–22.9%), penile indurations or narrowing (0%–16.7%), suture granuloma (0%–1.9%), and glans hypoesthesia (0%–21.4%).[20–22,28,30,31,33] Glans hypoesthesia is common postoperatively, though it frequently resolves after several months.

Of note, a new approach to plication has been recently suggested by Dugi and Morey.[40] In their practice they approach all dorsal and lateral plications through a penoscrotal incision, thereby avoiding degloving the penis. Dugi and Morey perform plication using polyester vertical mattress sutures arranged in parallel fashion on the convex side of the penis, and report excellent outcomes, with 93% satisfaction and 2% recurrence in 48 patients. Most notable, however, is their report of no loss of penile length postoperatively, though this measurement was only recorded on the most recent subset of their cohort.

TUNICA-LENGTHENING PROCEDURES

Plaque incision or excision with placement of grafts has been used successfully for patients with severe penile curvature, for complex hourglass deformity, and in men with preoperative significant penile shortening secondary to PD. In 1950, Lowsley and Boyce[41] first reported a series of patients with PD who underwent plaque excision with a fat graft, but there was no follow-up report of success.

Various materials have been used including dermis,[42] temporalis fascia,[43] vein,[44–47] cadaveric and bovine pericardium,[48–50] dura mater,[51] synthetic materials,[28] and porcine small intestine submucosa (SurgiSIS).[52] The ideal graft should be pliable, easy to handle, packaged in various sizes, have good tensile strength, a low inflammatory response, low risk of disease transmission, and low cost.[53]

The authors' group prefers porcine SurgiSIS Biograft (Cook Urological, Spencer, IN, USA). SurgiSIS is processed into a reliably packaged, acellular matrix, consistent in thickness and compliance. Patients should be made aware of the origin and nature of the graft material, and one drawback to the use of SurgiSIS is that some patients may not accept the use of the porcine graft material, on religious grounds. Although some surgeons have had less than satisfactory results, the authors' experience with SurgiSIS has been equivalent to or has exceeded that of other graft materials.[54,55]

Synthetic materials such as Dacron and Gore-Tex may cause severe postoperative inflammation, leading to fibrosis and postcorrection curvature. Licht and Lewis[28] reported poor patient satisfaction with synthetic grafts. Sampaio and colleagues[51] report that 95% of men achieved a straight penis using cadaveric dura mater; however, this material had not been widely accepted because of concerns over prion and slow virus transmission. Although prion transmission and transfer of infection from processed human tissue is exceedingly rare, the media and Internet have increased patients' concern over these modalities. Cadaveric pericardium has been widely used, with good postoperative results and excellent intraoperative tissue handling. The use of vein graft is well documented, with good results ranging from 60% to 95% in terms of straightening and from 88% to 92% in terms of satisfaction,[8,44–47] although these procedures do carry the additional morbidity of a second operative field, risks of harvest site infection and lymphatic leak, and longer operative times. Previously the deep dorsal penile vein has been used, but more recently vein grafts have used saphenous vein. Use of vein requires creation of a patchwork graft to fill larger tunical defects. Although the authors prefer SurgiSIS, no material has clearly emerged as the superior graft.[55]

Plaque Incision

The incision-excision straightening procedure begins with an artificial erection to assess penile curvature, as previously described. For dorsal plaques, a circumcising incision and degloving of the penis is performed. Ventral plaques may be accessed via a circumcision or a direct ventral incision longitudinally over the plaque. Dorsal penile incisions should again be avoided. The neurovascular bundles, located lateral to the deep dorsal vein of the penis, should be carefully dissected off the underlying tunica albuginea. The plaque can be approached through the bed of the deep dorsal vein if needed, with venous ligation 1 cm proximal and distal to the point of maximum curvature and excision of the venous segment. Buck's fascia can also be incised at the 3 o'clock and 9 o'clock positions, and dissected off of the tunica albuginea to retract the neurovascular structures from the plaque and curvature. Buck's fascia and the contained neurovascular bundles are then carefully dissected off of the tunica albuginea using sharp dissection. A relaxing H-shaped incision is then made in the plaque with subsequent grafting over it, a technique described by Lue and El-Sakka.[56] Egydio and colleagues[57] describe an incision using "tripod-shaped forks of 120°" to produce a geometrically optimized relaxing tunical defect for easy graft suturing. This "Mercedes-Benz" incision provides enhanced curvature correction for severe curvatures, especially when associated with an hourglass deformity at the location of curvature.

Plaque Excision

Larger or calcified plaques may require complete excision. The measurement of graft size can be estimated by measuring the convex and concave portions of the erect penis and using the difference for the first graft size estimate. After the curvature has been incised or the plaque excised, measurements are taken from the corners of the tunical incision. It is important to raise flaps of tunica at the H-shaped or Y-shaped incision to allow for full straightening.

The chosen graft material should be cut approximately 20% larger than the measured tunical defect, and sutured to the tunica albuginea with a running, locking 4-0 polydioxanone suture (PDS; Ethicon, Cincinnati, OH). Suture placement takes up approximately 3 to 5 mm of graft size along each edge. Tisseal (Baxter Healthcare, West Lake Village, CA, USA) can be applied as a spray under the graft material to promote further adherence to the underlying corporal tissue. After Tisseal has been applied and the graft has been sutured in place, an artificial erection should again be induced to check straightening and, when necessary, additional plications can be placed on the contralateral side of the penis to correct any residual curvature. Large residual curvatures may require a second incision and grafting, although this is rare. After straightening has been achieved, Buck's fascia and the skin are closed.

A penile block is again used, a fine suction drain (TLS) is left in the subcutaneous space overnight in selected cases, a noncompression dressing is applied, and the patient is discharged on the day of surgery or the following morning. Ice is maintained on the surgical site for 48 to 72 hours. As previously mentioned, the authors' patients are discharged home on 2 weeks of nightly benzodiazepines for suppression of nocturnal erections, and given amyl nitrate ampoules as needed to suppress daytime erections over that same period. Patients are advised to avoid sexual activity until their follow-up visit at 6 weeks.

Postoperative Considerations

If patients experience mild recurrence of curve in the postoperative period, a vacuum erection device (VED) may be employed for 10 minutes twice daily without the constriction ring once the patient has recovered from the discomfort of the surgery. This postoperative VED use is successful for mild to moderate curvature. Penile extender devices can also be used, and are a gentler stretching alternative. Many patients will experience "penile shock" for 3 to 9 months after surgery, so the authors' practice is to plan to use PDE-5 inhibitors in patients during that time. The authors prefer 5 mg tadalafil daily for postoperative care.

Reported satisfaction and straightening rates vary widely. Complications include worsening ED, with most studies reporting between 0% and 15%, though this takes up to 6 months to improve and may require the assistance of a vacuum device or PDE-5 inhibitors. Other complications include penile shortening (0%–40%), glans and penile hypoesthesia (0%–16.7%), curve recurrence (0%–16.7%), and hematoma.[8,28,44–52]

Although the risk for increased penile shortening is less with these procedures than with plication procedures, patients still need to be warned of this outcome. PD itself will cause shortening and may increase this complaint. Yurkanin and colleagues[46] reported average penile lengthening of 2.1 cm in the flaccid penis of men postoperatively in their study. In an interesting display of the psychosocial complexity of PD, more than half of the patients in this study reported postoperative subjective shortening.

PENILE PROSTHESIS IMPLANTATION

In patients found on preoperative assessment to have severe ED and PD, the best combined treatment is implantation of a penile prosthesis. The tunica-lengthening and tunica-shortening procedures described may provide a straight penis, but many will have some detrimental impact on erectile function. Patients are obviously not well served by a straightened penis that is incapable of becoming erect.

While all types of prostheses have been tried,[58] the 2-piece or 3-piece IPP has emerged as the standard of care in all but a select few cases.[50,59,60] In many patients the mechanical straightening provided by implantation of the prosthesis is enough to correct penile curvature. Patients with continued curvature should be treated with a modeling, plaque incision and grafting, or modified Nesbit procedure.

Wilson and Delk[61,62] first described modeling in a large, 138-patient retrospective study. Before pump placement in the scrotum, the cylinders are distended maximally and the connector tubing to the pump is clamped to prevent excessive back-pressure. In addition, digital pressure is placed over the corporotomy incisions to protect the suture lines. The penis is bent manually in the direction opposite the curve for 90 seconds, which results in plaque splitting and often an audible crack. Wilson and Delk[61] reported this technique as being successful in 118 of 138 patients, avoiding plaque excision and grafting; they also reported that modeling was associated with greater postoperative pain and swelling, and was possibly related to urethral perforation in 4 patients. Carson[63] described this technique in 30 patients, 28 of whom suffered no complications from modeling and all of whom had good penile straightening at a mean follow-up of 31.4 months. The remaining 2 patients in this study required additional plaque excision and grafting. Chaudhary and colleagues[59] reported the use of modeling in 28 of 46 patients undergoing prosthesis implantation for PD. The remaining 18 patients achieved adequate straightening merely with implantation of the prosthesis. Furthermore, studies have shown slightly higher patient (88% vs 81%) and partner (80% vs 72%) satisfaction rates for modeling than with corporoplasty with insertion of an IPP.[50] AMS 700CX InhibiZone (American Medical Systems, Minnetonka, MN, USA) and Coloplast Titan (Coloplast, Minneapolis, MN, USA) prostheses are best suited for patients with PD because these higher-pressure cylinders provide adequate rigidity to straighten the penis across the Peyronie plaque. AMS Ultrex cylinders are less likely to provide an adequate platform for modeling.[64]

Complications related to IPP implantation, such as infection and device breakdown, are certainly possible in these patients. Infection rates seem to be no more common in men with PD than in others undergoing IPP placement, although a recent small series has suggested that patients who undergo modeling do have a higher rate of long-term component malfunction requiring device replacement.[65] In an institutional cohort of 90 men, Levine and colleagues[66] report 7% mechanical failure, and 2% requiring revision for malposition, infection, and erosion, respectively. As mentioned earlier, 4 of 138 patients in the original study by Wilson and Delk suffered urethral perforation, possibly linked to modeling, though none of the patients in the series by Carson or Chaudhary and colleagues experienced urethral injury.[59,61,63] Regardless, all men undergoing prosthetic implantation should be warned before surgery of the risks for infection, device malfunction, urethral injury, penile shortening, and recurrent curvature.

SUMMARY

PD is an incurable, sexually debilitating disease resulting in penile deformity, coital failure, and significant psychological stress for patients and their partners. Urologists have an opportunity to help men suffering from PD to improve their lives and the lives of their partners.

Appropriate treatment should be individualized and tailored to the patient's goals and expectations, disease history, physical examination findings, and erectile function. After medical therapy is considered and the disease has stabilized, surgical correction is an excellent option for patients with functional impairment from their PD. Outcomes are satisfactory when proper treatment decisions are made, with the goal being expected return to normal sexual function following PD treatment.

REFERENCES

1. Devine CJ Jr, Somers KD, Jordan SG, et al. Proposal: trauma as the cause of the Peyronie's lesion. J Urol 1997;157:285–90.
2. Schwarzer U, Sommer F, Klotz T, et al. The prevalence of Peyronie's disease: results of a large survey. BJU Int 2001;88:727–30.
3. Mulhall JP, Creech SD, Boorjian SA, et al. Subjective and objective analysis of the prevalence of Peyronie's disease in a population of men presenting for prostate cancer screening. J Urol 2004;171:2350.
4. Gelbard MK, Dorey F, James K. The natural history of Peyronie's disease. J Urol 1990;144:1376–9.
5. Mulhall JP, Schiff J, Guhring P. An analysis of the natural history of Peyronie's disease. J Urol 2006; 175:2115–8.
6. Carson CC. Francois Gigot de la Peyronie (1678-1747). Invest Urol 1981;19:62–3.
7. Ralph D, Gonzalez-Cadavid N, Mirone V, et al. The management of Peyronie's disease: evidence-based 2010 guidelines. J Sex Med 2010;7:2359–74.
8. Montorsi F, Salonia A, Maga T, et al. Evidence-based assessment of long-term results in plaque incision and vein grafting for Peyronie's disease. J Urol 2000;163:1704–8.
9. Tornehl CK, Carson CC. Surgical alternatives for treating Peyronie's disease. BJU Int 2004;94:774–83.
10. Kim DH, Lesser TF, Aboseif SR. Subjective patient-reported experiences after surgery for Peyronie's disease: corporeal plication versus plaque incision with vein graft. Urology 2008;71(4):698–702.
11. Mulhall J, Anderson M, Parker M. A surgical algorithm for men with combined Peyronie's disease and erectile dysfunction: functional and satisfaction outcomes. J Sex Med 2005;2:132–8.
12. Schaeffer E, Jarow JJ, Vrablic J, et al. Duplex ultrasonography detects clinically significant anomalies of penile arterial vasculature affecting surgical approach to penile straightening. Urology 2006;67:166–9.
13. McMahon CG. Correlation of penile duplex ultrasonography, PBI, DICC, and angiography in the diagnosis of impotence. Int J Impot Res 1998;10:153–8.
14. Aversa A, Bruzziches R, Spera G. Diagnosing erectile dysfunction: the penile dynamic color duplex ultrasound revisited. Int J Androl 2005;28(Suppl 2):61–3.
15. Alphs HH, Navai N, Kohler TS, et al. Preoperative clinical and diagnostic characteristics of patients who require delayed IPP after primary Peyronie's repair. J Sex Med 2010;7:1262–8.
16. Levine LA, Greenfield JM, Estrada CR. Erectile dysfunction following surgical correction of Peyronie's disease and a pilot study of the use of Sildenafil citrate rehabilitation for post-operative erectile dysfunction. J Sex Med 2005;2:241–7.
17. Kadioglu A, Akman T, Sanli O, et al. Surgical treatment of Peyronie's disease: a critical analysis. Eur Urol 2006;50:235–48.
18. Nelson CJ, Diblasio C, Kendirci M, et al. The chronology of depression and distress in men with Peyronie's disease. J Sex Med 2008;5:1985–90.
19. Nesbit RM. Congenital curvature of the phallus: report on three cases with description of corrective operation. J Urol 1965;93:230–2.
20. Pryor JP, Fitzpatrick JM. A new approach to the correction of penile deformity in Peyronie's disease. J Urol 1979;122:622–3.
21. Rehman J, Benet A, Minsky LS, et al. Results of surgical treatment for abnormal penile curvature: Peyronie's disease and congenital deviation by modified Nesbit placation (tunical shaving and plication). J Urol 1997;157:1288–91.
22. Yachia D. Modified corporoplasty for the treatment of penile curvature. J Urol 1990;143:80–2.
23. Gholami SS, Lue TF. Correction of penile curvature using the 16-dot plication technique: a review of 132 patients. J Urol 2002;167:2066–9.

24. Dean RC, Lue TF. Penile plication using the 16-dot technique. In: Levine L, editor. Current clinical urology: Peyronie's disease: a guide to clinical management. 1st edition. Totowa (NJ): Humana Press Inc; 2006. p. 145–50.

25. van der Horst C, Martinez Portillo FJ, Melchior D, et al. Polytetrafluoroethylene versus polypropylene for Essed-Schroeder tunical plication. J Urol 2003; 170:472–5.

26. Baskin LS, Duckett JW. Dorsal tunica albuginea plication for hypospadias curvature. J Urol 1994; 151:1668–71.

27. Levine L. Penile straightening with tunica albuginea plication procedure. In: Levine L, editor. Current clinical urology: Peyronie's disease: a guide to clinical management. 1st edition. Totowa (NJ): Humana Press Inc; 2006. p. 151–9.

28. Licht MR, Lewis RW. Modified Nesbit procedure for the treatment of Peyronie's disease: a comparative outcome analysis. J Urol 1997;158:460–3.

29. Pryor JP. Correction of penile curvature and Peyronie's disease: why I prefer the Nesbit technique. Int J Impot Res 1998;10:129–31.

30. Savoca G, Trombetta C, Ciampalini S, et al. Long-term results with Nesbit's procedure as treatment of Peyronie's disease. Int J Impot Res 2000;12: 289–93.

31. Syeed AH, Abbasi Z, Hargreave TB. Nesbit procedure for disabling Peyronie's curvature: a median follow-up of 84 months. Urology 2003;61:999–1003.

32. Daitch JA, Angermeier KW, Montague DK. Modified corporoplasty for penile curvature: long-term results and patient satisfaction. J Urol 1999;162:2006–9.

33. Sulaiman MN, Gingell JC. Nesbit's procedure for penile curvature. J Androl 1994;15:54S–6S.

34. Greenfield JM, Lucas S, Levine LA. Factors affecting the loss of length associated with tunica albuginea plication for the correction of penile curvature. J Urol 2006;175:238–41.

35. van der Drift DG, Vroege JA, Groenendijk PM, et al. The plication procedure for penile curvature: surgical outcome and post-operative sexual function. Urol Int 2002;69:120–4.

36. Chahal R, Gogoi NK, Sundaram SK, et al. Corporal plication for penile curvature caused by Peyronie's disease: the patient's perspective. BJU Int 2001; 87:352–6.

37. Thiounn N, Missirliu A, Serbib M, et al. Corporal plication for surgical correction of penile curvature. Experience with 60 patients. Eur Urol 1998;33:401–4.

38. Geertsen UA, Brok KE, Andersen B, et al. Peyronie's curvature treated by plication of the penile fasciae. Br J Urol 1996;77:733–5.

39. Nooter RI, Bosch JL, Schroder FH. Peyronie's disease and congenital penile curvature: Long-term results of operative treatment with the plication procedure. Br J Urol 1994;74:497–500.

40. Dugi DD, Morey AF. Penoscrotal plication as a uniform approach to reconstruction of penile curvature. BJU Int 2009;105:1440–4.

41. Lowsley OS, Boyce WH. Further experiences with an operation for the cure of Peyronie's disease. J Urol 1950;63:888–902.

42. Devine CJ, Horton CE. Surgical treatment of Peyronie's disease with a dermal graft. J Urol 1974;111: 44–9.

43. Gelbard MK. Relaxing incisions in the correction of penile deformity due to Peyronie's disease. J Urol 1995;154:1457–60.

44. El-Sakka AI, Rashwan HM, Lue TF. Venous patch graft for Peyronie's disease. Part II: outcome analysis. J Urol 1998;160:2050–3.

45. Backhaus B, Muller S, Albers P. Corporoplasty for advanced Peyronie's disease using venous and/or dermis patch grafting: new surgical technique and long-term patient satisfaction. J Urol 2003;169: 981–4.

46. Yurkanin JP, Dean R, Wessells H. Effect of incision and saphenous vein grafting for Peyronie's disease on penile length and sexual satisfaction. J Urol 2001;166:1769–72 [discussion: 1772–3].

47. Adeniyi AA, Goorney SR, Pryor JP, et al. The Lue procedure: an analysis of the outcome in Peyronie's disease. BJU Int 2002;89:404–8.

48. Egydio PH, Lucon AM, Arap S. Treatment of Peyronie's disease by incomplete circumferential incision of the tunica albuginea and plaque with bovine pericardium graft. Urology 2002;59:570–4.

49. Chun JL, McGregor A, Krishnan R, et al. A comparison of dermal and cadaveric pericardial grafts in the modified Horton-Devine procedure for Peyronie's disease. J Urol 2001;166:185–8.

50. Usta MF, Bivalacqua TJ, Sanabria J, et al. Patient and partner satisfaction and long-term results after surgical treatment for Peyronie's disease. Urology 2003;62:105–9.

51. Sampaio JS, Fonseca J, Passarinho A, et al. Peyronie's disease: surgical correction of 40 patients with relaxing incision and dura mater graft. Eur Urol 2002;41:551–5.

52. Knoll LD. Use of porcine small intestinal submucosal graft in the surgical treatment of Peyronie's disease. Urology 2001;57:753–7.

53. Kadioglu A, Sanli O, Akman T, et al. Graft materials in Peyronie's disease surgery: a comprehensive review. J Sex Med 2007;4:581–95.

54. Breyer BN, Brant WO, Garcia MM, et al. Complications of porcine small intestine submucosa graft for Peyronie's disease. J Urol 2007;177:589–91.

55. Carson CC. Surgical treatment of Peyronie's disease. Can J Urol 2006;13:28–33.

56. Lue TF, El-Sakka AI. Venous patch graft for Peyronie's disease. Part I: technique. J Urol 1998;160: 2047–9.

57. Egydio PH, Lucon AM, Arap S. A single relaxing incision to correct different types of penile curvature: surgical technique based on geometrical principles. BJU Int 2004;94:1147–57.

58. Montorsi F, Guazzoni G, Bergamaschi F, et al. Patient-partner satisfaction with semirigid penile prostheses for Peyronie's disease: a 5-year followup study. J Urol 1993;150(6):1819–21.

59. Chaudhary M, Sheikh N, Asterling S, et al. Peyronie's disease with erectile dysfunction: penile modeling over inflatable prosthesis. Urology 2005;65:760–4.

60. Montorsi F, Guazzoni G, Barbieri L, et al. AMS 700 CX inflatable penile implants for Peyronie's disease: functional results, morbidity and patient-partner satisfaction. Int J Impot Res 1996;8:81–5.

61. Wilson SK, Delk JR II. A new treatment for Peyronie's disease: modeling the penis over an inflatable penile prosthesis. J Urol 1994;152:1121–3.

62. Wilson SK. Surgical techniques: modeling technique for penile curvature. J Sex Med 2007;4:231–4.

63. Carson CC. Penile prosthesis implantation in the treatment of Peyronie's disease. Int J Impot Res 1998;10:125–8.

64. Montague DK, Angermeier KW, Lakin MM, et al. AMS 3-piece inflatable penile prosthesis implantation in men with Peyronie's disease: comparison of CX and Ultrex cylinders. J Urol 1996;156:1633–5.

65. DiBlasio CJ, Kurta JM, Botta S, et al. Peyronie's disease compromises the durability and component-malfunction rates in patients implanted with an inflatable penile prosthesis. BJU Int 2010;106:691–4.

66. Levine LA, Benson J, Hoover C. Inflatable penile prosthesis placement in men with Peyronie's disease and drug-resistant erectile dysfunction: a single-center study. J Sex Med 2010;7(11):3775–883.

Penile Prosthesis Implantation in the Era of Medical Treatment for Erectile Dysfunction

Drogo K. Montague, MD

KEYWORDS
- Penile prosthesis • Penile prosthesis implantation
- Erectile dysfunction

As recently as the 1960s, erectile dysfunction (ED), then known as impotence, was considered to be invariably of psychogenic origin, and treatment was often empiric testosterone administration or psychiatric referral.[1] Three sentinel events define the history of our understanding and modern treatment of ED: inflatable penile prosthesis implantation (1973),[2] intracorporeal injection therapy (1982),[3] and effective systemic therapy, (1998).[4]

Nonsurgical therapies for ED are not always effective and, when they are effective, they are not always acceptable. For these reasons, although penile prosthesis implantation is the oldest of modern treatment options, it still plays a prominent role in the contemporary management of ED as evidenced by annual penile prosthesis implantation cases in the United States rising from 17,540 in 2000 to 22,420 in 2009.[5]

TYPES OF PENILE PROSTHESES
Noninflatable Penile Prostheses

Noninflatable penile prostheses are paired, solid malleable, or positional devices that fill each corpus cavernosum. Their advantages include low cost, little need for manual dexterity, and a relatively low rate of mechanical failure. Disadvantages include a constant prosthetic erection and increased chance of chronic pain and erosion.[6]

Inflatable Penile Prostheses

Inflatable penile prostheses are fluid filled devices that are either "two-piece," consisting of paired intracorporeal cylinders and a scrotal pump; or "three-piece," consisting of paired intracorporeal cylinders, a scrotal pump, and an abdominal fluid reservoir. In the United States, there are two inflatable penile prosthesis manufacturers: American Medical Systems (AMS), Minnetonka, MN and Coloplast, Minneapolis, MN.

Coloplast manufactures a two-piece inflatable prosthesis; however, it is not available in the United States. AMS has a two-piece inflatable prosthesis, the AMS Ambicor (**Fig. 1**), which is available in the United States. The Ambicor cylinders are nondistensible. When the device is deflated, the cylinders collapse and the penis, unlike that with a malleable prosthesis, is not rigid. When the scrotal pump is cycled, a small volume of fluid is transferred from the rear tips of the cylinders into the distal nondistensible chambers filling and then pressurizing them. With inflation, the Ambicor supplies rigidity comparable to that of a malleable prosthesis. Unlike the three-piece inflatable prostheses, however, the Ambicor does

The author is a consultant for American Medical Systems, Minnetonka, Minnesota.
Center for Genitourinary Reconstruction, Department of Urology, Glickman Urological and Kidney Institute, Cleveland Clinic Lerner College of Medicine of Case Western Reserve University, Q10-1, Cleveland Clinic, 9500 Euclid Avenue, Cleveland, OH 44195, USA
E-mail address: montagd@ccf.org

Urol Clin N Am 38 (2011) 217–225
doi:10.1016/j.ucl.2011.02.009

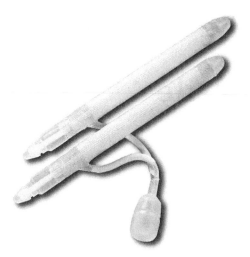

Fig. 1. AMS Ambicor Inflatable Penile Prosthesis. (*Courtesy of* American Medical Systems, Inc, Minnetonka, MN; www.AmericanMedicalSystems.com; with permission.)

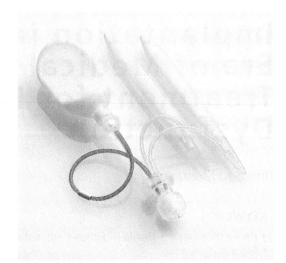

Fig. 2. Coloplast Titan Inflatable Penile Prosthesis. (*Courtesy of* Coloplast Corp, Minneapolis, MN; with permission.)

not increase in size with inflation. The advantage of this device is there is no abdominal fluid reservoir to implant. The disadvantage is that for many recipients, flaccidity and erection are not as good as those achieved with three-piece inflatable devices.

The ideal penile prosthesis would produce flaccidity and erection approaching that achieved naturally. Three-piece inflatable penile prostheses, which transfer a large volume of fluid into expandable cylinders for erection and out of the cylinders for flaccidity, approach this ideal. These devices require a fluid reservoir that is too large for the scrotum and needs to be implanted in the abdomen.

Coloplast manufactures the Titan Inflatable Penile Prosthesis (**Fig. 2**) and the Titan Narrowbase Inflatable Penile Prosthesis. The Narrowbase implant is for small penises or for cases in which dilation is limited because of scarring from disease or previous surgery.

AMS manufactures the AMS 700 CX Inflatable Penile Prosthesis (**Fig. 3**), the AMS 700 LGX Inflatable Penile Prosthesis, and the AMS 700 CXR Inflatable Penile Prosthesis. The CXR device, like the Titan Narrow-base prosthesis, has smaller diameter cylinders and is used in revision cases and less commonly in men with small penises.

The paired corpora cavernosa of the penis consist of an outer fibroelastic tunica albuginea filled with cavernosal smooth muscle. The tunica albuginea has both inner circular and outer longitudinal elastic fibers (**Fig. 4**). With normal erection, cavernosal smooth muscle relaxation occurs and the corpora fill with blood. The elastic fibers of

the tunica albuginea allow the corpora to expand both in diameter and in length. When the elastic limits of these fibers are reached, the corpora and the penis become rigid. The ideal penile prosthesis would be undetectable while deflated, allowing a man to feel comfortable in locker rooms. With inflation, the prosthesis would create girth expansion, length expansion, and rigidity comparable to that of a normal erection. One device, the AMS 700 LGX Inflatable Prosthesis, comes closest to meeting this ideal because, in addition to girth expansion with inflation like the other three-piece inflatable devices, it also provides length expansion. In **Fig. 5**, one LGX cylinder of a pair is deflated and the other is inflated. After AMS 700 LGX implantation in one patient, the pubis-to-glans tip length with the device deflated

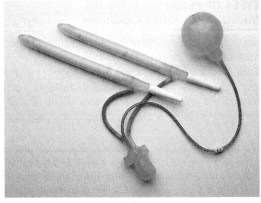

Fig. 3. AMS 700 CX Inflatable Penile Prosthesis. (*Courtesy of* American Medical Systems, Inc, Minnetonka, MN; www.AmericanMedicalSystems.com; with permission.)

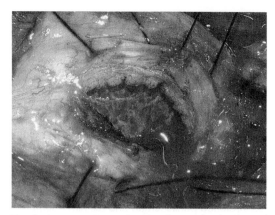

Fig. 4. A corporotomy showing inner circular (round bundles) and outer longitudinal layers of the tunica albuginea.

is 10.5 cm (**Fig. 6**) and after inflation 12.5 cm (**Fig. 7**).

Although the AMS 700 LGX prosthesis approaches the ideal, its use is not indicated for every patient. In patients with organic ED and erectile deformity or curvature, girth only expanding CX or CXR cylinders provide better correction of deformity.[7] In men with small penises or men with scarring due to ischemic priapism or previous penile surgery where corporeal dilation is limited, smaller diameter CXR cylinders often fit better.[8] These cylinder applications are summarized in **Table 1**.

PATIENT SELECTION

Formerly, specialized diagnostic testing for ED such as nocturnal penile tumescence testing, color duplex ultrasonography, and cavernosometry-cavernosography were in vogue, and their use helped provide a better understanding of the pathophysiology of ED. In 1990, Lue[9] introduced the

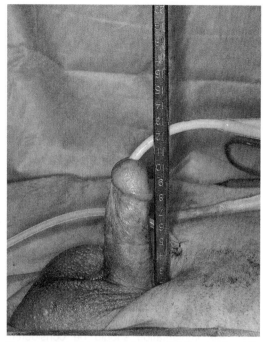

Fig. 6. Deflated length of penis (10.5 cm) after LGX implantation.

concept of "patient goal-directed therapy" and, since then, these tests have been largely restricted to patients who want more specific information regarding the cause of their ED.

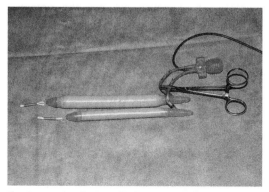

Fig. 5. A pair of LGX cylinders: one deflated and one inflated.

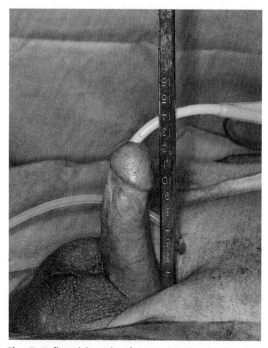

Fig. 7. Inflated length of penis (12.5 cm) after LGX implantation.

Table 1
AMS cylinder selection

	Small Penis	Fibrosis	Curvature	Most Others
CXR	X	X	X	—
CX	—	X	X	—
LGX	—	—	—	X

Today, the diagnosis of ED is based largely on history. Unless there is a contraindication, such as the use of nitrates, most patients have a therapy trial with one or more of the type 5 phosphodiesterase inhibitors. If this first line of treatment is not satisfactory, patients are offered the use of a vacuum erection device, intraurethral medication, or intracavernous injection therapy. These second-line treatment options may be explored by the patient and, if satisfactory, continued. If first- and second-line treatments are not effective or the patient chooses not to try them, then penile prosthesis implantation should be considered. Penile prosthesis implantation, however, should not be done for ED that is likely to be temporary, the result of a relationship problem, or otherwise potentially reversible.

Whenever possible, it is desirable to have the partner included in these treatment discussions. In considering a man for penile prosthesis implantation, his fitness for an elective surgical procedure, his ability to give informed consent, and his manual dexterity are all issues to be considered.

Additional considerations in prospective penile prosthesis recipients include previous surgical history, a history of ischemic priapism, or the presence of erectile deformity such as Peyronie disease. Regarding the surgical history, the elements of specific importance include previous genital or penile prosthesis-related surgery; surgery for inguinal hernia repair and whether mesh was used; history of radical prostatectomy and whether it was open, laparoscopic, or robotic-assisted laparoscopic (intraperitoneal) prostatectomy; or a history of radical cystoprostatectomy.

Since penile prosthesis implantation is capable of providing only a prosthetic erection, the patient should be questioned preoperatively about his libido and the presence of orgasm with or without ejaculation.

INFORMED CONSENT

As in all surgical procedures, the type of anesthesia, the length of stay, postoperative morbidity, and length of disability are discussed. There is also a discussion of the various types of penile prostheses. Most patients in my practice choose a three-piece inflatable device and, although these provide flaccidity and erection coming closest to the natural states, there are important differences. The penile prosthesis will only treat ED. If libido, orgasm, or ejaculation are impaired, they may be absent or impaired after the implant. I tell the patient that most men with three-piece inflatable devices will feel comfortable in a locker room. The erection produced by a three-piece device differs from a normal erection in that the glans does not increase in size. In the examination room, I demonstrate, for the patient and partner, his stretched penile length and tell him (them) that this will be the approximate length of his prosthetic erection. For most men, this is somewhat shorter than he would expect and for some men it is much shorter. Men in the latter category include those after radical prostatectomy where loss of penile length has been well documented.[10–12] Also in this category are men who have a history of ischemic priapism, Peyronie disease, removal of an infected penile implant, and some men who are obese. This issue of length is most important because, in my experience, if a man has had a successful implant and is unhappy, it is usually because the prosthetic erection is shorter than he expected.

Infection is the bane of penile prosthesis surgery because, if it is present in the space around the implant, total removal of all prosthetic material will be required. Penile prosthesis reimplantation in these men is frequently difficult due to fibrosis of corporeal smooth muscle, which also makes the penis permanently smaller. Internal erosion of the cylinders often requires revision surgery. External erosion of the prosthesis is usually the result of infection. Although men who have a penile prosthesis removed for reasons other than infection might still be able to have successful treatment for their ED using a vacuum erection device or intracavernous injection therapy, penile prosthesis implantation still has the potential, especially if infection occurs, of destroying any residual erectile tissue. Penile prostheses can fail mechanically, and the likelihood of this occurring is discussed below.

PREOPERATIVE PREPARATION

Penile prosthesis implantation should be delayed until bacteriuria or urinary tract infection are eliminated, and should not be performed if the patient has a systemic infection or if there is local infection in the operative field. Broad-spectrum antibiotics (gentamicin and vancomycin) covering both gram-positive and gram-negative organisms should be administered 1 hour before the procedure. I continue these antibiotics until the patient is released from the outpatient surgical area the morning after surgery; I do not use antibiotics beyond this point.

Shaving is done in the operating room immediately before the procedure to avoid colonization of skin breaks that might occur with earlier shaving. I do a 10-minute skin preparation. Paper drapes are preferable over cloth drapes; the latter are permeable to bacteria when wet. Irrigation with an antibiotic solution (100,000 units of bacitracin in 1 L of normal saline) is important. Rather than frequent random irrigation, I irrigate at specific times, such as while the cylinders and reservoir are inserted and before closing tissues over portions of the prosthesis. Silicone has a positive charge and attracts airborne particles. The rationale for irrigation is that it washes these particles off the surface of the prosthesis.

InhibiZone, a surface coating of minocycline and rifampin, is available for the AMS 700 Inflatable Penile Prosthesis product line, and I routinely implant devices coated with these antibiotics. Once the components have been prepared for implantation, they should be kept in a dry, covered basin (not soaked in a solution). Irrigation of these components as described above is permissible and encouraged. All these issues in preoperative preparation are related efforts to avoid infection.

SURGICAL APPROACHES

Surgical approaches for inflatable penile prosthesis implantation include infrapubic and penoscrotal approaches. The infrapubic approach has a single advantage: reservoir insertion under direct vision. Its disadvantages include limited corporeal exposure, possible dorsal nerve injury, and inability to anchor the pump. The penoscrotal approach provides much better and, if necessary, nearly complete corporeal exposure. The structure that might be injured with this approach is the urethra, and avoidance of urethral injury is much easier than avoidance of dorsal nerve injury with the infrapubic approach. Finally, the pump can be contained within a sub dartos pouch.

Many physicians use a transverse upper scrotal incision because this provides a transverse dartos flap to cover tubing and the connector, making the device less detectable and protecting the prosthesis against infection should there be superficial wound infection or dehiscence. I am concerned about this incision because the resultant scar is not along normal skin lines and thus is more prominent. Instead, I use a vertical penoscrotal skin incision along the penoscrotal raphe dividing dartos fascia

completely in the upper half and partially in the lower half. I then dissect the lower transverse dartos flap off the proximal corpora and urethra. This lower flap later buries the tubing and connector, and the subcuticular, vertical skin closure leaves a scar along the raphe that is barely visible.

Reservoir implantation is often done blindly through the penoscrotal approach. This can be done safely if the retropubic space contains only the bladder or the bladder and prostate. The bladder must be emptied by inserting a Foley catheter, which is attached to closed gravity drainage. The fascia in the medial aspect of the floor of the external inguinal ring is punctured and this fascial opening is maintained with a long-blade nasal speculum while the empty reservoir is inserted. If the external ring is not palpable, I choose a point above the pubic tubercle for this fascial puncture. While the fascia is thickened after open radical prostatectomy, the retropubic space is maintained by the full bladder and it opens up when the bladder is emptied. We reported successful reservoir implantation through the penoscrotal incision in 115 consecutive men who had undergone radical retropubic prostatectomy.[13]

After robotic-assisted laparoscopic radical prostatectomy or after cystectomy, there may be bowel in the retropubic space. In these patients, I implant the reservoir through a second incision placing it between the rectus muscle and the posterior fascia. Reservoir implantation is facilitated in these cases by using the flat Conceal AMS reservoir (**Fig. 8**).

KEY ASPECTS OF PENILE PROSTHESIS IMPLANTATION
Cylinder Sizing

The conventional technique for cylinder sizing uses a reference suture at the midpoint of the corporotomy, makes distal and proximal measurements from this reference point, and then adds them together to obtain the cylinder size. Because a solid measuring tool is used to make these two surface measurements, the resultant combined measurement is often 2 cm longer than the actual length along the center of the corpus cavernosum. This is not obvious to most implanters because they evacuate fluid from the cylinders before implantation, making the flat cylinders easy to push down and close over.

The consequences of oversizing the cylinder are twofold. First, with the LGX (formerly Ultrex) cylinder, which expands both in girth and in length, oversizing results in the "S-shaped penile deformity" described by Wilson and colleagues.[14] Secondly, when failure occurs in most cylinders,

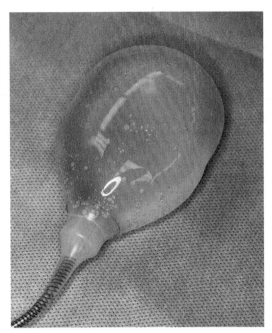

Fig. 8. Conceal reservoir.

it is usually just in front of the input tubing. This site for cylinder failure may exist because this is where the cylinder flexes or moves when the patient walks; however, when a cylinder is oversized, this is also the site of a small S-shaped curve in the cylinder that, theoretically, would cause increased wear and early cylinder failure.

To avoid this measurement error, I omit the 2 cm corporotomy from my surface measurements.[15] I also implant cylinders that are rounded (full of fluid but not under pressure). After the cylinders are in place, the portion viewed through the corporotomy should be flat. Within the incision, I palpate proximally to determine that the proximal cylinders fill the crura. I then release the penis from the ring retractor and check the position of the cylinder tips and glans support. Most of the time, the initial cylinder length determined in this fashion is correct. If it is too short, I remove the proximal cylinder and add an additional 1 cm of rear tip extension.

Corporotomy Closure

I place two pair of horizontal mattress sutures of 2-0 PDS in the corporotomy to serve initially as guy sutures during dilation and measurement. These sutures are also used to close the corporotomy over the cylinder eliminating the need to suture over a cylinder. An air knot is tied between the proximal ends of opposing sutures. This knot is pulled down and the distal strands are then tied. This is repeated with the second set of sutures.[16]

Pump Placement

Another disadvantage of the infrapubic approach for penile prosthesis implantation is that the pump needs to be placed in a lateral sub dartos pouch. This makes pump manipulation somewhat more difficult in that the patient needs to get his thumb or finger between the medial aspect of the pump and the ipsilateral testicle. With the septal sub dartos pouch pump placement, possible with the penoscrotal approach, it is usually possible to lift the pump forward allowing both testes to drop back. This allows the patient to easily access both sides of the pump.

The deep layers of dartos fascia are punctured and the septal pouch is created (I find the use of a ring forceps ideal for this). If the surgeon then takes the preconnected pump and drops it into this pouch, the pump tubing will end up being covered only by scrotal skin and subcutaneous tissue. This results in tubing that is often visible and readily palpable; this is undesirable from a cosmetic standpoint. More importantly, if a superficial wound infection or a wound dehiscence occurs, the entire device is potentially infected.

To avoid these two problems, I use a right-angle clamp to make a puncture deep through the back wall of the sub dartos pouch. A long-blade nasal speculum is used to hold this puncture open and the pump is brought through the opening into the pouch. The opening at the top of the pouch is then closed with running 3-0 absorbable suture.

The incision and reservoir placement are discussed above.

POSTOPERATIVE CARE

Penile prosthesis implantation is done as an outpatient procedure usually with a 23-hour stay. After removal of the Foley catheter and drain the morning following surgery, the patient is sent home. Although it is not always possible, I encourage the patient to wear the penis up on the lower abdomen to avoid downward curvature as healing takes place. This downward curvature is more likely in men with longer penises. If it occurs, repeated gentle bending (modeling) of the penis when the device is inflated will usually satisfactorily straighten it.

Most men require oral narcotic pain medication for up to 1 week following surgery. Heavy lifting and other activities that might result in displacement of the reservoir into the inguinal canal are proscribed for 4 weeks. Instruction on the use of the device and return to sexual activity is done at a postoperative visit in 4 to 6 weeks.

Initial inflation of the prosthesis may be difficult; I instruct the patient to inflate and deflate the device twice daily for 1 month after the initial instruction period. During this time, the implant becomes easier to inflate. When coitus is first resumed, I suggest the initial use of a lubricant. I also tell the male partner that foreplay is now important for him; if he has coitus without being aroused, achieving orgasm may not occur.

RESULTS
Freedom from Mechanical Failure

In the early days of inflatable penile prosthesis surgery mechanical failure occurred often and early. Failed devices were, and have continued to be, returned to manufacturers for examination by their biomedical engineers. Based on these examinations, many design improvements were developed and these collective changes over time have resulted in greatly improved device survival.

Early reporting of device survival usually gave the range and mean follow-up, and then the total number of mechanical failures that had occurred in that series at the time of reporting. Because this method of reporting fails to take into consideration differences in follow-up, it did not allow meaningful comparisons among various reported series. American Urological Association Guidelines for the Management of Erectile Dysfunction recommends that Kaplan-Meier projections[17,18] be used to report freedom from mechanical failure for urologic prosthetic devices.[19]

Because the AMS 700 CX and CXM (now CXR) devices were introduced in 1986 and have not had design changes that significantly impact device survival, there are numerous studies of these devices with Kaplan-Meier reporting (**Table 2**). Five-year survival, free of mechanical failure, ranges from 83.9% to 93.2%. There are two studies with 10-year projections: 78.2% and 81.3%.

Mentor Alpha-1 three-piece inflatable penile prosthesis (forerunner of the Coloplast Titan) underwent major design change affecting mechanical survival in 1992.[20] The AMS 700 Ultrex (forerunner of the AMS 700 LGX) underwent major design change affecting mechanical survival in 1993.[21] Five-year freedom from mechanical failure after these changes for the Alpha-1 device was 92.6%; and for the Ultrex it was 93.7% (see **Table 2**).

Freedom-from-mechanical-failure projections beyond 10 years are not available for any single device. However, in a series of 2,384 patients with four different models of inflatable penile prostheses, Wilson and colleagues[22] found by Kaplan-Meier projections revision-free survivals for all reasons to be 68.5% at 10 years and 59.7% at 15 years. For freedom from mechanical failure, the results were 79.4% at 10 years and 71.2% at 15 years.

Table 2
Percent freedom from mechanical failure (Kaplan-Meier projections)

References	Number of Patients CX/CXM	5 Years	10 Years
Deuk Choi et al[31]	273	90.4	—
Carson et al[32]	372	86.2	—
Montorsi et al[33]	90	93.1	—
Daitch et al[34]	111	90.8	—
Dubocq et al[35]	103	83.9	—
Dhar et al[36]	455	—	81.3
Kim et al[37]	397 AMS Ultrex	93.2 —	78.2 —
Milbank et al[21]	52 Mentor Alpha-1	93.7 —	— —
Wilson et al[20]	971	92.6	—

Patient and Partner Satisfaction

Early satisfaction studies were retrospective and did not use standardized questionnaires. McLaren and Barrett[23] reported on 272 AMS Inflatable penile prosthesis recipients and noted that 83% of the men and 70% of their partners were satisfied. In another study of 145 AMS Inflatable penile prosthesis recipients, Holloway and Farah[24] reported a similar 85% of recipients and 76% of their partners as being satisfied.

In later prospective studies, Tefilli and colleagues,[25] reported that 35 inflatable penile prosthesis recipients showed significant improvements in their psychosexual wellbeing. In another study, Mulhall and colleagues,[26] reported that 96 inflatable penile prosthesis recipients had significant improvements at 12 months over baseline scores on the International Index of Erectile Function (IIEF) and the Inventory of Treatment Satisfaction (EDITS) surveys.

Sexton and colleagues[27] compared 115 intracavernosal injection patients to 65 penile prosthesis recipients. At a mean follow up of 5.4 years, 41% of penile injection patients were still using this therapy whereas 70% of penile prosthesis recipients were still sexually active. Rajpurkar and Dhabuwala,[28] compared 31 patients receiving sildenafil citrate, 22 using penile injection therapy, and 32 penile prosthesis recipients. The penile prosthesis recipients had significantly higher scores on the erectile function domain of the IIEF and satisfaction scores on EDITS than did patients in the other two groups.

Akin-Olugbade and colleagues,[29] showed significant improvement in IIEF and EDITS scores in 114 penile prosthesis recipients. However, the following subgroups had lower satisfaction than the overall group: men with Peyronie disease, body mass index greater than 30, and radical prostatectomy. It is noteworthy that men in these three subgroups all have shortened penises, and their dissatisfaction is likely at least in part due to a failure of penile prosthesis implantation to restore lost penile length. The study by Kramer and Schweber[30] reinforces this by showing that low preoperative expectations correlated with high postoperative satisfaction scores.

RECOMMENDATIONS FOR THE FUTURE

Overall prosthesis survival and survival free of mechanical failure should always continue to be reported in terms of Kaplan-Meier projections. Studies of patient satisfaction should include partners, be prospective, and use standardized questionnaires. More studies should be done showing the overall effect of penile prosthesis implantation on quality of life factors such as improvements in relationships, self esteem, and depression. Finally, more prospective studies need to be done comparing penile prosthesis implantation to other forms of ED treatments.

SUMMARY

Penile prosthesis implantation, the oldest of the modern treatment options for ED, continues to play an important role in ED management in spite of the advent of less invasive alternatives. For some men with ED, penile prosthesis implantation is the only effective treatment; for others it may be the most acceptable. Improvements in both prosthesis design as well as implantation techniques have resulted in significant increases in device survival as well as patient satisfaction.

REFERENCES

1. Smith DR. General urology. 5th edition. Los Altos (CA): Lange Medical Publications; 1966.
2. Scott FB, Bradley WE, Timm GW. Management of erectile impotence: use of implantable inflatable prosthesis. Urology 1973;2:80–2.
3. Virag R. Intracavernous injection of papaverine for erectile failure. Lancet 1982;2:938.
4. Goldstein I, Lue TF, Padma-Nathan H, et al. Oral sildenafil in the treatment of erectile dysfunction. Sildenafil Study Group. N Engl J Med 1998;338: 1397–404.
5. Available at: http://www.marketresearch.com. Accessed October 11, 2010.
6. Zermann DH, Kutzenberger J, Sauerwein D, et al. Penile prosthetic surgery in neurologically impaired patients: long-term followup. J Urol 2006;175: 1041–4.
7. Montague DK, Angermeier KW, Lakin MM, et al. AMS 3-piece inflatable penile prosthesis implantation in men with Peyronie's disease: comparison of CX and Ultrex cylinders. J Urol 1996;156:1633–5.
8. Montague DK, Angermeier KW. Corporeal excavation: new technique for penile prosthesis implantation in men with severe corporeal fibrosis. Urology 2006;67:1072–5.
9. Lue TF. Impotence: a patient's goal-directed approach to treatment. World J Urol 1990;8:67–74.
10. Savoie M, Kim SS, Soloway MS. A prospective study measuring penile length in men treated with radical prostatectomy for prostate cancer. J Urol 2003;169: 1462–4.
11. Mulhall JP. Penile length changes after radical prostatectomy. BJU Int 2005;96:472–4.
12. Gontero P, Galzerano M, Bartoletti R, et al. New insights into the pathogenesis of penile shortening after radical prostatectomy and the role of postoperative sexual function. J Urol 2007;178:602–7.
13. Lane BR, Abouassaly R, Angermeier KW, et al. Three-piece inflatable penile prostheses can be safely implanted after radical prostatectomy through a transverse scrotal incision. Urology 2007;70:539–42.
14. Wilson SK, Cleves MA, Delk JR 2nd. Ultrex cylinders: problems with uncontrolled lengthening (the S-shaped deformity). J Urol 1996;155:135–7.
15. Montague DK, Angermeier KW. Cylinder sizing: less is more. Int J Impot Res 2003;15(Suppl 5):S132–3.
16. Montague DK. Penile prosthesis corporotomy closure: a new technique. J Urol 1993;150:924–5.
17. Kaplan E, Meier P. Nonparametric estimations from incomplete observations. J Am Stat Assoc 1958; 53:457–81.
18. Sur RL, Dahm P. Evidence-based urology in practice: Kaplan-Meier analysis. BJU Int 2009;105(10): 1360–2.
19. Montague DK, Jarow JP, Broderick GA, et al. Chapter 1: The management of erectile dysfunction: an AUA update. J Urol 2005;174:230–9.
20. Wilson SK, Cleves MA, Delk JR 2nd. Comparison of mechanical reliability of original and enhanced Mentor Alpha I penile prosthesis. J Urol 1999;162: 715–8.
21. Milbank AJ, Montague DK, Angermeier KW, et al. Mechanical failure of the American Medical Systems Ultrex inflatable penile prosthesis: before and after 1993 structural modification. J Urol 2002;167:2502–6.
22. Wilson SK, Delk JR, Salem EA, et al. Long-term survival of inflatable penile prostheses: single

surgical group experience with 2,384 first-time implants spanning two decades. J Sex Med 2007; 4:1074–9.

23. McLaren RH, Barrett DM. Patient and partner satisfaction with the AMS 700 penile prosthesis. J Urol 1992;147:62–5.

24. Holloway FB, Farah RN. Intermediate term assessment of the reliability, function and patient satisfaction with the AMS700 Ultrex penile prosthesis. J Urol 1997;157:1687–91.

25. Tefilli MV, Dubocq F, Rajpurkar A, et al. Assessment of psychosexual adjustment after insertion of inflatable penile prosthesis. Urology 1998;52:1106–12.

26. Mulhall JP, Ahmed A, Branch J, et al. Serial assessment of efficacy and satisfaction profiles following penile prosthesis surgery. J Urol 2003; 169:1429–33.

27. Sexton WJ, Benedict JF, Jarow JP. Comparison of long-term outcomes of penile prostheses and intracavernosal injection therapy. J Urol 1998;159:811–5.

28. Rajpurkar A, Dhabuwala CB. Comparison of satisfaction rates and erectile function in patients treated with sildenafil, intracavernous prostaglandin E1 and penile implant surgery for erectile dysfunction in urology practice. J Urol 2003;170:159–63.

29. Akin-Olugbade O, Parker M, Guhring P, et al. Determinants of patient satisfaction following penile prosthesis surgery. J Sex Med 2006;3:743–8.

30. Kramer AC, Schweber A. Patient expectations prior to Coloplast Titan penile prosthesis implant predicts postoperative satisfaction. J Sex Med 2010;7:2261–6.

31. Deuk Choi Y, Jin Choi Y, Hwan Kim J, et al. Mechanical reliability of the AMS 700CXM inflatable penile prosthesis for the treatment of male erectile dysfunction. J Urol 2001;165:822–4.

32. Carson CC, Mulcahy JJ, Govier FE. Efficacy, safety and patient satisfaction outcomes of the AMS 700CX inflatable penile prosthesis: results of a long-term multicenter study. AMS 700CX Study Group. J Urol 2000;164:376–80.

33. Montorsi F, Rigatti P, Carmignani G, et al. AMS three-piece inflatable implants for erectile dysfunction: a long-term multi-institutional study in 200 consecutive patients. Eur Urol 2000;37:50–5.

34. Daitch JA, Angermeier KW, Lakin MM, et al. Long-term mechanical reliability of AMS 700 series inflatable penile prostheses: comparison of CX/CXM and Ultrex cylinders. J Urol 1997;158:1400–2.

35. Dubocq F, Tefilli MV, Gheiler EL, et al. Long-term mechanical reliability of multicomponent inflatable penile prosthesis: comparison of device survival. Urology 1998;52:277–81.

36. Dhar NB, Angermeier KW, Montague DK. Long-term mechanical reliability of AMS 700CX/CXM inflatable penile prosthesis. J Urol 2006;176:2599–601.

37. Kim DS, Yang KM, Chung HJ, et al. AMS 700CX/CXM inflatable penile prosthesis has high mechanical reliability at long-term follow-up. J Sex Med 2010;7:2602–7.

Penile Prosthesis Infection: Approaches to Prevention and Treatment

J. Patrick Selph, MD, Culley C. Carson III, MD*

KEYWORDS

• Penile prosthesis • Infection • Prevention • Treatment

Epidemiologic studies have estimated that more than 50% of men ages 40 to 70 have some form of erectile dysfunction, with nearly half of men ages 60 to 70 having moderate to severe erectile dysfunction.[1] Among 40- to 69-year-old white men, it is estimated that nearly 620,000 will develop erectile dysfunction each year in the United States.[2] Penile prosthesis implantation remains a mainstay for treatment of erectile dysfunction unresponsive to other less-invasive methods. An estimate of the number of penile prostheses implanted each year in the United States approaches 15,000 devices.[3] Since the introduction of the inflatable penile prosthesis (IPP) by Scott and colleagues[4] in 1973, inflatable prostheses have become the most commonly placed implant,[5,6] and improvements in penile prosthesis design have extended the long-term survival of implants, with 5-year mechanical survival estimates ranging from 86% to 96%[7–10] and longer-term studies suggesting 10-year mechanical survival of 67% to 88%.[7,8,11,12] As the improved design of prostheses has led to their increased mechanical survival, other complications, such as infection, have emerged as the leading causes of implant failure.[6] This article focuses on approaches to prevention and treatment of penile prosthesis infection.

PATHOGENS AND RISK FACTORS FOR INFECTION

Infection rates for virgin IPPs have typically been approximately 1% to 3%, but published rates have been significantly higher in revision surgery or when reconstructive procedures are involved.[6,13] Compared with a 1.8% risk of infection in virgin penile prosthesis implantations, Jarow[14] noted a 13.3% risk of infection after revision surgery for an uninfected malfunctioning penile prosthesis and a 21.7% risk if a penile reconstructive procedure was involved. The only significant difference between the three groups was mean operating time (98, 110, and 255 minutes for the primary, revision, and reconstructive groups, respectively), so the length of the operation was thought to have played a role in infection risk. Other studies have shown the risk for infection in revision surgery to range from 6.7% to 18.8%.[15–18] The higher risk of infection during revision surgery is thought related to factors that impair host resistance to infection, including poor antibiotic penetration due to capsule formation around the previous implant and poor wound healing.[14,19]

The source for infection is usually skin flora introduced at the time of the operation.[20] The most common offending organism is *Staphylococcus epidermidis* in both primary and revision surgery, although gram-negative fecal pathogens can cause infection.[20–22] Other organisms implicated include *Pseudomonas aeruginosa*, *Escherichia coli*, *Serratia marcescens*, *Enterococcus* species, *Proteus mirabilis*, and methicillin-resistant *Staphylococcus aureus* (MRSA).[22] Several studies have suggested that the higher rate of infection during revision surgery may be explained by the fact that

Division of Urologic Surgery, Department of Surgery, University of North Carolina, 2113 Physician's Office Building, Chapel Hill, NC 27599-7235, USA
* Corresponding author.
E-mail address: culley_carson@med.unc.edu

Urol Clin N Am 38 (2011) 227–235
doi:10.1016/j.ucl.2011.02.007
0094-0143/11/$ – see front matter © 2011 Published by Elsevier Inc.

even clinically uninfected prostheses are often colonized by bacteria. This was suggested by Licht and colleagues,[21] who noted that 40% of clinically uninfected penile prostheses were culture positive at the time of revision. Although three of the patients with positive cultures went on to develop infection requiring prosthesis removal, none of the patients with negative cultures developed infection. Henry and colleagues[19] published a multicenter study in which 54 of 77 (70%) clinically uninfected patients had a culture-positive penile prosthesis at the time of revision surgery. Furthermore, of the 48 patients who had time to revision data culture results and underwent revision due to mechanical failure, those who had positive cultures had significantly shorter revision-free times: 6.3 years for positive cultures versus 8.9 years for negative cultures. The reason for this finding is unclear, but it suggests colonization may play a role in mechanical failure.

Persistent bacterial adherence to implanted medical devices is mediated by bacterial production of biofilm, a survival mechanism by which bacteria produce a slimy matrix that reduces phagocytosis, prevents antibiotic diffusion, and traps nutrients.[23] The National Institutes of Health estimates that 80% of all infections are caused by biofilms.[24] Henry and colleagues[19] noted the visible presence of biofilm on some of the clinically uninfected prostheses removed in their multicenter study, and, using laser microscopy, Silverstein's group[25] noted biofilm on 8 of 10 clinically uninfected prosthesis removed for mechanical failure. They also suggested that it is likely that essentially all implants have some biofilm matrix formation. A patient begins to experience symptoms of infection when the bacteria in the biofilm propagate and become free-floating or planktonic, and currently, the only mechanism to eradicate biofilms is by removing the prosthetic.[23] Antibiotics are able to suppress these planktonic bacteria, but the bacteria imbedded in the biofilm remain untouched. It is postulated that revision surgery could be a stimulus that activates the bacteria in these biofilms to become planktonic, and this theory has been the basis for the salvage protocols developed by surgeons.[19,26,27] Future directions in preventing and treating prosthetic infections may involve disrupting the communication of bacteria in biofilms and administration of antibiotics concomitantly with drugs that can disperse biofilms into a planktonic state.[28,29]

Other documented risk factors for infection include diabetes mellitus, spinal cord injury, urinary tract infection, immunosuppression, and distant sites of infection. The literature on the risk of infection in diabetic patients is mixed. Fallon and Ghanem[30] had a 3-fold higher incidence of infection in their diabetic population. Bishop and colleagues[31] suggested that elevated hemoglobin A1c (HgbA1c) levels in diabetics may predict a higher incidence of infection in this population. In a series of 90 patients in which 5 of 32 diabetics had postoperative infections, diabetics with an HgbA1c of greater than 11.5% had a 31% risk of infection compared with 5% in patients with an HgbA1c less than 11.5%. The investigators suggested better diabetes control preoperatively might help lower the risk of infection. In response to the Bishop and colleagues' findings, one group noted in their series of 389 implants that diabetics had an 8.7% infection rate compared with 4.0% in nondiabetics, but there was no difference in the mean or median HgbA1c levels in the infected versus uninfected diabetic.[32] Although the study suggested diabetics had higher rates of infection, they concluded that neither glycosylated hemoglobin levels, fasting sugar levels, nor insulin dependence increased the risk of infection in diabetics undergoing prosthesis implantation. Conversely, in Jarow's[14] series, diabetics had no increased incidence of infection in either the primary or revision implant group. In a series of 1251 operations, Wilson and Delk[16] noted no significant increase in infections in diabetics receiving an initial implant. Other studies have shown that usage of antibiotic-coated penile prostheses can reduce the risk of infection in diabetics to 0% to 1%.[33,34]

Spinal cord injury has been documented in numerous studies to increase the risk of IPP infection,[16,35–39] although others have shown no increased incidence of infection in the spinal cord injury population.[40] The spinal cord–injured population has unique risk factors, including a higher rate of urinary tract infections and decreased sensation that predisposes to implant erosion. Literature on studies of immunosuppressed patients has been mixed as well. In Wilson and Delk's[16] large series, 5 of 10 patients on chronic steroids developed infections; however, in a series of 13 diabetic patients on immunosuppression after organ transplantation who received a penile prosthesis for impotence, there was no increased incidence of infection.[41] Cuellar and Sklar[42] found no increased risk of infection in their series of organ transplant recipients who had penile implants placed. Barry[43] suggested transplant recipients meet certain criteria before penile prosthesis implantation, including stable graft function for greater than 6 months, avoiding an intra-abdominal reservoir, and low-dose immunosuppression. Postorgan transplant patients with erectile dysfunction should appropriately be offered a penile prosthesis without undue risk for infection.

Prolonged hospitalization is a risk factor for infection due to skin flora changes to more virulent organisms; thus, same-day admission is advantageous. Others have shown that late hematogenous spread is possible, and one case of a *Salmonella* infection of an IPP in a renal transplant recipient has been reported.[44,45] Although the risk of late spread should be considered rare, ruling out distant infection should be part of the workup before performing surgery.

Most infections of penile prostheses are caused by skin flora introduced at the time of surgery. Spinal cord injury, poorly controlled diabetes, distant active infections, prolonged hospitalization, and prior implantation can increase the risk of developing infection. Although these factors may increase the risk of infection in certain subsets of patients, appropriate perioperative planning and operative technique can minimize these risks.

SURGICAL PLANNING

Having discussed preoperative risk factors associated with infection, other perioperative considerations are important for reducing the risk of infection. Patients should be assessed for genital skin lesions preoperatively to rule out active infections, and remote infections should be eliminated. Sterile urine cultures are an imperative measure to reduce the risk of infection from urine spillage, and placing a urethral catheter is advisable in patients with neurogenic bladder. Same-day admission is warranted to reduce the risk of skin flora changes to more virulent and resistant organisms. Increased risk of infection from performing simultaneous procedures at the time as IPP placement should be considered. Some investigators have suggested simultaneous circumcision and IPP increases risk of infection,[30] whereas other investigators have suggested that closing the incisions related to the implant before performing concomitant minor genital procedures does not increase risk.[13] Carson and Noh[46] documented an increased risk of infection when additional foreign bodies, such as Gore-Tex or Dacron, were implanted at the same time as a penile prosthesis, whereas Jarow[14] found a 21.7% incidence of infection when reconstructive procedures were involved. Simultaneous placement of an IPP and artificial urethral sphincter has been suggested to decrease infection risk due to the decrease in operative time and avoidance of reoperation in a surgical field that may have an asymptomatic colonized prosthetic.[47] Thus, if multiple procedures are being considered, the benefit of a single course of anesthesia must be weighed against the possible increased risk of infection in some settings.

Preoperative bathing with an antibacterial shower has been suggested by several investigators to reduce risk of infection.[13,48,49] Bathing with chlorhexidine has been shown to decrease colony counts on skin but has not been shown to reduce surgical site infection rates.[50–52] At the authors' institution, any preoperative antiseptic bath is not used for penile prosthesis patients. On the contrary, skin preparation with antimicrobial agents has been shown to reduce the incidence of surgical site infections. A recent prospective, randomized study showed that chlorhexidine-alcohol–based preparations were superior to povidone-iodine–based preparations in preventing surgical site infections in clean-contaminated surgery, and a meta-analysis by Noorani and colleagues noted similar findings.[53,54] Consequently, the authors' institution has mandated the use of chlorhexidine-alcohol–based solutions for preoperative surgical skin preparation. An no-touch technique devised by Siegrist and colleagues[55] involves placing a drape over the incision that limits the contact between the skin and surgical field. The rate of infection in the no-touch group was 0.73% compared with 2.23% in the standard technique group.

Various studies have shown that clipping hair in the operating room significantly reduces the risk of infection compared with shaving the night before, and current recommendations are to perform clipping, if needed, immediately before the operation.[56,57] The Sexual Medicine Society of North America (SMSNA) maintains that surgeons should be given the option of shaving with a razor as opposed to the more ubiquitous clippers mandated by most hospitals, because there is less tissue trauma with no increased risk of infection.[58] No matter the method chosen, it should be performed immediately preceding the operation.

With the increasing rates of MRSA isolates in hospitals, preoperative measures to reduce MRSA colonization have been suggested. Prospective, randomized, controlled trials have shown no benefit to preoperative decolonization with mupirocin in unselected patients.[57] Although current recommendations do not advise decolonization of unselected patients with mupirocin nasal ointment, recent studies in the cardiothoracic and orthopedic literature have shown a reduction in the rate of MRSA surgical site infections when mupirocin ointment applied to the nares was part of a regimen designed to decrease the risk of these infections.[59,60] The generalizability of these results is unclear, and further study of this topic is needed before definitive recommendations can be made. Other mechanisms to minimize the risk of postoperative infection include limiting operating traffic, appropriate hemostasis of bleeding tissues, avoiding flashing of instruments, maintaining postoperative glucose levels below 200, and preventing intraoperative hypothermia.

Preoperative administration of prophylactic antibiotics is recommended by the American Urological Association for open procedures involving the placement of prosthetic implants.[61] Antimicrobials of choice include an aminoglycoside plus a first-generation or second-generation cephalosporin or vancomycin administered within 1 to 2 hours before incision and given for a duration of 24 hours or less. This regimen targets the commonly implicated gram-positive skin flora and urinary tract pathogens most likely to cause infection. Although there are no recommendations on the practice, most urologists discharge postoperative IPP patients with oral prophylactic antibiotics. One abstract looking at practice patterns among urologists who perform penile prosthesis surgery noted that 94% of SMSNA urologists prescribe postoperative home oral antibiotics compared with 88% of non-SMSNA members.[62] The same survey noted that 100% of SMSNA members and 92% of non-SMSNA urologists irrigate intraoperatively with antibiotic solution. Although it may seem prudent to irrigate with antibiotic solution during primary implantation, there are currently no recommendations on the practice to guide urologists. For revision surgery due to noninfectious reasons, a group of urologists at three institutions recommended using an antibiotic washout procedure because they found a rate of infection of 2.86% for the washout group versus 11.6% for the nonwashout group.[63] The same group also noted that the rate of positive tissue capsule cultures performed during revision surgery decreased from 43% to 25% after the washout.[64] Although this group used antibiotic irrigation, they postulated that the most important part of the washout may be the mechanical débridement of the biofilm, and some of the agents used in the washout (eg, hydrogen peroxide) may actually increase the risk of infection. A study of washout procedures comparing antibiotic irrigation with saline irrigation may shed some light on the issue and potentially provide urologists with guidelines on whether or not to irrigate with antibiotics. Caution should be advised when implanting a prosthesis coated with antibiotics because copious irrigation may cause elution of the antibiotics before insertion.

Although meticulous sterile technique is critical to reducing the risk of prosthetic infection, recent advances in prosthetic technology have further decreased the incidence of implant infection. American Medical Systems (AMS) (Minnetonka, MN, USA) and Coloplast Corporation (Minneapolis, MN, USA) each manufacture three-component prostheses that allow incorporation of antibiotics into the implant. The AMS 700 Series of IPPs is impregnated with InhibiZone, a coating on the external surface of the device that elutes rifampin and minocycline to create a zone of inhibition for bacterial growth. The amount of drug is less than a single oral dose, with a large drop-off in drug levels occurring at approximately 7 days. Coloplast manufactures the Titan IPP, which has a hydrophilic polyvinylpyrrolidone coating that can be soaked in antibiotics intraoperatively. Surgeons have the advantage of choosing the antibiotics in which to soak the Titan, and these then diffuse into the tissue around the implant to neutralize bacteria.

Many studies have documented the decreased incidence of infection associated with these implants. In 2004, Carson[65] published retrospective data on 2261 men who received InhibiZone prostheses compared with 1944 men who received untreated prostheses; the InhibiZone group had an 82.4% reduction in infection at 60 days and a 57.8% reduction in infection at 180 days. Wilson and colleagues[34] published data on InhibiZone-coated prostheses, showing a reduction in the rate of infection in virgin nondiabetic, virgin diabetic, and revision implants with washout compared with their historical rates. Furthermore, of the 223 nondiabetic patients who received virgin implants, none developed infection. In a similar study, a second group also noted no infections in 58 patients (0%) who had InhibiZone-coated prostheses placed compared with 3.2% (3/94) of patients who had uncoated prostheses.[33] A retrospective study of patient information forms filed with the AMS covering 7 years and more than 40,000 IPPs (36,659 InhibiZone prostheses and 3456 noncoated prostheses) showed an infection rate of 1.77% for InhibiZone-coated prostheses and 3.09% for noncoated prostheses at 84 months.[66] A study of 2357 implants of the Coloplast Titan and 482 Alpha-1 IPPs (Coloplast Corporation, Minneapolis, MN, USA) showed an infection rate of 1.06% in the antibiotic-coated Titan compared with 2.07% in the noncoated Alpha-1.[67] An even larger study of 17,900 Titan implants showed an infection rate of 1.6% compared with 8825 Alpha-1 implants with an infection rate of 4%.[68] Dhabuwala and colleagues[69] recently compared the antibiotic-soaked Coloplast Titan to the InhibiZone-coated AMS prosthesis. The rates of infection for the vancomycin/gentamicin-coated Titan, the rifampin/gentamicin-coated Titan, and InhibiZone-coated AMS were 4.4%, 0%, and 1.3%, respectively. The investigators suggested that the infection rate between the rifampin/gentamicin-coated Titan and the AMS InhibiZone models were comparable and that all Titan prostheses should be coated with rifampin/gentamicin solution. Wilson[70] recently presented an abstract in which he prefers coating the Titan with Bactrim due to its low cost, broad-spectrum activity, and ease of handling. Revision implants have shown similar trends. In one study of 55 patients who underwent revision surgery for mechanical failure and had an InhibiZone-coated prosthesis implanted, only one (1.8%) developed infection compared with the historical standard of 10%.[71]

A final consideration to prevent complications is whether or not to place a drain, which some investigators have argued increases the risk of infection. Sadeghi-Najed and colleagues[72] retrospectively reviewed data on 425 consecutive nonantibiotic-coated implants placed at three separate institutions. Each patient had a closed-suction drain placed for 12 to 24 hours postoperatively and the overall infection rate was 3.3%, which was similar to published historical rates. Garber[73] used a closed-suction drain in 50 patients for 24 hours postoperatively and had one periprosthetic infection. Using a closed-suction drain does not seem to increase the risk of infection, and advocates recommend placing the drain through a separate incision and not the surgical incision to avoid bacterial migration into the dissection site.

TREATMENT OF PROSTHESIS INFECTION

As discussed previously, most prosthetic infections are thought to occur because of bacterial contamination at the time of surgery. Although less virulent than other organisms, S epidermidis is the most common offending organism, because it is a commensal skin flora capable of forming a biofilm. More virulent organisms, such as Pseudomonas and Proteus mirabilis, can cause clinically apparent infections in 20% of cases, often occurring within 1 month of surgery.[74] Penile prosthesis infections can be divided into clinically apparent and subclinical infections. Symptoms of a clinically apparent infection include fever, pain, erythema, induration over a component, drainage, and eventually extrusion. Most infections occur within 1 year, but late infections have been reported.[44] Care should be taken to rule out a more severe infection causing gangrene of the penis, a rare but dreaded complication.[75] Fishman

and colleagues[76] noted that 56% of infections occur within 7 months of surgery, 36% between 7 and 12 months, and 2.5% after 5 years.

Most infections fall into the subclinical category. These infections are difficult to diagnose and treat, and they are often associated with chronic device-related pain. Continued pain after surgery that does not subside and device migration both suggest infection, which may eventually warrant implant removal. Parsons and colleagues[77] recommended an initial trial of oral antibiotic therapy for this subset of patients. If the pain improves with treatment, then antibiotics are continued for 10 to 12 weeks. With ciprofloxacin (500 mg twice a day for 10 to 12 weeks), a 60% success rate was noted. Cephalexin (500 mg 4 times daily) can also be used. For those who fail to have resolution of pain, or if the pain returns on cessation of antibiotics, surgical intervention is needed. Mulcahy[78] recommends using Bactrim DS twice a day for 4 weeks to see if symptoms resolve, and if not, then proceed to surgery.

The grossly infected penile prosthesis warrants surgical intervention along with systemic antibiotics. The most conservative approach involves explanting the prosthesis with the intention of reinsertion several months later. Thorough irrigation of the component spaces is undertaken after removal and culture of the component spaces. Drains are then placed in a method similar to abscess drainage, including intracorporeal drains and an intrascrotal drain at the site of the pump. The drains are left to suction and irrigated with antibiotics (eg, vancomycin and gentamicin) every 8 hours.[79–81] Once cultures have returned, antibiotic irrigation can be tailored to the pathogen, and drains can be removed after 72 hours of irrigation with culture-appropriate antibiotics.[82] It is then recommended to use a vacuum erection device without the constrictive ring to limit the penile shortening and ventral curvature that occur.[78]

Various salvage approaches have been developed with the aim of preventing corporal fibrosis that makes subsequent reimplantation more difficult. Patients who are severely ill (eg, patients with sepsis or diabetics with severe ketoacidosis) or who have significant necrotic tissue or a rapidly developing infection; diabetics with significant purulence; and cases of significant cylinder extrusion should not be considered candidates for salvage. A thorough discussion of risks and benefits of salvage surgery should be done with patients before proceeding with salvage measures. If the salvage route is chosen, perioperative antibiotics are administered and all components of the penile prosthesis and other foreign bodies, such as Gore-Tex and Dacron, should be removed. Cultures from each of the spaces should be taken followed by irrigation in each area where the prosthetic resided, which can be aided by a red rubber catheter advanced into each component space. Brant and colleagues[26] recommend a sequence of irrigation as follows: kanamycin (80 mg/L) and bacitracin (1 g/L) in normal saline followed by half-strength hydrogen peroxide, half-strength povidone-iodine solution, pressurized normal saline (5 L) containing vancomycin (1 g) and gentamicin (80 mg), half-strength povidone-iodine, half-strength hydrogen peroxide, and lastly the kanamycin/bacitracin irrigation (**Box 1**). The pressurized irrigation is important to help disrupt any biofilm that may have formed. Once this step is complete, gloves, instruments, and drapes are changed and a new prosthesis is inserted. Wounds are closed and no drain is left in place, and patients are placed on 1 month of oral antibiotics with good tissue penetration. This initial report involved 11 patients in which 9 of 12 cultures grew *S epidermidis*, with a documented success rate of 91% (10/11 patients) at a mean follow-up of 21 months. Later studies documented an 84% (85/101 patients) success rate for men undergoing the salvage procedure.[81] Failures in this series were more likely to have happened when a short incubation period was present, there was significant cellulitis involved, and more virulent organisms were cultured. These symptoms likely indicate tissue infection along with implant cavity infection. In two later cases with these presenting symptoms, successful salvage was performed when the abscess cavities were drained and at least a 48- hour course of systemic antibiotics was administered before surgery. It is thus recommended, in cases such as these, to give a 3-day course of systemic antibiotics before salvage to treat the tissue infection.[81]

Other options include delayed or partial salvage. Knoll[27] described a delayed salvage procedure in which 31 of 41 patients who presented with an infected IPP underwent removal of the prosthesis followed by drain placement and antibiotic irrigation for 72 hours before replacement. The success rate was 71% for the delayed salvage procedure and 80% for the 10 patients who underwent immediate salvage. Although the results are similar to immediate salvage, the increased cost associated with two procedures and a longer hospital stay led the investigator to conclude that immediate salvage was superior, and other investigators have agreed.[27,78] The partial salvage approach involves removing the single infected or eroded component of the prosthesis and then implanting a new replacement component in an unoperated space.[82] The authors were successful in 16 of 22 scrotal pump erosions and 7 of 9 cases of cylinder erosion. This technique is somewhat riskier in that other components of the prosthesis are likely to be coated with biofilm, and bacterial migration to this new component can occur and potentially cause later infection.[19,21,25,78] Consequently, many surgeons advise against this technique.[77,83,84]

SUMMARY

Although the rate of penile prosthesis infections is generally low, they are devastating complications for patients that lead to increased morbidity and health care costs. Understanding the pathogenesis of infection and the risk factors that predispose for infection can reduce the incidence of this complication. Proper sterile technique is critical to preventing infection, and recent technological advances in antibiotic-coated prostheses have aided urologists in further reducing the incidence of infection. Novel agents targeting biofilms may continue to bring infection rates down even further. When infections do occur, salvage techniques can treat infection and provide potentially better outcomes for patients. Future directions should include developing guidelines for using postoperative antibiotics and intraoperative antibiotic irrigation.

Box 1
Salvage protocol for infected penile prosthesis

1. Remove infected prosthesis
2. Sequential irrigation

   a. Kanamycin (80 mg/L) and bacitracin (1 g/L)
   b. Half-strength hydrogen peroxide
   c. Half-strength povidone-iodine solution
   d. Pressurized washing with normal saline (5 L) containing vancomycin (1g) and gentamicin (80 mg)
   e. Half-strength povidone-iodine solution
   f. Half-strength hydrogen peroxide
   g. Kanamycin (80 mg/L) and bacitracin (1 g/L)

3. Change gloves, drapes, and instruments
4. Place new prosthesis

REFERENCES

1. Feldman HA, Goldstein I, Hatzichristou DG, et al. Impotence and its medical and psychosocial correlates: results of the Massachusetts male aging study. J Urol 1994;151:54.

2. Johannes CB, Araujo AB, Feldman HA, et al. Incidence of erectile dysfunction in men 40 to 69 years old: longitudinal results from the Massachusetts male aging study. J Urol 2000;163:2.

3. Darouiche RO. Device-associated infections: a macroproblem that starts with microadherence. Clin Infect Dis 2001;33(9):1567–72.

4. Scott FB, Bradley WE, Timm GW. Management of erectile impotence: use of implantable inflatable prosthesis. Urology 1973;2:80.

5. Jhaveri F, Rutledge R, Carson C. Penile prosthesis implantation surgery: a statewide population based analysis of 2354 patients. Int J Impot Res 1998; 10(4):251.

6. Henry GD, Wilson SK. Updates in inflatable penile prostheses. Urol Clin North Am 2007;34:535–47.

7. Carson CC, Mulcahy JJ, Govier FE. Efficacy, saftety and patient satisfaction outcomes of the AMS 700 CX inflatable penile prosthesis: results of a long term multicenter study. AMS 700 CX study group. J Urol 2000;164:376–80.

8. Wilson SK, Delk JR, Salem EA, et al. Long-Term survival of inflatable penile prostheses: single surgical group experience with 2,384 first-time implants spanning two decades. J Sex Med 2007; 4:1074–9.

9. Montague DK, Angermeier KW. Contemporary aspects of penile prosthesis implantation. Urol Int 2003;70(2):141–6.

10. Montorsi F, Rigatti P, Carmignani G, et al. AMS three-piece inflatable implants for erectile dysfunction: a long-term multi-institutional study in 200 consecutive patients. Eur Urol 2000;37(1):50–5.

11. Dhar NB, Angermeier KW, Montague DK. Long-term mechanical reliability of AMS 700CX/CXM inflatable penile prosthesis. J Urol 2006;176(6 Pt 1):2599–601.

12. Kim DS, Yang KM, Chung HJ, et al. AMS 700CX/CXM inflatable penile prosthesis has high mechanical reliability at long-term follow-up. J Sex Med 2010 Jul;7(7):2602–7.

13. Mulcahy JJ. Penile implant infections: prevention and treatment. Curr Urol Rep 2008;9(6):487–91.

14. Jarow JP. Risk factors for penile prosthesis infection. J Urol 1996;156:402–4.

15. Quesada ET, Light JK. The AMS 700 inflatable penile prosthesis: long-term experience with the controlled expansion cylinders. J Urol 1993;149(1):46–8.

16. Wilson SK, Delk JR 2nd. Inflatable penile implant infection: predisposing factors and treatment suggestions. J Urol 1995;153:659–61.

17. Thomalla JV, Thompson ST, Rowland RG, et al. Infectious complications of penile prosthetic implants. J Urol 1987;138:65–7.

18. Lotan Y, Roehrborn CG, McConnell JD, et al. Factors influencing the outcomes of penile prosthesis surgery at a teaching institution. Urology 2003;62: 918–21.

19. Henry GD, Wilson SK, Delk JR, et al. Penile prosthesis cultures during revision surgery: a multicenter study. J Urol 2004;172:153–6.

20. Carson CC. Infections in genitourinary prostheses. Urol Clin North Am 1989;16:139.

21. Licht MR, Montague DK, Angermeier KW, et al. Cultures from genitourinary prostheses at reoperation: questioning the role of Staphylococcus epidermidis in periprosthetic infection. J Urol 1995;154:387.

22. Mulcahy JJ. Long-term experience with salvage of infected penile implants. J Urol 2000;183:481–2.

23. Stewart PS, Costerton JW. Antibiotic resistance of bacteria in biofilms. Lancet 2001;358(9276):135–8.

24. National Institutes of Health (NIDCR, NIAID). Targeted research on oral microbial biofilms (DE-98-006). 1998. Available at: http://grants.nih. gov.libproxy.lib.unc.edu/grants/guide/rfa-files/RFA-DE-98-006.html. Accessed March 6, 1998.

25. Silverstein AD, Henry GD, Evans B, et al. Biofilm formation on clinically noninfected penile prostheses. J Urol 2006;176(3):1008–11.

26. Brant MD, Ludlow JK, Mulcahy JJ. The Prosthesis salvage operation: immediate replacement of the infected penile prosthesis. J Urol 1996;155:155–7.

27. Knoll DK. Penile prosthetic Infection: management by delayed and immediate salvage technique. Urology 1998;52:287–90.

28. Costerton JW, Montanaro L, Arciola CR. Bacterial communications in implant infections: a target for an intelligence war. Int J Artif Organs 2007;30(9):757–63.

29. Davies DG, Marques CN. A fatty acid messenger is responsible for inducing dispersion in microbial biofilms. J Bacteriol 2009;191(5):1393–403.

30. Fallon B, Ghanem H. Sexual performance and satisfaction with penile prostheses in impotence of various etiologies. Int J Impot Res 1990;2:35–42.

31. Bishop JU, Moul JW, Sihelnik SA, et al. Use of glycosylated hemoglobin to identify diabetics at high risk for penile periprosthetic infections. J Urol 1992; 147(2):386–8.

32. Wilson SK, Carson CC, Cleves MA, et al. Quantifying risk of penile prosthesis infection with elevated glycosylated hemoglobin. J Urol 1998;159:1537–46.

33. Droggin D, Shabsigh R, Anastasiadis AG. Antibiotic coating reduces penile prosthesis infection. J Sex Med 2005;2:565–8.

34. Wilson SK, Zumbe J, Henry GD, et al. Infection reduction using antibiotic-coated inflatable penile prosthesis. J Urol 2007;70:337–40.

35. Radomski SB, Herschorn S. Risk factors associated with penile prosthesis infection. J Urol 1992;147(2): 383–5.

36. Collins KP, Hackler RH. Complications of penile prostheses in the spinal cord injury population. J Urol 1988;140(5):984–5.

37. Golgi H. Experience with penile prosthesis in spinal cord injury patients. J Urol 1979 Mar;121(3):288–9.

38. Rossier AB, Fam BA. Indication and results of semi-rigid penile prostheses in spinal cord injury patients: long-term followup. J Urol 1984;131(1):59–62.

39. Dietzen CJ, Lloyd LK. Complications of intracavernous injections and penile prostheses in spinal cord injured me. Arch Phys Med Rehabil 1992; 73(7):652–5.

40. Diokno AC, Sonda LP. Compatibility of genitourinary prostheses and intermittent self-catheterization. J Urol 1981;125(5):659–60.

41. Sidi AA, Peng W, Sanseau C, et al. Penile prosthesis surgery in the treatment of impotence in the immunosuppressed man. J Urol 1987;137(4):681–2.

42. Cuellar DC, Sklar GN. Penile prosthesis in the organ transplant recipient. Urology 2001;57(1):138–41.

43. Barry JM. Treating erectile dysfunction in renal transplant recipients. Drugs 2007;67(7):975–83.

44. Carson CC, Robertson CN. Late hematogenous infection of penile prostheses. J Urol 1988;139(1):50–2.

45. Sausville J, Gupta G, Forrest G, et al. Salmonella infection of a penile prosthesis. J Sex Med 2009; 6(5):1487–90.

46. Carson CC, Noh CH. Distal prosthesis extrusion: treatment with distal corporoplasty or Gortex windsock reinforcement. Int J Impot Res 2002;14:81–4.

47. Kumar R, Nehra A. Dual implantation of penile and sphincter implants in the post-prostatectomy patient. Curr Urol Rep 2007;8:477–81.

48. Sadeghi-Najed H. Penile prosthesis surgery: a review of prosthetic devices and associated complications. J Sex Med 2007;4:296–309.

49. Fallon B, Ghanem H. Infection control in outpatient unicomponent penile prosthesis surgery. Int J Impot Res 1999;11:25–7.

50. Mangram AJ, Horan TC, Pearson ML, et al. Guideline for prevention of surgical site infection, 1999. Centers for disease control and prevention infection control practices advisory committee. Am J Infect Control 1999;27(2):97–132.

51. Rotter ML, Larsen SO, Cooke EM, et al. A comparison of the effects of preoperative whole-body bathing with detergent alone and with detergent containing chlorhexidine gluconate on the frequency of wound infections after clean surgery. The European Working Party on Control of Hospital Infections. J Hosp Infect 1988;11(4):310–20.

52. Leigh DA, Stronge JL, Marriner J, et al. Total body bathing with 'Hibiscrub' (chlorhexidine) in surgical patients: a controlled trial. J Hosp Infect 1983;4(3):229–35.

53. Darouiche RO, Wall MJ Jr, Itani KM, et al. Chlorhexidine-alcohol versus povidone-iodine for surgical-site antisepsis. N Eng J Med 2010;362(1):18–26.

54. Noorani A, Rabey N, Walsh SR, et al. Systematic review and meta-analysis of preoperative antisepsis with chlorhexidine versus povidone-iodine in clean contaminated surgery. Br J Surg 2010;97(11): 1614–20.

55. Siegrist TC, Kwon EO, Fracchia JA, et al. The "no-touch" technique: a novel technique for reducing post-operative infections in patients receiving multi-component inflatable penile prostheses. J Urol 2008; 179(Suppl 4):404.

56. Kjonniksen I, Andersen BM, Sondenaa VG, et al. Preoperative hair removal-a systematic literature review. AORN J 2002;75:928–38 940.

57. Kirby JP, Mazuski JE. Prevention of surgical site infection. Surg Clin North Am 2009;89:365–89.

58. Domes T, Grober E. Pre-operative hair removal on the male genitala—clippers versus razors: support for the SMSNA position [abstract 104]. In: Program book for the 16th annual fall scientific meeting of the Sexual Medicine Society of North America, Inc. Miami (Fl), November 11–14, 2010. p. 247.

59. Rao N, Cannella B, Crossett LS, et al. A preoperative decolonization protocol for staphylococcus aureus prevents orthopedic infections. Clin Orthop Relat Res 2008;466(6):1343–8.

60. Walsh EE, Greene L, Kirshner R. Sustained reduction in methicillin-resistant Staphylococcus aureus wound infections after cardiothoracic surgery. Arch Intern Med 2011;171(1):68–73.

61. Wolf JS, Bennett CJ, Dmochowski RR, et al. Best practice policy statement on urologic surgery antimicrobial prophylaxis. J Urol 2008;179:1379–90.

62. Wosnitzer M, Greenfield J. Antibiotic patterns among urologists who perform inflatable penile prosthesis insertion. J Sex Med 2010;7(Suppl 1):12.

63. Henry GD, Wilson SK, Delk JR, et al. Revision washout decreases penile prosthesis infection in revision surgery: a multicenter study. J Urol 2005; 173:89–92.

64. Henry GD, Carson CC, Wilson SK, et al. Revision washout decreases implant capsule tissue culture positivity: a multicenter study. J Urol 2008;179:186–90.

65. Carson CC. Efficacy of antibiotic impregnation of inflatable penile prostheses in decreasing infection in original implants. J Urol 2004;171(4):1611–4.

66. Carson CC, Mulcahy JJ, Harsch MR. Long-term infection outcomes after original antibiotic impregnated inflatable penile prosthesis implants: up to 7.7 years of followup. J Urol 2011;185(2):614–8.

67. Wolter CE, Hellstrom WJ. The hydrophilic-coated inflatable penile prosthesis: 1-year experience. J Sex Med 2004;1(2):221–4.

68. Richardson B, Caire A, Hellstrom W. Retrospective long-term analysis of Titan hydrophilic coating: positive reduction of infection compared to non-coated device. J Sex Med 2010;7(Suppl 1):28.

69. Dhabuwala C, Sheth S, Zamzow B. Infection rate of rifampin/gentamicin-coated titan coloplast penile implants. Comparison with Inhibizone-impregnated AMS penile implants. J Sex Med 2011;8(1):315–20.

70. Wilson SK. The ideal antibiotic dip for the Coloplast Titan prosthesis [abstract: 99]. In: Program book of

the 16th annual fall scientific meeting of the Sexual Medicine Society of North America, Inc. Miami (Fl), November 11–14, 2010. p. 242.

71. Abouassaly R, Angermeier KW, Montague DK. Risk of infection with an antibiotic coated inflatable penile prosthesis at device replacement for mechanical failure. J Urol 2006;176:2471–3.

72. Sadeghi-Najed H, Ilbeigi P, Wilson SK, et al. Multi-institutional outcome study on the efficacy of closed-suction drainage of the scrotum in three-piece inflatable penile prosthesis surgery. Int J Impot Res 2005;17:535–8.

73. Garber BB. Mentor Alpha 1 inflatable penile prosthesis: patient satisfaction and device reliability. Urology 1994;43(2):214–7.

74. Montague DK, Angermeier KW, Lakin MM. Penile prosthesis infection. Int J Impot Res 2001;13:326–8.

75. McClellan DS, Masih BK. Gangrene of the penis as a complication of penile prosthesis. J Urol 1985;133(5):862–3.

76. Fishman IJ, Scott FB, Selam IN. Rescue procedure: an alternative to complete removal for treatment of infected penile prosthesis. J Urol 1987;137:202A.

77. Parsons CL, Stein PC, Dobke MK, et al. Diagnosis and therapy of subclinically infected prostheses. Surg Gynecol Obstet 1993;177:504–6.

78. Mulcahy JJ. Penile prosthesis infection: progress in prevention and treatment. Curr Urol Rep 2010;11:400–4.

79. Maatman TJ, Montague DK. Intracorporeal drainage after removal of infected penile prostheses. Urology 1984;23(2):184–5.

80. Kim JC, Lunati FP, Khan SA, et al. T-tube drainage of infected penile corporeal chambers. Urology 1995;45(3):514–5.

81. Mulcahy JJ. Treatment alternatives for the infected penile implant. Int J Impot Res 2003;15(Suppl 5):S147–9.

82. Furlow WF, Goldwasser B. Salvage of the eroded inflatable penile prosthesis: a new concept. J Urol 1987;138:312–6.

83. Carson CC. Diagnosis, treatment, and prevention of penile prosthesis infection. Int J Impot Res 2003;15(Suppl 5):S139–46.

84. Lue TF. Penile prosthetic infections: management by delayed and immediate salvage techniques. J Urol 1999;161(5):1727–8.

Index

Note: Page numbers of article titles are in **boldface** type.

Urol Clin N Am 38 (2011) 237–241
doi:10.1016/S0094-0143(11)00040-1
0094-0143/11/$ – see front matter © 2011 Elsevier Inc. All rights reserved.

urologic.theclinics.com

Printed and bound by CPI Group (UK) Ltd, Croydon, CR0 4YY

03/10/2024

01040355-0013